LEARNING

ABOUT

Sexuality

Compliments of:

The Population Council
Monteverde Mansions 2A3
85 Xavier Street, Greenhills
San Juan, Metro Manila
Tel. no. 722-6886
Fax no. 721-2786

LEARNING

ABOUT

Sexuality

A PRACTICAL

BEGINNING

SONDRA ZEIDENSTEIN AND KIRSTEN MOORE
EDITORS

THE POPULATION COUNCIL
INTERNATIONAL WOMEN'S HEALTH COALITION
NEW YORK

*We dedicate this book
to the memory of
Elisa Jiménez Armas*

Grateful acknowledgment is made for permission to reprint the following:

Adriana Baban and Henry David, *Voices of Romanian Women: Perceptions of Sexuality, Reproductive and Partner Relations During the Ceausescu Era.* Bethesda, MD: Trans-national Family Research Institute.

Ruth Dixon-Mueller, "The Sexuality Connection in Reproductive Health," excerpted with permission of the Population Council from *Studies in Family Planning* 24, no. 5:269–82.

Production supervised by Jenna Dixon
Copyedited by Linda Lotz   *Typeset by Sarah Albert*
Proofread by Beth Richards   *Index by Mary Neumann*
Cover design by Diana Hrisinko

Printed in the United States of America
on acid-free paper by Edwards Brothers.

Library of Congress Cataloging-in-Publication Data

Learning about sexuality : a practical beginning / Sondra Zeidenstein, Kirsten
    Moore, editors.
        p.   cm.
    Includes index.
    ISBN 0-87834-085-8 (pbk. : alk. paper)
    1. Birth control clinics. 2. Community health services.
3. Hygiene, Sexual—Study and teaching. 4. Sex customs—Study and
teaching.   I. Zeidenstein, Sondra. II. Moore, Kirsten.
HQ 763.5.L43   1995
363.9'6—dc20   95-40084

96   97   98   99   00   01   02   03   6   5   4   3   2   1

Contents

Foreword

The timeliness of this publication needs no emphasis. The Conference on Population and Development in Cairo in 1994, the Social Summit in Copenhagen in 1995, and the Fourth World Conference on Women in Beijing in 1995 show how those who are interested in women and gender issues, in family planning, in working with young people, and in addressing the problems of AIDS and sexually transmitted diseases have all come to the same conclusion: that sexual health is an area on which they should be concentrating in order to meet their differing objectives.

It should never have taken so much work for us all to recognize sexuality as a central part of our lives—it relates strongly to our behavior, our interactions with one another, our decisions, and our social environment. This recognition has been portrayed by artists, writers, musicians, and even in jokes for as long as we know. Yet it seems that this realization has only just begun among those whose work it is to promote health and development in whatever form.

This book's title is important: *Learning about Sexuality: A Practical Beginning*. The chapters in the book show us how far and how little we have progressed in articulating the relationship between sexuality, people's concerns, and the programs that many of us try to provide for their support. It is comprehensive in scope. It deals with boys, girls, men, and women; with the difficulties of researchers; with participatory approaches to learning; with the importance of understanding sexuality for family planning programs; with training; with research; with the darker side of sexuality and power; and with the attempts by people themselves to articulate their own understandings and concerns. It brings experience from a wide variety of cultures. Throughout, it outlines areas of human interest that, so far, we have failed to relate to in a programmatic way.

The standard pattern of the majority of health programs has been to prescribe action—either as a result of the provision of information, motivation, or exhortation to action, or as a result of the demand that people use a particular service provided. The program areas mentioned above all have their own agendas and domains of political correctness. But the use of the word "learning" brings us back to the understanding that programs that want to relate to sexuality (or perhaps in some cases it might be more correct to say that want to *use* sexuality) are deluding themselves if they think that they have messages to deliver or advice to provide about sexuality or sexual interaction. It is well known in social development that when programmers try to use their biased knowledge to manipulate people into predefined actions, without first reflecting on their own values, little real change can occur. This book shows how important it is, first, to help those responsible for the provision of services and programs to come to an understanding of the role that their own sexuality plays in their decisions and how their services are delivered; and second, to help people articulate their own concerns and then choose the paths of action that will improve their situations.

It has been a constant worry to many people that programs that address sexuality will carry a message about morality or culture or may facilitate what they refer to as "promiscuity" or amount to an encouragement to have sex. This book makes it plain that there should never be any question of imposing the values of one person or culture on another in programs in which sexuality is explored. Each of us, whether we provide or receive programs, has concerns about and interests relating to sexuality that can only be better dealt with as a result of exploration with others. Concerns about sexual interaction are worldwide—each of them articulated in ways defined by the particular culture. To date, people have been relatively silent about those concerns because there have been few forums in which it is safe to explore them. As a result, many of us have found a variety of coping mechanisms to deal with situations we do not really like. This book may help us in facilitating the development of forums for achieving better understanding and communication, where people everywhere can articulate in their own ways what they feel about sexual interaction.

At a recent IPPF workshop that was preparing health personnel for community work, the workers were asked to analyze various methods of coping in relation to sexual health by writing poems related to their own feelings. The men and women produced statements that immediately revealed how strongly they felt. Take a look at just two of these poems:

I'm Stanley, with a wife and three kids.
I love my woman but what can I do.
She has no job and I don't too.
So John who has a job is striking, and is taking his chance,
And all I have to give is acceptance.

Harry was almost everything
A woman could want
But anal sex was a disaster.
So we discussed it and we compromised.
We went from 52 to 4 times a year.

These statements were made by people whose concerns and attitudes are rarely explored by programmers or supervisors in the rush to work with "communities." Yet how important these feelings are!

An understanding of the importance of sexuality, and the willingness to learn about it both with others and for ourselves, is therefore central to the development of sexual health programs—whatever the agenda that drives them.

This book is exactly what its title implies: it is a supremely practical beginning for all of us in learning about sexuality. It provides us with a focus point while we develop our approaches for the betterment of sexual health, wherever we are.

HALDFAN MAHLER
Secretary-General
International Planned Parenthood Federation
February 1995

Acknowledgments

Learning about Sexuality: A Practical Beginning is an outgrowth of a process that began at the 1992 annual meeting of the National Council of International Health. It is the result of a collaboration between the Population Council and the International Women's Health Coalition (PC/IWHC) to bring attention to the lack of awareness about the role of sexuality in population and family planning disciplines. This project received financial and moral support from both institutions, as well as funding from the Ford Foundation and the Swiss Development Corporation.

This book builds on the discussions and presentations of the PC/IWHC working group on sexuality and gender, most notably on the contributions of some of its earliest members, including Ruth Dixon-Mueller, John Gagnon, Jacqueline Pitanguy, and Nicole Ridgway, who helped inform our understanding of the theoretical constructs of sexuality and the practicalities of research on sexual behavior and its meanings for individuals. Dixon-Mueller's work, in particular, established a useful framework for conceptualizing the links between sexuality and family planning and reproductive health services.

The Ford Foundation is one of the more thoughtful and supportive donors in the reproductive health field today. We are grateful to Margaret Hempel, programs officer, for comments and suggestions that were always constructive; her commitment to integrating sexuality into family planning programs and research kept us focused on the important links to be made. In addition, many of the Ford Foundation's reproductive health staff, including Lucile Atkin, Maggie Bangser, Mary Ann Burris, and Sandra

Vallenas, introduced us to a wide range of researchers and practitioners in this field, some of whom contributed to this book.

Diane Rubino and Emmy Kondo of the Population Council were dedicated stewards of the manuscript during various stages of the drafting and production process. Similarly, Valerie Hull, Chris Elias, and Guille Herrera from the Population Council, and Andrea Irvin of IWHC, helped facilitate communication with potential contributors, ensuring that a balance was maintained between the needs and goals of the authors and those of the editors. Also, Paul Constance and Len Holness were instrumental in helping us overcome language barriers by providing careful translations of several chapters from Spanish and French into English.

We benefited from the insights and guidance of our editorial committee—Judith Bruce, Andrea Eschen, Adrienne Germain, Sia Nowrojee, Debbie Rogow, and Nahid Toubia. They helped us define the goals and scope of this book and expanded our network of contributors. Furthermore, each played a critical role at various points in the process. Nahid Toubia helped set the stage for this work within the Population Council and encouraged us to be explicit about our own attitudes and values concerning sexuality. Judith Bruce's insight that we two would work well together on this project foretold the magical influence we were to have on each other, both professionally and personally. Andrea Eschen consistently provided timely and thoughtful responses to drafts of numerous chapters. Adrienne Germain's tireless work to include women's voices and women's issues on international agendas helped open the door for the experiences included in this book.

We want to acknowledge the contributions of two members of our editorial committee, Debbie Rogow and Sia Nowrojee. They provided critical feedback on many of the chapters. In several cases, they worked closely with authors to draw out and shape their material to be more relevant to the audience for this book. Their professionalism and good sense, along with their keen interest in the topic of sexuality, were indispensable in shaping the overall framework of this book.

Finally, we are grateful to the many authors who contributed to this book for their good humor and compelling frankness in engaging in the sometimes difficult process of telling their stories to editors who were far away and, in some cases, unknown to them.

*I*ntroduction

Sondra Zeidenstein and Kirsten Moore

*F*amily planning and reproductive health programs have rarely considered sexuality, gender roles, and power in designing and providing services. Sex has been perceived as too "private" and gender roles as "impossible to change" and socially and politically "sensitive," at least within the context of clinically oriented service delivery programs. Although a large body of research tells us about the many factors affecting contraceptive use and choice, risk of sexually transmitted disease (STD) and cervical cancer, and unwanted pregnancy, we are just beginning to understand how these outcomes are profoundly affected by dynamics of sexuality and gender. Increasingly, family planning providers are becoming vocal about the critical, if undefined, role that sexuality and gender play in their work.

Learning about Sexuality: A Practical Beginning is intended to stimulate further thinking and action about these issues within the fields of family planning and reproductive health. Through concrete examples of authors' program and research experiences, it explores the very construction of sexuality and how this differs for men and for women, the ways sexuality and power differences between men and women shape contraceptive practice

1

and reproductive health, the influence providers' own attitudes toward sexuality have on provision of services, the possibility of changing sexual attitudes and behavior, and what it takes for programs to help clients move toward more satisfactory sexual lives and greater well-being.

Learning about Sexuality is a descriptive rather than prescriptive volume, practical rather than theoretical. It makes more widely available accounts of innovative, often small-scale efforts that illuminate how people have learned about sexuality, efforts that have, in many cases, not been written about or recorded, that have often been considered inappropriate or awkward to write about. Their insights suggest ways in which the field of reproductive health and family planning can include a focus on sexuality.

The authors are social and biomedical scientists, family planning and reproductive health care providers, health activists, and others whose names came to us from an ever-expanding network. Their experiences illustrate the dynamics of sexuality and gender-based power differences and how they influence women's and men's reproductive health and their utilization of services. They share not only data and experiences but also the processes by which they became interested in the subject, how they pursued that interest, and the difficulties they encountered along the way. Experts in their fields, they present their experiences in a narrative style and personal voice that is one of the hallmarks of this resource volume, which is intended to support others in their efforts to make changes.

Learning about Sexuality has twenty-four chapters, three of which are excerpts from already published works. The chapters feature program and research work in all regions of the world with women, men, girls, and boys. They are written by women and men from over a dozen countries, with over half the contributions coming from authors in developing countries. Collectively, these chapters represent an exploration of the relationship of sexuality to reproductive health, contraceptive practice, and overall well-being. For all their variety of place, approach, and focus, a number of common themes emerge.

A central theme is that sexuality is a social construction of a biological drive; it is multidimensional and dynamic. An individual's experience of sexuality, therefore, is mediated by biology, gender roles, and power relations, as well as by factors such as age and social and economic conditions. Perhaps the most profound societal influence on an individual's sexuality comes from prescribed gender roles—the social norms and values that shape the relative power, responsibilities, and behavior of women and men. Since gender roles typically support an imbalance of power between men and women, an individual's experience of sexuality is likely to express that imbalance. These roles impose a framework that at best leaves women and men ill prepared for mutually satisfying intimate relationships.

For example, broadly speaking, women's prescribed role in sexual relations is often to be passive. Women are not encouraged or given the support to make decisions regarding their choice of sexual partners, to negotiate with their partners the timing and nature of sexual activity, to protect themselves from unwanted pregnancy and disease, and least of all to acknowledge their own sexual desire. For men, sexual conquest is almost universally prescribed as a way of proving one's manhood. Men are encouraged to think primarily of sexual performance; women's sexual pleasure is valued usually as proof of male performance. Also, the socially prescribed roles that demand a sexually domineering male mean that men face risks for not acting like "a man"; in many cases, this translates into a fear of being labeled "homosexual." In many parts of the world, as our chapters suggest, homophobia is an integral part of the social construction of male sexuality; it leads to patterns of behavior such as early, often risk-taking sex or coercive and abusive sex. Homophobia is destructive for men and women, homosexual and heterosexual.

Men's and women's mutually reinforcing gender roles have particularly debilitating consequences for reproductive health and contraceptive practice. They place a woman's health at risk when they lead her to have unwanted pregnancies and unsafe abortions. They subject her to morbidity from neglected health, gender-based abuse and violence, genital mutilation, harmful practices such as rape and other forced sex, and STDs, including HIV and AIDS. Given the pressure to start sexual activity early and the social approval of multiple partners, men too are at risk for STDs and HIV and AIDS, although to a lesser extent than women. The emphasis on the reproductive role of women, to the exclusion of men, means that often men do not have access to reproductive health services and cannot participate in responsible reproductive decision making. The consequences of such norms for reproductive ill health—unwanted or too early pregnancy, abuse, risk of AIDS—are cyclical and are perpetuated through the generations.

Another important theme that emerges from the chapters is that, as a social construct, sexuality can be influenced and changed. Too often, men and women act compulsively, as if driven by their societally prescribed roles. This is partly because they have no language for these matters. Talking, finding language for what has not been expressed, is a key way for individuals to change their perceptions of themselves and to come to understand the relationship between their individual behavior and the social and cultural context in which they live. Such awareness can transform individuals by raising their self-esteem and increasing their sense of control over their own sexuality and their own lives—in other words, by empowering them.

Over and over again, the experiences recounted in this collection demonstrate that people appreciate the opportunity to talk and ask questions about their sexual experiences; institutional, not individual, constraints keep sexuality hidden. For the most part, women and men have not had opportunities to talk about their sexuality with nonjudgmental and informed listeners on a one-to-one basis, in groups, or even as couples. Indeed, the phrase "I've never told anyone else this" is often repeated in the chapters that follow. Contrary to the expectations of many, when women are in a private and comfortable environment, with trusted facilitators or professionals who value their knowledge and experience and treat them with respect, they are comfortable talking about sex. The same is true for men in the few experiences that document their involvement.

Therefore, a final key theme is that it is necessary to create an atmosphere of trust that allows people to talk intimately and freely. Such an atmosphere is as necessary for collecting data on sexuality and sexual behavior as it is for providing services. Social scientists and biomedical researchers need to be cognizant of their own biases and judgments about sexuality to make their agendas, the questions they ask, how they listen and respond, and the completeness of what they learn more accurate. In order to create such an environment, providers, counselors, facilitators, and researchers need to examine their own attitudes, biases,

judgments, and values about sexuality and achieve some understanding of their *own* sexuality.

Links to Family Planning Services

Learning about Sexuality: A Practical Beginning demonstrates that
change is possible. It is a hopeful book because it shows that we
are not locked into destructive behaviors that are biologically
controlled. And since family planning programs regularly deal
with fundamental questions of sexual and reproductive choice,
they are an appropriate place to begin to address the imbalance
of power between intimate partners.

Chapters in this book demonstrate that women—and, to a
lesser extent, men—are not in a position to make autonomous,
"rational" decisions about their sexual behavior, fertility, and contraceptive practice, that their choices are implicitly and explicitly
controlled by their gender identity and sexual partners. They
demonstrate that women and men are constrained in their decision-making abilities by a lack of basic knowledge about their
bodies and about how different contraceptive methods can affect
their sexual relationships. They lack the opportunities, and often
even the language, to discuss with their partners critical issues
related to their sexual activity—from what is pleasurable to what
happens if they are faced with an unwanted pregnancy. Although
they may understand how a variety of institutions—including
families—within their culture shape and reinforce their gender
role identity, they are frustrated by a lack of opportunity to challenge those roles.

The chapters in this book also demonstrate that family planning and reproductive health services, and even research itself,
can create a *process* that helps individuals understand the links
between their gender roles, sexuality, and sexual behavior and
take action to improve their health and well-being. There are a
number of challenges that family planning and reproductive
health programs face in trying to support such a process. Do policymakers and program managers have the will and the resources
to design services that invest in such a process? Can they create
the necessary opportunities for providers to explore their own

attitudes, values, prejudices, and experiences regarding sexuality? Do they have an adequate understanding of who has sex with whom and under what circumstances? Do providers have the skills and the openness to be able to hear that clients are engaging in sexual behavior that is outside the traditional reproductive model, including homosexual or same-sex encounters among otherwise heterosexual individuals, or that young people, even children, may be engaging in a range of sexual activities? Can they facilitate communication between partners and help them challenge behaviors that jeopardize their own or their partners' health? Can they be comfortable in the knowledge that they will not always be able to meet all their clients' reproductive health and family planning needs and understand that by treating clients with respect and sympathy as they engage in a dialogue of exploration, they provide an invaluable service?

These are just some of the challenges that face the family planning and reproductive health field as it begins to incorporate an awareness of the critical influences that gender power and men's and women's sexual roles have on clients' choices regarding fertility and contraceptive practice. And yet, as the following chapters illustrate, these challenges are being met in a variety of ways, ways that can be deeply satisfying for both the practitioner and the participant.

Overview of Chapters

Learning about Sexuality is divided into three main parts. The first part includes approaches that program staff, activists, and researchers are taking to understand people's experiences of sexuality. The second explores the explicit and implicit links among health-seeking behavior, contraceptive practice, reproductive health, and sexuality. The chapters in the third part focus on activities that challenge entrenched attitudes and behavior about sexuality that have real and potentially harmful effects on women's and men's reproductive health.

In spite of the wealth of relevant experience described in the pages that follow, there are several gaps that we are aware of. In particular, although the relationship between violence and reproductive ill health is mentioned implicitly and explicitly in many chapters, we regret that we could find no material about how family planning and reproductive health services are addressing sexuality-related violence perpetrated against women, how to identify those at risk, what can be done to protect and help victims of abuse, or how programs can address issues such as male responsibility and violence. To stimulate action, we have included in the appendixes a list of papers that provide background material about these questions and a guide to help health care providers screen and counsel abused women.

We were also unsuccessful in finding papers that dealt with aspects of reproductive, gynecological, or sexual health services that are important for the well-being of lesbian women and homosexual men. Nor could we find examples of programs that are meeting such clients' needs in innovative ways. Appendix I includes a reference to a paper that suggests issues that reproductive health care workers and researchers should be aware of in making their services useful to lesbian women. We hope that this book stimulates readers to work on these and other gaps.

Approaches to Understanding the Experience of Sexuality

Talking and Listening. The first four chapters provide accounts of the process of talking and listening about sexuality—a process of change that requires that each person's experience be validated and that facilitators develop an egalitarian rather than authoritarian relationship to participants.

In the chapter by Baban and David, three Romanian women, interviewed with great skill and empathy, discuss their reproductive and sexual lives under a rigidly enforced pronatalist regime in which reproductive health services and information about sex were unavailable, contraceptives were not available publicly, abortions were illegal, and women's reproduction was policed by enforced gynecological examinations. At the same time, the state reinforced gender inequalities that resulted in women bearing the entire responsibility for reproduction. The chapter draws a particularly stark picture of what happens when women and their partners are unable to make free and fully informed decisions about sexuality and reproduction.

In her chapter, Jiménez narrates the process of how she learned, from talking and listening to women, that the social construction of sexuality in Venezuela keeps women ignorant of their own bodies, subject to discrimination and violence, and without self-esteem. Jiménez helped establish the Venezuelan Association for Alternative Sexual Education (AVESA) to fill the gap in available services and information on sexuality and reproduction. She explains how she came to see consciousness-raising—a process through which women share their personal stories in a nonjudgmental atmosphere and begin to understand how their behavior is prescribed by society—as a central way to support women's sexual and reproductive rights and health.

Schultz and Hedges's chapter is an edited transcript of a guided roundtable discussion—a sort of consciousness-raising—among several college-age men in the United States about their experiences and feelings concerning sexuality and its links to reproduction, including their roles as partners and potential parents. For many readers, this will be the first opportunity to hear how complex and vulnerable the process of men's coming of age is and how such discussion can itself be a process of change.

Researchers on Researching Sexuality. These chapters look at how research about sexuality, especially as it pertains to reproductive health and contraceptive use, has been and is being done.

Ericksen and Steffen's chapter traces the history of sexual behavior surveys in the United States and draws implications for comparable research in other settings. They show how unquestioned acceptance of dominant constructions of sexuality—for example, differences in male and female sex drive and behavior—has affected survey questions and analysis of data.

Amuchástegui candidly examines the personal biases and ethical dilemmas she experienced in conducting a study on sexual initiation among youth in three Mexican communities. By being explicit about her own feelings and biases and being aware of their influence on her research behavior and interpretation of interviews, she posits that her research can better elicit people's complex sexual realities.

Ali's chapter on his research on contraceptive decision-making processes among poor urban and rural households in Egypt describes differences in the kinds of information he was able to gather when he moved from focus group discussions to being a participant-observer. Living in a village, where there were extensive opportunities for give-and-take, he was able to develop a more contextualized understanding of men's fertility decision-making processes and, of key importance, the continually negotiated nature of masculinity and its relation to power.

Havanon describes the research process in a study she conducted on sexual networking in provincial Thailand, as well as personal insights that this work evoked. Initially, Havanon anticipated difficulties in eliciting responses from men and women on sexual attitudes and behavior, especially from women, as they are not supposed to discuss sexual matters openly. But she found that once they understood how the information would help lead to a better understanding of sexual behavior in the general population, female respondents answered willingly. From their responses, she came to appreciate the dangers that all Thai women face because they are not permitted to interfere with their partners' sexual behavior.

Worth's chapter reflects her experiences studying women at high risk of HIV infection from drug injections and sex with drug injectors. Looking for factors in their life histories that make them vulnerable to infection, she found a high prevalence of emotional, physical, and sexual abuse in their early lives. Developing and refining her questions from one study to the next, looking for explanations of why they knowingly put their lives at risk through unprotected sex with infected partners, she gradually came to see the role of a longing for romantic love in supporting sexual risk-taking behavior.

Understanding and Acting on the Links among Sexuality, Contraception, and Reproductive Health

Bringing Sexuality into Family Planning Services. Authors in this part explore such issues as how to learn about the connections between family planning and reproductive health and sexuality, what changes to make in services, and how to make them.

Dixon-Mueller's chapter develops a definition of sexuality and sexual behavior that is more multidimensional than the model of mutually monogamous, penile-vaginal intercourse that most providers base their services on. She shows how sexuality and sexual behavior are directly related to contraception and reproductive health.

Widyantoro writes about how her experiences providing sexuality counseling in family planning settings in Indonesia refute widely held beliefs that women are reluctant to talk about their sexuality, are always passive in sexual activities, or are unaware of or unconcerned about the sexual side effects of contraceptives. In her experience, it is natural and common for women to raise the most intimate issues of sexuality, including maximizing pleasure, when the atmosphere is sympathetic.

Plata documents the evolution of PROFAMILIA, the largest family planning service in Colombia, toward its proactive approach in supporting noncoercive sexual relationships. When staff became aware that women's ability to make decisions about their fertility and reproductive health was undermined by their lack of sexual decision-making power, PROFAMILIA called on the expertise of women's groups. Their input led to a series of changes to better support women's self-esteem and communication between couples, including workshops to retrain staff and directors in understanding how women's inequality in sexual relationships affected their contraceptive use and reproductive health as well as changes in the ways services were delivered.

Rogow describes her experience in helping to develop and introduce fertility awareness classes in a public family planning clinic in California. Participants were taught how to observe bodily changes that indicate when they are fertile, allowing them to assess their own contraceptive needs more accurately. Such information, which was not available in the local sex education programs, increased women's communication with their sexual partners, their sexual decision-making power, their enjoyment of sex, and their self-esteem.

Reproductive Health Interventions. Research on matters of reproductive health and contraception can itself be an important intervention. Research that is interactive with informants can raise their self-esteem through respect for what they know, provide new information in ways that answer their questions, and help them become more aware of the causes and consequences of their own behavior.

Diaz, interviewed by Moore, details how a sex education program in a family planning clinic in Brazil evolved from a small research project. A survey identified a high proportion of family planning clients who reported sexual dysfunction problems that they thought were related to contraceptives. The clinic began a sex education program to create an opportunity for women to speak about their own sexual histories in an atmosphere of trust. It soon became evident that, for many women, a lack of communication and respect in their intimate relationships was more significant than sexual dysfunction. The real problems, Diaz observes, arose from gender role imbalances and the social repression of female sexuality.

Niang's chapter describes an intervention that is part of a research program to identify factors that influence women's risk of HIV infection and ways to prevent infection. His study focused on Laobe women, an ethnic group in Senegal, who are traditional providers of sexual products and advice and are sought out as wives or occasional sex partners. Laobe women were approached for their expertise as informants about sexual behavior and practices. In exchange, they were taught about STDs and AIDS prevention and were supported in integrating condoms for men into the range of erotic products they promote.

The Bangs' chapter details the research process of a pioneer study of gynecological disease prevalence in two rural communities in India. It revealed that a high proportion of the women suffered from gynecological diseases, although only a small percentage had previously sought medical care. The process of entering the villages to do a study that included taking sexual and reproductive histories and performing pelvic examinations was full of lessons for the researchers, including how to deal with problems of nonparticipation. The Bangs share their experiences candidly in the hopes of helping others who do such studies.

In a chapter complementary to the Bangs', Khattab, Zurayk, Younis, and Kamal describe the efforts taken to ensure high participation in a study of reproductive morbidity, which included a gynecological exam, in two rural villages in Egypt. The project depended on a team of field-workers who were given special training and preparation for working within a community. The participation rate of 91 percent was attributed to the effective involvement of the field-workers as intermediaries between the women and the research team and health professionals.

Biomedical research. When deciding how to test, measure, and interpret sexual interest, activity, and behavior, biomedical scientists need to take into consideration more than clinical data. They must incorporate into their study design and analysis an understanding of the social construction of sexuality and its elements, including gender and power.

Dennerstein's chapter reviews what is known about changes in women's sexual interest during the course of their menstrual cycles and what is being learned about how synthetic hormones used in oral contraceptives affect sexual response. She describes research problems, challenges in measuring sexual interest, and interpretation of research findings, all of which require an awareness of gender power imbalances.

The chapter by Anderson-Hunt and associates narrates a process of conceptualizing and carrying out research on the role of the hormone oxytocin in female sexual arousal. This took place within an academic center that promotes a research model whose content is defined by women and informed by feminist, social, biomedical, and community perspectives. The process involved acknowledging the existence of social forces and gender and power issues in what is usually considered a purely "scientific" or biomedical arena. It produced a model that can be used for incorporating ethical and social dimensions into other biomedical research about sexuality.

Robbins's chapter looks at the effect of hormones, especially the androgen testosterone, on male sexual behavior. Tracing what has been learned from animal studies and, more recently, from clinical trials on hormonal methods of contraception for men, she concludes that although male libido and sexual behavior are closely linked to androgen, there are technical and ethical aspects of this research that make it difficult to systematically analyze and interpret the biological influences on male sexual behavior. She also provides some insights into the similarities and differences in the design and analysis of findings between male and female contraceptive trials.

Challenging Entrenched Attitudes and Behavior Related to Sexuality

Learning about sexuality requires a willingness to listen with an open mind in an atmosphere of trust and equality so that people can explain and explore their feelings and behavior. Judgmental attitudes in matters of sexuality force people into defensive postures or isolate and stigmatize them and reinforce low self-esteem.

Rajani and Kudrati's chapter describes a Tanzanian NGO's research on the sexual behavior of street children in order to promote their sexual health. To be able to learn, *kuleana* staff had to let go of "moral baggage" about how children should behave sexually. Their research shows that children are more likely to engage in risky sexual activities with one another—behavior that they do not consider sexual—than they are to engage in commercial or transactional sex with adults. The research also highlights the complex links among power, social support, and affection and their impacts on the sexual behavior of street children.

Simonetti, Simonetti, Arruda, and Rogow describe how Studies and Communication on Human Sexuality and Reproduction (ECOS), a Brazilian nongovernmental organization (NGO), is seeking to understand adolescent male culture as a way to help boys develop satisfying and respectful sexual lives. They describe a series of group discussions on the topic of sexuality in which safe group dynamics enable boys to reveal their confusion and the conflict between wanting to be themselves and feeling that they have to respond to strong pressure from peers, fathers, and older male family members to demonstrate their heterosexuality by having sex early.

Wilson's interview with Chantawipa Apisuk explains the program approach of Empower, a Thai grassroots advocacy organization for sex workers in Thailand. Chantawipa's analysis of the situation of sex workers, which underlies the vision of Empower, is that sexual exploitation is not the dominant problem that sex workers face; rather, it is their marginalization from society and from social services. Working with sex workers in relationships of friendship and trust, Empower helps meet needs and priorities identified by sex workers.

Stewart's chapter describes the work of a small Zimbabwean NGO, Musasa, with a mandate to change attitudes about violence toward women in Zimbabwe. Stewart analyzes the particular variants of universal rape culture that Zimbabwean culture manifests—the assumptions that women are at fault for being raped and that male needs for sex are incontrovertible. Musasa's initial work has been to change police behavior at both individual and systemic levels when dealing with rape.

Gordon's chapter, which fittingly concludes this volume, takes a realistic and somewhat daunting look at the gap that exists between the services provided by several West African Family Planning Associations of International Planned Parenthood Federation and clients' contraceptive and safe-sex needs. The gap is described as the difference between providers' attitudes about sexuality and sexual behavior and the realities of clients' lives. The chapter describes how safer-sex options of condom use, abstinence, fidelity within marriage, and nonpenetrative sex are being presented by service providers and the obstacles to their use that arise from the sexual and gender power realities of clients' lives.

———————

Learning about sexuality—including our own—is an iterative and challenging process. And yet, the more we engage in this process, the richer our understanding becomes, and the more satisfying the results for our work. Sexuality is complex, but the complexity begins to unfold as we listen in nonjudgmental ways to what people have to say about their own sexual realities. This information guides us in learning how to offer services and information in ways that enhance equality and fairness between sexual partners, support partner communication, and address the gender inequality that is the root of much reproductive ill health.

PART ONE

*Approaches
to Understanding
the Experience
of Sexuality*

Talking and Listening

*V*oices of Romanian Women

Perceptions of Sexuality, Reproductive Behavior, and Partner Relations during the Ceauşescu Era

Adriana Baban and Henry P. David

*A*lthough several surveys of reproductive behavior have been and are being conducted in Romania, few if any have focused on how individual women of varied ages and circumstances coped with the pronatalist edicts of the Ceauşescu era. On October 1, 1966, without prior warning, Ceauşescu restricted legal abortion to women who were over forty-five years of age, or who already supported four or more children, or whose lives would be endangered by pregnancy, or who met other very narrowly defined medical criteria (Ceauşescu 1966). At the same time, the importation of contraceptives was prohibited, divorce was severely restricted, and illegal abortion became a punishable offense for women and their service providers. In December 1985, Ceauşescu again restricted access to legal abortion to women over forty-five years of age who had five living children, all under the age of eighteen (Ceauşescu 1985). Official importation of contraceptives had virtually ceased, and the sale of contraceptives in pharmacies was prohibited. Employed women between the ages of sixteen and forty-five were required to undergo regular gynecological examinations.

We thought it important to document actual events in the lives

19

of some women, how Romanian cultural traditions interacted with governmental policies, and what the effects were on private reproductive behavior and partner relations. The true situation of women in Romania was carefully concealed by the regime. From a public health perspective, it was important to identify the impact of Ceaușescu's policy on psychological well-being and reproductive health. From a sexuality education perspective, further knowledge of sexual life is needed to strengthen the developing Romanian programs in reproductive health. From a psychological perspective, an in-depth study held the promise of obtaining a better understanding of cognitive and emotional determinants that influence sexual behavior under specific circumstances. And, from a cross-cultural perspective, it was hoped that the study would facilitate an explanation of similarities and differences in partner relationships under differing conditions.

Beyond the general objectives, the study, which was conducted in 1992–93, endeavored to explore, through selected in-depth interviews, the effects of a rigidly enforced pronatalist policy on women's lives, sexual and reproductive behavior, and partner relations.[1] Among the topics discussed were:

- Perceptions of sexuality in the parental home;
- Perceptions of sexuality before marriage;
- Contraceptive practices;
- Resolution of unwanted pregnancies; and
- Perceptions of partner relations.

Because the purpose of the study was exploration rather than hypothesis testing, we used in-depth, random interviews to highlight personal experiences believed to have been characteristic for many Romanian women who lived through the Ceaușescu era.[2] We ensured their confidentiality and explained to each woman that her name and address would not be recorded; our interest was solely in her personal experiences. Confidentiality was necessary both for purposes of scientific integrity and to assure women that the information they were sharing would not be turned over to the state. The length of the interview was open-ended; every woman was free to stop at any time. The interviews usually lasted from fifty to ninety minutes, depending on the woman's desire to talk. All interviews were in Romanian and tape-recorded for subsequent qualitative analysis. Although an extensive structured interview guide was developed, specific questions were asked only when a woman did not spontaneously mention an important topic. Each woman was paid 2,000 lei, equal to about U.S.$5 at the time.

In all the interviews, there was considerable overlap in discussing perceptions of sexuality before and within marriage, contraceptive practices, and resolution of unwanted pregnancies. However, the partner relationship emerged as an important aspect in a woman's sexual decision making throughout her life. Following are three of the five interviews included in the original paper.[3]

Interview with a thirty-six-year-old Romanian Orthodox unskilled laborer, with a basic level of education. She has been married for sixteen years and has three children, aged fifteen, fourteen, and twelve. Her husband is forty and is a worker.

I was a child when my father died and I found myself, all of a sudden, fatherless. I had three older brothers. Mother was overwhelmed with the hardships of life, as she had to work in the field (she was a peasant) from early morning till late at night. She had no idea of preparing me for life. I think she was not aware of very many things herself. So, I found my way by myself. Mother didn't even prepare me for my period. It all came when I was eleven and it was a shocking experience for me. I was ashamed to tell her and she pretended not to see. As I had only brothers, I didn't have anybody to talk to.

When I grew up, my brothers would forbid me to go out on dates. They told me that boys only wanted to abuse girls and, thereafter, no other man would ever accept them for a wife. "Boys have sex with girls they do not respect and they usually marry the respectable ones," they kept on telling me. Anyway, I was overloaded with work, and I didn't want to incur shame in the village. I wanted to find a good husband, to have my own home, and to live a happier life, as my childhood had been full of hardships.

I married when I was twenty. Because I was too young and ignorant or because that's the way I am, I have been most unfortunate ever since. I can say that it has been as bad as possible. My husband likes drinking and kicking up a fuss. I have been living such a life since the beginning of my marriage. It's my fate! He is callous whenever he drinks; he is callous when he doesn't. I have never liked to have sex with him, neither have I ever met another man. In fact, I think that all men are the same. I also talk, sometimes, to my colleagues. I am not really interested in sex. I have never been one of "those" who make eyes at everybody. I simply have sex with him because I must. If I ever reject him because I'm tired, and I usually tell him, "Man, I'm tired," he makes such a fuss that I give in. And, when he is drunk, it's an agony to have sex. I torture myself because I cannot really cope with him in preventing unwanted pregnancies. He thinks that all these are none of his business and that it is the woman who is supposed to take care of herself not to get pregnant. I wished to have only two children. There is not enough money for one, let alone three!

He doesn't always agree to withdrawal and tells me that it disturbs him. I cannot rely on him, anyway, when he is drunk. At the beginning, I had no knowledge about rhythm. Somebody taught me to insert some soap into the vagina before having sex. It was awfully unpleasant. Later on I started to introduce vitamin C and, after sex, I used vaginal douches with vinegar. I remember that once, spending a lot of money, I bought condoms for him. He threw them all away and told me never to dare to tell him what to do. That's the way he is. I think I was unlucky because I got pregnant frequently. I just didn't know what to do to avoid pregnancies. He always told me, "The only thing you can do is to bear children."

When I gave birth to my third daughter, he refused to come to take us home from the maternity hospital because I had another girl. I was pregnant seven times in Ceaușescu's time. I could have killed myself every time I realized I was pregnant again. Besides, I was aware that I couldn't have done anything to prevent it. There were times when I wished him to go for a date with other women and to leave me alone. I could face everything only because of my girls. Only me and God know how I found my way with all my pregnancies. I had no one to rely on. If you did not have money, nobody would ever help you!

As a woman, I had to learn not only to cook, to sew, and to raise my children, but also how to bring about an abortion. I always started with hot baths and lifting weights. Then I used to drink yeast; once I got rid of a pregnancy by drinking photochemical substances. I tried everything that I was told to do. It did not matter how much I suffered. What was important was to get rid of the pregnancy, and that something unfortunate wouldn't happen to me, and to be able to take care of my girls. They needed their mother more than they needed other brothers. I swallowed quinine several times and in huge quantities, but I never succeeded to abort this way. However, I couldn't hear for a couple of days. I remember that one of my neighbors, who worked for a vet, once gave me oxytocin, an injection they used for cows in a similar situation, and she told me that I could abort using it. I had no one to help me make the injection. So, I tried to learn to do it myself, and I used a potato for it. When I grew more skillful, I did it myself. It's hard to believe what somebody can do when she is desperate. Most of the time, I aborted with a urinary catheter, which I used on myself. I went with it inside me to my working place, to go shopping, and to do housework until I started to bleed. A couple of times I thought I'd pass away. I lost so much blood and then a month passed and I couldn't stand or walk. I only knew that, for a while, my husband was going to leave me alone and he didn't insist on having sex with me. However, there were moments when he told me that I was pretending and that I couldn't feel so sick. Because of so many abortions, I was anemic.

Even if I had four days to tell you my story, it wouldn't be enough to tell you all my troubles. It isn't easy for me now. From 1990 until now, I have had five abortions in the clinic. Ever since he knows that abortion is legal, my husband doesn't protect me at all. He doesn't allow me to insert an IUD because I'd have sex with other men, he says. I never had an eye for men when I was younger, how could I have one now that I'm old and had such experiences! I only hope that he would curb his desires as he is old enough. He is forty, and he has grown-up daughters! What else can I do? Good or good-for-nothing as he is, I have a husband of my own. Wherever I go, I am a married woman and not a divorced one. My brothers wouldn't let me divorce, not for the world. And where else could I go? What could a lonely woman with three children do? Everybody would mock me. This was my fate and I can't help it. That's my fortune! If only my girls are luckier than me!

Interview with a forty-three-year-old skilled worker with a secondary school education. She has been married for seventeen years to a technician (aged forty-three) and has two children, ages fourteen and thirteen. She is Romanian Orthodox.

When I was a young girl, mothers didn't know how to become friends to their daughters. They didn't talk about sex or sexuality, particularly in the village where I grew up. As if there weren't such a problem! Only when my present husband began to woo me, my mother started to tell me to be careful not to commit a sin and that a respectable girl is led to the altar only if she is immaculate. It is only when you are immaculate that your husband honors you. That's the way I wanted to be! Even if times have changed, it is the way I think about it today as well.

When I married, I almost didn't know anything, except that I was in love with my husband. At the beginning, I had no idea about preventive methods, neither did I ask myself about it, because I wanted children as soon as possible. I married rather late, when I was twenty-six, and in the country one is considered a spinster at that age. I was terribly shy at the beginning. You can't get accustomed immediately to a man, even if he is your husband. I don't know why, but when we made love, I seldom felt pleasure. I have a cool nature, I think, but for me sex is not important in marriage. What really matters is to understand each other. It also matters that your children have a father who can help you to make a living and, as you are for him, he is for you, a real support when you are old.

My husband would have liked to have had sex more often. Men are different; they think of sex more often than women. We are busy with our work, housework, and children. My husband is very kind and sympathetic. He gives all his salary for the house, he doesn't drink, he loves us all, but he doesn't help with the housework. It is the way he got used to from his mother: to be taken care of, to be always assisted, to be helped to the dish as if he were a child. He is so helpless, he cannot even make tea for himself! When he comes home from work, he puts on his pajamas and sits in the armchair, reading the newspapers or watching television.

I have never told him I didn't like to make love. You are not allowed to reject men because they are weak and frivolous. If other women make eyes at them, men lose their heads so foolishly.

But a wise woman always knows how to keep her man.

In my first two years of marriage, I was awfully desperate that I couldn't get pregnant. I had been told by my colleagues that if one likes making love, one gets pregnant easily. It suddenly came to my mind that I didn't get pregnant because I felt no pleasure. Marriage without children is no marriage. Children strengthen any marriage. Without children, life has no aim, you have no one to work with and to earn a living for!

After giving birth to my two children, I got pregnant twice more. I didn't want any more children because we wanted to provide as much as possible for those we had. My husband would have easily accepted the third child, but I decided to abort. I got pregnant while I breast-fed my youngest child. I had an idea that one is absolutely safe then, that one couldn't get pregnant. I simply couldn't believe that I was pregnant. Therefore, I aborted when I was in the third month. I went to a midwife, in a village some 180 kilometers from Cluj, sent by an intermediary who was one of my colleagues. I had to reach that place late in the evening so that nobody could see me. There she did the abortion for me, by an oil lamp so that nobody could see anything from outside. I was terrorized with fear, and I thought that I could never ever go back home safe. Fear appeared again, a couple of months later, when I found out from my colleague that the midwife had been arrested, caught in the act. It crossed my mind that I could have been that woman, only I had been luckier. For a while I always shuddered when I heard the doorbell. I was afraid that the police had forced her to denounce all the women she had aborted. It was a nightmare. My husband reproached me that if I had kept the baby, we wouldn't be so stressed. But I thought that my way was better for my family. When everything ended, I felt myself free, although, being a believer, I'll die with this sin on my soul.

After that experience, I was awfully scared to get pregnant again. I shuddered every month. My husband was kind and sympathetic and, on dangerous days, we didn't make love and, on the other days, we used withdrawal. I trusted him completely because he had absolute self-control. He tried once with a condom, but he didn't like it and he told me, "as long as I live, I won't have sex with a condom." Withdrawal didn't bother me, but I think that it wasn't very healthy for him. I have never talked about it with him, and he has never mentioned anything to me.

When I got pregnant once again, I went to another woman to abort. While she was bringing about the abortion with a urinary catheter, I felt, all of a sudden, that my whole body was terribly hot. When I asked her what she was doing, she told me that she had poured 90 percent alcohol into my uterus.

Actually, whenever you found yourself pregnant, you were happy to find someone to help you and, being at their mercy, you had to give them a lot of money, but had no idea what to expect. You were simply happy to have gotten rid of it. But I think I needed a hysterectomy at forty-two because of what they'd done to me. After the second abortion I felt pain and I bled whenever I made love. But for several years, I was ashamed to go to a gynecologist and, in the end, I had to have a surgical operation. I asked the doctor not to tell my husband that he took away my uterus. I didn't want him to believe that I was not a woman anymore. Perhaps I wouldn't be in this situation if I didn't have the two abortions. Who knows? What is important for me now is to be healthy, to raise my children.

I didn't educate my boys sexually because they know much more than we did—with these movies and magazines one can find to buy everywhere now!

Interview with a thirty-four-year-old economist with a university degree. Her husband, who is thirty-five, is an engineer. They have a nine-year-old child. She is Orthodox.

Although both my parents had completed university studies (they were both pharmaceutical chemists), my mother accepted my father's domination. Whatever he said was considered brilliant. Whatever my mother said was worthless, but nevertheless indulgently and contemptuously accepted by Father.

My family background and the sexual education I got were completely different for me as compared to my brother. I was told that getting pregnant meant to ruin my future, and, therefore, I had to be very strictly supervised. Father decided that every month I had to prove to my mother that I was having my period. Good care prevents deadly peril, he used to tell me. My brother, in contrast, was being encouraged to initiate sexual relationships with girls. They considered it part of a boy's education, and good for his health. Moreover, he was told that if he had problems with a girl whom he had gotten pregnant, he should immediately inform Father so he could help solve the problem.

My parents destroyed any trace of femininity in me. I was always brought impersonal gray clothes, and they didn't allow me to show any sign of coquetry. I was told that I was skinny and that I had crooked legs; they did whatever they could to ruin my self-esteem and self-trust as a woman. And now, when I am having disagreements with my husband because I am more interested in my profession than in household problems, they reproach my lack of femininity. Father told me that this is the most important feature that any man values in a woman. As I know him very well, I know, for sure, what femininity means to him.

I began my sexual life at twenty-one, because my friend exerted pressure upon me. I did it out of fear of being abandoned, and I experienced no sexual pleasure. Although fear of getting pregnant was always present, I used no preventive methods, only that I had sex on the so-called safe days. I read in books how one could find out which those days were. This method protected me for only a year. When I realized that I was pregnant, I thought I was the most unfortunate being in the world. One couldn't think of something worse to happen to a girl! I had in mind doing anything to get rid of it. I told myself that it was better to risk my life than to ruin it. I was about to render justice to my parents! It was beyond question to talk to them about my troubles.

I couldn't rely on my friend as he was completely helpless and ignorant; he was more scared than I had been. One of my friends took me to a medical student who brought about the abortion with a catheter. I had to pay her with my gold necklace and, at home, I told everybody that I had lost it. I was terribly scared that something might happen to me, but my friend said that I'd be all right because the same student had done it to her four times and with no consequences whatsoever; she was a real specialist.

After getting rid of the pregnancy, I told myself that no man in the world is worth having such tormenting experiences. One is happy for a minute or two and then one endures a month, if one is not miserable for the rest of one's life. . . . Once more I realized that fate is more unjust with women than with men.

When I got acquainted with my husband and when I made love with him, he suspected that I was not a virgin. He told me that with a lost virginity, any woman might pretend she is with a second partner. I felt offended that he did not trust me and that he had tried to make me feel guilty for having had a previous boyfriend.

When I married, I realized that my parents felt relief and were happy, not necessarily because of my marriage but because they had feared I would become a spinster. In contrast, my brother was told that there was enough time for him to get married and that it was a foolish thing to hasten that. No girl seemed good enough for him. In their opinion, what seemed important for me was simply to be married.

After two months of marriage, I got pregnant, although we used withdrawal. We had decided not to have children so quickly because my working place was in another town. I was afraid to tell my husband that I was pregnant and have him decide to keep the child. It would have been very hard for me and not for him. I asked one of my cousins for help because she told me that she had more than ten abortions with some Arabic medicine she had bought from some sailors in Constanza. She provided some for me—I don't know what pills they were. I had to take nine pills a day for a couple of days. They proved ineffective with me, so I decided not to have an abortion and to keep the baby. I was really terrorized for nine months. I was afraid to give birth to a malformed baby. I have never told anyone what I had done. Only my cousin knew about it and now it is you. When I gave birth, I asked the doctor three times if my baby had everything it was supposed to have. In fact, I didn't settle down until my child started to walk and to talk, and I was convinced that his intellect was not affected. God helped me that everything ended well!

When I succeeded in changing my job and I was in Cluj, I wanted to have another child. But I couldn't convince my husband, not a bit. He kept on telling me that we didn't live in an age when it is worthwhile giving birth to children. It is true we were struggling hard to get food. That took all our time.

When I got pregnant again I thought that I could convince him, but he didn't even listen to the idea of having another child. At last I agreed to an abortion on condition that he should find a way. I secretly hoped that he couldn't find a way out. But he planned with a gynecologist to perform the abortion at our home in exchange for a great amount of money. Although it was my husband who settled everything, it was I who suffered from pain and fear.

Several months passed until I was able to have sex again. Having sex by withdrawal was always the same; when I was about to feel pleasure, he ejaculated and I was left frustrated. I have never known whether there is something wrong with me or with my husband because I had an orgasm so seldom! I cannot talk to him about it because he has a cold nature. If I wished to make love, I would have been ashamed to tell my husband because he would have thought bad things about me!

I was quivering every month waiting for my period. Once, I wished I had my menopause and was finished with that dreadful monthly fear. Anyway, I had so little happiness with my sexual life!

In comparison to other families, I might say that I have a good family life. And yet, I don't think that's the way a real couple should be! My husband is very reproachful to me that I am too involved professionally. He says that in a family, the two members of the couple cannot achieve equally. It is not normal that a woman is professionally ambitious. I was obviously to be the one who would give up ambition so as to offer him support for his achievements. This would mean that housework and the child's education were supposed to be only on my shoulders and he would have the psychic comfort to concentrate on his profession. When things do not go his way he makes me feel guilty for being an undevoted mother and wife. He is not happy with my professional growth.

We don't have serious disputes in the family, but I feel that both of us, in the depth of our hearts, are dissatisfied with each other, and we don't even tell each other. We only know that we have a child to raise!

After the revolution I put in an IUD, but our sexual life is not much better, although I got rid of the fear of pregnancy.

A Final Note

The women's narratives about clandestine abortions were often told in a context of trauma and tragedy, creating an emotionally charged atmosphere that was sometimes as difficult for the interviewer as for the subject. Although it seemed to be a therapeutic experience for some women, it was a painful recollection for others—one that they wanted to forget but could not. Still, when recalling the terror of an unwanted pregnancy, the women generally reasserted their strong will to terminate at whatever cost or risk to their well-being.

The words uttered by one of the subjects were typical for the study group, and they were repeated by most women: "I did not want children anymore. Nobody and nothing could stop me from making the decision to abort. I would have done anything to get rid of my pregnancy. I assumed all risks involved, but I consciously and voluntarily kept trying not to think about them. The only thought was to solve my terrible problem that had plunged me into a catastrophic situation, no matter how."

Notes

1. This study was graciously funded by grants from the International Health Foundation and the Population Council to the Transnational Family Research Institute.

2. The study group consisted of fifty women who were between eighteen and fifty-five years of age in 1988, the year before the December 1989 revolution. They lived in Cluj-Napoca, a large city in Transylvania, located near the border with Hungary. There were ten women each in the age groups twenty-one to twenty-five, twenty-six to thirty, thirty-one to thirty-five, and thirty-six to forty, and five women each in the age groups eighteen to twenty and fifty to fifty-five. Women aged fifty to fifty-five were included in the study group to assess the impact of the 1966 law, which restricted legal abortion to women over age forty-five. Forty women were married, four were divorced, two were remarried or cohabiting with a partner, and four were unmarried. Thirty-six women had one or two children, eight women had no children, and six women had three or more children. Most of the women, thirty-eight, were Romanian Orthodox; twelve were Catholic.

3. Further interviews and an analysis are presented in the complete monograph, which is available for US$10 from the Transnational Family Research Institute, 8307 Whitman Drive, Bethesda, MD 20817 USA.

References

Battiata, M. 1990. A Ceauşescu legacy: Warehouses for children. *Washington Post,* June 7.

Ceauşescu, N. 1966. Decret no. 770, 29.IX.

———. 1985. Decret no. 411, 26.XII. In *Official Bulletin* no. 76, December 26, 1985.

———. 1986. *Der Spiegel,* October 20, pp. 217–18.

David, H. P. 1970. *Family planning and abortion in the socialist countries of Central and Eastern Europe.* New York: Population Council.

———. 1990a. Ceauşescu's psychological legacy: A generation of unwanted children. *Psychology International* 1(2):6–7.

———. 1990b. Romania ends compulsory childbearing. *Entre Nous* 14(15):9–10.

———. 1990c. Romania ends compulsory childbearing. *Population Today* 18(3):4–10.

———. 1992. Abortion in Europe, 1920–1991: A public health perspective. *Studies in Family Planning* 23(1):1–22.

David, H. P., and R. J. McIntyre. 1981. *Reproductive behavior: Central and Eastern European experience.* New York: Springer.

David, H. P., and N. Wright. 1971. Abortion legislation: The Romanian experience. *Studies in Family Planning* 2:205–10.

Gilberg, T. 1979. Rural transformation in Romania. In *The peasantry of Eastern Europe,* edited by I. Volgyes. New York: Pergamon.

Grigoroiu-Serbanescu, M. 1990. How a restrictive abortion policy affected child mental health. *Entre Nous* 14(15):6.

Harsanyi, D. P. 1993. Women in Romania. In *Gender politics and postcommunism,* edited by N. Funk and M. Mueller. New York: Routledge.

Hord, C., H. P. David, F. Donnay, and M. Wolf. 1991. Reproductive health in Romania: Reversing the Ceauşescu legacy. *Studies in Family Planning* 22(4):231–40.

Johnson, B. R., M. Horga, and L. Andronache. 1993. Contraception and abortion in Romania. *The Lancet* April 3;341(8849):875–878.

Johnson, B. R., M. Horga, and L. Andronache. 1995. Women's perspective on abortion in Romania. *Social Science and Medicine* (in press).

Kligman, G. 1991a. Women and reproductive legislation in Romania: Implications for the transition. In *Dilemmas of transition in the Soviet Union and Eastern Europe,* edited by G. Breslauer. Berkeley: University of California Press.

Kligman, G. 1991b. *The wedding of the dead.* Berkeley: University of California Press.

Kligman, G. 1992. The politics of reproduction in Ceauşescu's Romania: A case study in political culture. *East European Politics and Societies* 6(3):364–418.

Kligman, G., and S. Mezei. (forthcoming). *When abortion is banned: Politics of reproduction in Ceauşescu's Romania.* (Working title).

Legge, J. S. 1985. *Abortion policy: An evaluation of the consequences for maternal and infant health.* Albany: State University of New York Press.

Mehlan, K. H. 1965. Legal abortions in Romania. *Journal of Sex Research* 1(1):31–38.

Muresan, P., and I. M. Copil. 1974. Romania. *Population policy in developed countries,* edited by B. Berelson. New York: McGraw-Hill.

Mutler, A. 1994. Confusion about sex, birth control in Romania. *Chicago Tribune,* 17 May.

Puia, S., and C. Hirtopeanu. 1990. Coming out of the dark: Family planning in Romania. *Planned Parenthood in Europe* 19(2):5–6.

Rochat, R. 1991. *Women's health, family planning, and institutionalized children in Romania.* USAID/Trust Through Health.

Romania. Ministry of Health. 1957. Decree No. 463, 25 November.

Romania. Ministry of Health. 1989. Decree No. 605, 27 December.

Serbanescu, F. 1994. Personal communication, 3 May.

Serbanescu, F., and L. Morris. 1994. Reproductive health survey Romania 1993. Preliminary Report, Institute for Mother and Child Care, Ministry of Health, Bucharest and Division of Reproductive Health; Centers for Disease Control and Prevention, Atlanta.

Stephenson, P., M. Wagner, M. Badea, and F. Serbanescu. 1992. Commentary: The public health consequences of restricted induced abortion— lessons from Romania. *American Journal of Public Health* 82(10): 1328–31.

United Nations Population Fund (UNFPA). 1990. Report on mission to Romania 5–15 March 1990. Unpublished.

*L*earning Together

A Woman's Story

Elisa Jiménez Armas

This is a story about women—myself and possibly thousands more—who have shared in an effort to discover, build, and transform our lives. Specifically, my account has to do with women's experience of sexuality and childbearing. It takes place within a broader educational process through which I was able to make sense of my own existence. It is a story about consciousness-raising, starting from my own experience as an educator and building on a constant process of dialogue, reflection, and action with other women.

I lived thirty years of my life perfectly encased in the mold that I inherited. Until then, living as a woman meant obeying guidelines that had been prescribed for my gender by the Venezuelan upper middle class into which I was born. I fulfilled the ritual roles of daughter, girlfriend, wife, and, finally, mother. Lucky enough to have a father and a husband who "permitted" me to study, I managed to complete a degree. I was determined to be a good modern mother—well-informed, familiar with the latest pediatric and psychological trends, and devoted to the task of child rearing. But I often felt guilty for my lack of enthusiasm in carrying out the duties of a responsible wife and for my shortcomings as a mother.

I would daydream, either because I was bored with my insular world or because of a growing unconscious need to have my own dreams and to fulfill them. The long-coveted completion of my psychology degree went part of the way toward meeting this need. But I was still not completely happy. I was still anxious and eager to escape. Why? What motivated my desire to do something more?

The answers to these questions came suddenly when I had a chance to compare my story with that of other women. In my first job as a psychologist, I was asked to join a team that would develop a state-run program to provide psychosocial and educational support to pregnant working-class women at the nation's largest maternity hospital in the heart of Caracas. Part of the program was a course on sexuality, contraception, child care, education, pediatrics, and related topics. Participating women also received pregnancy and labor training, along with one-on-one psychological counseling. Some of the women we served in this clinic were being treated for incomplete abortions and also needed clinical and counseling care.

Early in this work, I discovered that as soon as women began to interact in a group, they would look inward and become conscious of the fact that things were not going well. They began to communicate their desires, needs, and frustrations. Listening to women's stories, I began to have a profound sense of how they lived and experienced sexuality and childbirth. By comparing their stories with mine, I began a process (ongoing to this day) of becoming conscious of the social and cultural implications of being a woman. Through my contact with these women, I began to grasp the fact that we were discriminated against and oppressed as a gender, and to see the obstacles that get in the way of our development as individuals.

The more I confronted thoughts about myself and my life and compared them with those of other women, the more I realized that the conflicts and struggles we had in common could be traced to our presumed destiny as women. This destiny is understood strictly in terms of what we do for others; it was the equivalent of not "being" at all.

Defining the Problem

Abortion is illegal in Venezuela, even in cases of rape and when the life of the woman is in danger. In the hospital, we met desperately poor women who had come to the emergency room to complete an abortion they had started at home, generally with a dangerous method. These women were resigned to being stigmatized and mistreated in the "abortion ward." None of them thought that they could demand respectful treatment.

We understood that women resort to abortion to resolve an intractable situation. However, we were puzzled that although these women apparently made rational decisions based on their knowledge and assessment of their situations, they strove to forget the incident. The women did not have the slightest notion of their right to make decisions about sexuality and reproduction. Even women who were urgently seeking abortions because they had been raped came to doubt whether they had the right to do so. We came to see this tendency to avoid a rational, critical assessment of such an event, which can never be insignificant in a woman's life, as a consequence of the sexual ideology that prevails in our culture. Through our work, we sought to dismantle the myths that allow this subjugation to be perceived as natural.

To remember that period of my life is to hear those women reconstructing their personal histories and recognizing themselves as part of a single common history—one of violence and discrimination.

Their Voices

The women arrived at the hospital to blindly fulfill the destiny they believed was naturally theirs. I remember the essence of our conversations. Though their body language was defiant, their faces revealed the fear, guilt, frustration, and lack of communication that corrupt women's experience of sex:

> *"I can't tell him that I don't feel any pleasure; he'll think I'm a no-good woman and that I'm probably seeing someone else. . . . It will*

wound his sense of manhood." . . . *"If I show him that he excites me, if I'm assertive with him, he might think I know too much, he'll start to ask me where I learned it."* . . . *"He won't forgive me because I didn't bleed on the first night, and he won't believe that I was still a virgin."* . . . *"He thinks he can do whatever he wants to me because I had a previous boyfriend."* . . . *"I dreamed that I was masturbating and I woke up crying because I felt so guilty."*

Their feelings about maternity:

"I'm already eighteen years old—it's high time I had a child." . . . *"You've got to have kids to be a real woman."* . . . *"He asked me for that proof of my love."* . . . *"He's never had children and he wanted to see if he was capable."* . . . *"I didn't want one, but what can you do? Once you have it inside you you've got to love it."* . . . *"He never wants to use protection and I have to take precautions in hiding."*

Their shame, guilt, and self-loathing following an abortion:

"When that bastard raped me my husband almost left me; imagine what would have happened if I had told him that I was pregnant. He wouldn't have forgiven me. It wasn't my fault, I know that it's a sin to kill a child, but is it still a sin when you've been raped?" . . . *"A girlfriend helped me when I went to abort the first one. It hadn't even been a real relationship, it was really stupid on my part. I don't know why I let myself get carried away. But I'm going to have this one, even if I am alone. I won't be at peace until I have that child that I denied myself earlier."* . . . *"I just wanted to protect the children that I already have, I can't have a single one more; no one knows about it; don't tell anyone, let me forget it."*

The surprise, pain, and anger they feel when they are brutalized, manipulated, negated:

"He always treated me like a little girl, in the sense that he made all the decisions. He even thought he could decide the sex of our children in advance. His reaction when he found out it was a girl was so violent that I have never been able to forgive him." . . . *"Men like my boss have a very clear sense of their power, and when they decide to go for one of their female subordinates no one stops them. It nearly cost me my life to put him in his place. I'm exhausted, but now I know that I also have power."*

Over time, I also witnessed the awakening of their conscious-ness, their joy in discovering that they too could be protagonists and control the outcome of their own lives:

"I stayed in the course, I kept coming after the first session, because here with the rest of you it dawned on me that I am a person, that the world moves because of the influence of thinking people, and that I am such a person." . . . *"Now I feel like I have hopes, I feel a kind of happy tiredness, do you know what I mean?"* . . . *"No one will be able to shut my eyes again, nor my mind, to say nothing of my heart."* . . . *"I never understood what it meant to say that one existed in the world."* . . . *"I am now able to give my child the most important thing he can possibly have: I want him to think, to have his eyes open."*

The Evolution of a Framework

Those of us who ran the hospital-based program (mostly profes-sional women in the health, education, and psychology fields) came to believe that the possibility of a fulfilling and enjoyable sexual and reproductive life (that is, one that allows for planned births and a dignified existence) is conditioned by a complex interplay of factors.

In addition to various biological and socioeconomic character-istics, a woman's sexual and reproductive health is determined by her self-esteem, her capacity for self-determination, and her free-dom to make choices. If she is prevented from realizing her poten-tial as an individual and kept alienated from her own body and sexuality, she will remain ignorant and powerless to become an agent of change in her own well-being.

We therefore decided to focus our educational efforts on con-sciousness-raising, or the process through which individuals change their view of themselves and of their surrounding reality. This process requires an ongoing dialogue, whereby a critical understanding of reality leads to personal transformation and the creation of a new social identity. We viewed consciousness as the sum of a woman's self-image—which is the product of her per-sonal history—*and* her concept of the role she plays in society. We also believed that a woman's understanding of that role is often subconscious, inarticulate, and not necessarily reflective of her objective reality. As opposed to viewing a woman's personal history as an isolated event, consciousness-raising attempts to place that history within the framework of social values and norms. For example, a woman cannot understand her sexual experience without first analyzing key formative experiences that determine her gender identity, her relationship to her body, and her concept of pleasure. Although this analysis should be centered on her particular experience, it should also constantly refer to the circumstances of her family and culture and to the sexual values and social norms that have made sexuality itself a problem. Personal decisions should be seen within the context of social and historical factors that have determined them.

Our goal was to counteract the effects of the prevailing sexual ideology in Venezuela,[1] which denies the creative and humanizing power of sexuality and instead links natural instincts to sin. It attempts to make sex a purely private moral issue, ignoring its links to psychological, political, and historical determinants. In short, it defines people's sex lives as a problem area. The specific rules or "sexual mores" that underlie this ideology are assimilated by children from the very beginning of the socialization process. Ironically, what children learn about sex is the importance of denying it, because the topic is barred from everyday conversation. This repression affects a child's entire development, typically creating sexual conflicts later in life.

We believe that the psychosocial and material conditions that characterize most women's lives, along with their typically negative sexual and reproductive experiences, amount to nothing less than a pattern of social violence against women. We concluded that this violence is rooted in the power relationship between men and women and is embedded in the very structure of society. The power inequities in male–female relationships, in turn, are perpetuated by specific cultural constructs of "masculinity" and "femininity." Such constructs promote the idea that men's and women's sexual needs are inherently "different" and have particular characteristics. For example, men are supposed to require immediate sexual satisfaction to remain physically healthy, a concept that is vaguely attributed to virility. Women, in contrast, are supposed to be able to control or postpone their sexual needs in order to remain faithful.

Although such stereotypes are equally prevalent in all social classes, they are potentially more potent among socioeconomically deprived sectors, where they are linked to the notion of motherhood as destiny, of poorer women's greater vulnerability to "machismo," and to the general absence of sexual information even of a purely physiological nature. These factors mean that a pleasurable sex life becomes something of a rare privilege for most of the women in our program.

We concluded that gender-based violence and underlying sexual repression are the primary obstacles to reaching satisfactory levels of sexual and reproductive health among women. This understanding was confirmed by numerous accounts of the deep guilt experienced by women who have suffered the trauma of unplanned pregnancies and, in the worst cases, of rape.

An Alternative Approach: AVESA's Unplanned Pregnancy Crisis Care Program

Based on this critical assessment of the problems surrounding sex education, sexual and reproductive health, and sexual violence against women, we determined to offer women alternative services, including counseling and education in their own communities. We thought it essential to find the means by which women could develop a critical awareness of themselves and of the reality that determines their subjugation. This shared goal of those of us in the hospital-based program led to a practical commitment to form the first Venezuelan nongovernmental organization that approaches sexual and reproductive health and violence against women from a critical perspective and that proposes alternatives to give women greater control of their health and sexuality. We realized that we had learned a lot about what women need and what we needed to do. So in 1984, a group of us decided to take all we had learned and create AVESA (see box).

We designed AVESA's Unplanned Pregnancy Crisis Care Program to meet the needs of women or couples who were living through that crisis. Based on our earlier experience in the hospital, we set out to provide a combination of empathy and support and start a process of consciousness-raising. This included providing information on sexual and reproductive health and explaining the

AVESA: An Overview

In 1984, a group of psychologists, students, and friends came together to create the nongovernmental organization AVESA. AVESA's purpose was to fill the gap in available services and information on sexuality and reproduction. Located centrally in the city of Caracas, AVESA was the first national organization created to critically examine reproductive and sexual health by addressing the following:

- the lack of access to therapeutic treatment and support for female rape victims

- the complex problem of unwanted pregnancy and the impact of clandestine abortion and mortality

- the role of men in the family (abandonment and irresponsible fatherhood affect more than 50 percent of Venezuelan homes)

- the lack of research, information, treatment, and services related to sex education, pre- and postnatal care, and sexual and reproductive health

Programs

AVESA addresses these issues through a structure of "action units" or programs: Sex Education and Awareness Program; Unplanned Pregnancy Crisis Care Program; Pre- and Postnatal Education Unit; Female Rape Victim Assistance Program; and Reproductive and Sexual Health Program. Counseling is an important aspect of all these programs. Today, in addition to clinical services, AVESA conducts research, training, and advocacy related to these issues.

Membership and Financial Support

AVESA gathers both political and financial support through a broad-based membership system that includes active members who are responsible for the daily activities of AVESA; collaborating members who are in training and are occasionally active in AVESA; and honorary members representing national scientific, cultural, and political spheres.

The work of AVESA is made possible by the voluntary efforts of its members, modest contributions from the private sector, and income produced by the program's modest and sliding-scale fees.

Outreach

Community outreach. As the only national organization to actively place sexual and reproductive rights in the public arena, AVESA has an impact in the broader community. Additionally, AVESA has played an important role as a maturing influence on the women's movement in Venezuela. It has fostered the transfer of information and support into the women's movement through public forums, workshops with clients, lobbying with influential individuals and political leaders, and work through the mass media (newspapers and television). AVESA is currently working on increasing the visibility of and the legitimate leadership for the national campaign for reproductive rights.

Men. Although there is no specific outreach to men, male partners (mainly university students) often participate in the counseling sessions and are encouraged to continue to participate. AVESA has also initiated a research project on men and violence.

concept of sexual and reproductive rights. Counseling is an important aspect of all of AVESA's programs, especially the Unplanned Pregnancy Crisis Care Program. We also sought to create a support network of men and women who had participated in the program.

Counseling

In Venezuela, many women are reluctant to go to a provider for follow-up care after having secured an abortion, because of the illegality of the procedure. However, because of our sympathetic and respectful approach, many women come to AVESA for counseling and contraceptive and clinical services after they have had abortions.

In the beginning, we provided personal counseling to women or couples before and after pregnancy termination. Later, we decided that there were benefits to holding postabortion counseling in group sessions. We believed that the opportunity to share one's individual story with others was an important step in understanding a personal experience in its broader social and political context.

When a woman comes to AVESA, she (and her partner, if he accompanies her) goes through a two-hour workshop, during which she gets information and counseling on sexual and repro-ductive health. If requested, individual counseling is offered. The woman also receives a physical exam, to ensure that she is in good health after the abortion.

The group counseling session is structured like a workshop. It is facilitated by a team—one man (often a doctor) and one woman (often a psychologist). This ensures that clinical and psy-chosocial information is integrated. The session takes about two hours. About five to six women attend each session, and some-times their partners come along. There are a few structured activi-ties, but basically the sessions are free-flowing and informal. To give the women an opportunity to learn factual information and grapple with issues related to sexual and reproductive decision making, the group discusses a range of issues related to the ques-tion How did you get pregnant?

The facilitators provide basic information and answer ques-tions on sexuality, anatomy, reproduction, and birth control. They also facilitate discussion and lead some exercises to help women understand where they got their views about sex, pregnancy, and related issues and how this understanding can help them in their future reproductive and sexual decisions.

We are very satisfied with the results of this counseling. We find that women who participate develop a significantly different way of dealing with feelings of guilt and are able to reach a critical understanding of the factors that led to their current crisis and determine their behavior. We also see changes in both men's and women's attitudes toward contraception, which they now tend to see as a right and a responsibility shared by both partners.

What the Program Means to Our Clients

In a country where abortion is illegal, even when a woman has been raped, we were able to create a space and time where women (some alone, some with their partners) could find companionship and support during a personal crisis. What this opportunity means for the participating women is best expressed in their own words.

"For me it was very important to share with other women the kind of feelings that this experience provoked, both before and after. We were able to understand the entirety of what we had lived and we all felt the strength of our courage at having been able to make that decision. I think that we will go on from here with a better sense of who we are, and with the will to fight for our rights." —Isabel

"It amounts to feeling that I am taking part in my own liberation, to seeing that along with me, other women have been able to learn that we do matter, because we are capable of making our own decisions." —Teresa

"What I've been able to share today has helped me to placate that sense of guilt. . . . I see clearly now that our inaccurately named 'weak sex' is the one responsible for choosing and making decisions in spite of what has been imposed on us. I feel that this is also our power." —Luisa

"It has been a fundamentally human, noble experience. It has been a kind of rebirth through the opening of new ideas and perspectives. It has been a way of exercising liberty. It means that I feel myself capable of determining the direction of my own life, and that I recognize my duty to fight in order to make change possible." —Rebeca

"This last step has been necessary, because we have to confront our experiences in order to see clearly to our future. I am another man now; I feel more complete." —Pablo

"It was a very intense experience; I lived emotions that I didn't know I was capable of. It has humanized my life." —Rafael

"It was an opportunity to understand the world as it really is, to discover myself playing a role as man that I was not previously aware of. I felt tremendously happy at being able to reaffirm who I am." —Andres

What Did We Learn?

We learned that women can be liberated through an educational consciousness-raising process that allows them to see and comprehend the power mechanisms that create inequality and gender discrimination. The Unplanned Pregnancy Crisis Care Program also reaffirmed our conviction that we as women have to gain control of our sexuality and our reproductive lives if we are to reach equality in other spheres.

We gained new understanding into the importance of male participation in crisis situations related to contraception or unwanted pregnancy. Through their participation, men can become conscious of their own responsibility in the fight for reproductive rights.

The program has been one of AVESA's most important activities because we have created a network of thousands of men and women who are committed to fighting for reproductive rights, which are completely ignored in our country.

Finally, we developed a methodology for treating the personal crisis caused by an unwanted pregnancy that has two key advantages: it can be used in countries where abortion is illegal, and it promotes a process of critical reflection that can fuel action for social change.

Note

1. I speak of ideology as the means by which the nature of particular social relations (for example, those between men and women) are falsified, hidden or misrepresented in order to protect prevailing social interests.

*H*earing Ourselves Talk

Links between Male Sexuality and Reproductive Responsibilities

Jason Schultz and Warren Hedges

*L*ike other programs in the United States, Men Acting for Change (MAC), a group of Duke University students, staff, and alumni, has worked with men on questions of male gender and sexual identity. In a safe yet challenging environment, men can explore their ideas, experiences, and fears in a way that encourages self-reflection and change. We have learned that there is no homogeneous male—rather, men have a range of questions, concerns, backgrounds, lifestyles, and needs.

What follows is a discussion within MAC about reproduction. It suggests that understanding and challenging men's attitudes about sex and reproductive technologies is a long and complex process because men's attitudes are themselves complex. It proved impossible, and probably undesirable, to discuss reproduction without considering other, ostensibly unrelated, issues from which the men's underlying motivations and beliefs about sexuality, masculinity, and relationships gradually emerged.

Although every man's perspective was different, some common themes and experiences surfaced. First and most striking is the extraordinary difficulty most of us had getting information about reproductive choices when we were younger; typically, learning about sex and reproductive choices was a solitary affair. Second, and not unrelated, there was a pronounced disconnection between information available about pleasure and information available about preventing pregnancy; our information about reproduction was usually ancillary to (often misleading) information about sex. Typically, sexuality was presented as having *nothing to do* with reproduction, and reproductive choices, especially condoms, took away from the pleasure of sexuality. Third, attitudes about reproductive choices nonetheless remain inextricably tethered to attitudes about sex and sexual practices, whether they are about "trophy" girlfriends, abortion, the heterosexist tilt in sex education, or how a man would feel about getting NORPLANT® if it was available for men. Throughout the discussion, it was difficult to talk about reproduction without talking about sex, but it was not, perhaps unfortunately, difficult to talk about sex without talking about reproduction.

Finally, we'd like to point out that some of the most innovative and promising ideas about reproductive education came from group members familiar with gay culture. Many gay people, after all, think of themselves as distinctive from "breeders"—those heterosexual couples who reproduce. Already historically defined as "unnatural" by a homophobic culture, many gay people show little investment in believing that unprotected vaginal intercourse between a man and a woman is the most natural or satisfying form of sexuality. Consequently, they are often more open to other forms of sexual expression, a flexibility that has intensified due to the high degree of awareness about HIV and AIDS in the gay community.

Unfortunately, aside from sporadic paranoia about the consequences of sexually transmitted diseases (STDs), most mainstream public commentary about sexuality and reproductive technology in the United States is split between the clinical and the illicit—between dry medical discussions that are anything but sexy and pornography that is anything but educational. HIV and AIDS activism is one of the few areas that successfully bridges (and eroticizes) this gap, often with latex. In many segments of the gay community, in everything from high art to pornography to sexual practice, condoms and dental dams are portrayed as sexy *in and of themselves*. In some gay people's view, unprotected penetrative sex is not only dangerous, it's unimaginative.

If MAC goes on to develop programs to educate students about reproductive choices and STD prevention, chances are that we will follow this lead by attempting to create a new language of sexuality that is less invested in the "naturalness" of unprotected, potentially procreative sex. This sort of educational program might include less about prevention and more about pleasure; fewer physiological diagrams and more information on dental dams. As one of us put it as we reflected on our discussion, "So people complain that a condom is like a raincoat, do they? Well, some of us *like* raincoats."

Hearing Ourselves Talk

Perhaps the most significant thing about the conversation that follows is that it illustrates a process that is valuable in and of itself. The *tone* of this discussion is a process of change. It is the sort of dialogue MAC goes through prior to developing projects to encourage other men to reflect on their own attitudes and behavior. In our discussions, we try to maintain an atmosphere that encourages honesty over posturing, support over defensiveness, and the process of learning over a scramble for the moral high ground. The most important thing that the transcript should convey is that men's attitudes change most profoundly in an atmosphere where they are comfortable and secure enough to be honest about their feelings. Although many of the issues we address are culturally specific, we hope that our methodology (the same one that Paulo Freire used to educate peasants in Brazil) will translate well: *we establish a comfortable, egalitarian atmosphere, treat concrete experiences as a valuable source of knowledge, and then use those experiences to reflect on the world at large and our own behavior in it.*

Because of the complicated nature of male sexuality and men's attitudes, at times this conversation may seem to wander to topics that are not ostensibly about "reproductive choices." These are perhaps the passages that should command the greatest attention, because they invariably provide the opening for us to talk and think about reproduction. They function as safety nets and brainstorming sessions, moments to pause and compare experiences, rediscover memories, and find the courage to speak and to share. During these interludes, men are able to focus on how they feel and what they believe (which may be different from what they "think") about an issue. It is also a time when important connections surface that may not be apparent. A high school boy's need to sleep with several women, for example, may turn out to have had more to do with a need to demonstrate his heterosexuality than with a desire for the women themselves.

Here are a few techniques we used to ensure that the conversation kept moving forward:

- Everyone's experiences were treated as worthy objects of attention and reflection. Sharing experiences was perceived to be more important than articulating and defending opinions, especially in the early stages of the discussion.

- The all-male setting helped encourage honesty instead of posturing, especially considering that most of the men had feminist beliefs.

- Initially, the men often had greater access to their feelings when they talked about past experiences, especially about how they first learned or experienced something.

- This focus on past experiences also encouraged people to reflect on how they had acquired their current attitudes rather than suggesting that those attitudes were wrong and needed to be defended.

- We, as facilitators, often reflected on our own experiences and attitudes. We were participants and learners instead of experts. (In the following dialogue, our contributions are italicized when we are strictly "facilitating.")

- People felt comfortable disagreeing, but they didn't put one another down when they did so, even when their disagreement was an ethical one.

It should also be noted that this discussion was never really completed. Issues arose that we had not previously considered, and we had additional questions that were not explored. We left wanting more.

The Transcript

Jason: What sources of information on sexuality and reproduction were available to you during your sexual development as a male?

Jeremy: The first information I got was talking with friends and hearing dirty jokes but not really understanding what they meant. I had some gross misconceptions about the act of sex.

Jason: What kind of misconceptions?

Jeremy: I didn't know the function of the vagina. And I thought the man would put his penis in the anus of the woman. It just wasn't very clear early on. These were cleared up in due time, but I don't think my father ever said, "son, let's have the talk about the birds and the bees."

Jason: Yeah, I know what you mean. I had a similar experience. I was waiting for this enlightening talk and it never happened.

Jeremy: My father just said, "You know, son, if you ever have any questions, I'm here." And that was the extent of that. Another early memory was that my uncle used to get *Playboy,* so I would look through those. He didn't try to hide them from me. He would just laugh as I looked through them.

Joe: For me, it was a little different. I had the sort of family where sex wasn't taboo. When my parents went upstairs and locked the door to the bedroom, I knew exactly what they were doing. In my family, we couldn't watch violent horror films, which was the opposite from most families. My parents felt that would scar us in some way, but they believed that sexuality and the body were natural things.

I don't know where I learned the specific information, but I knew that sex had to do with reproduction. I think from early on, we were always allowed to watch movies. So for me, sex became a very stylized thing. It was more involved with passion and romance than with any sort of health issues. And it could lead to reproduction, but I guess the predominant theme related to sex was the sensuality of it. Not so much its taboo nature.

Linnie: I was caught between two opposing forces: between my mother, who favored sex after marriage and love, and friends who thought I should experiment. From one angle, my older uncles and their friends were always pushing me, saying, "You should have sex." But at home my mom, being a single parent, always stressed that sex is love. And to me, love meant something to do with religion and had a wedding and a church. So I was really confused.

I knew sex had to do with reproduction. Being young, I had cousins being born and I wondered where babies came from. I figured there was no such thing as a stork. So actually, I had this misconception that when couples were in love and God condoned it, they would have sex and he would use his powers to create a baby within the womb, and that's how babies would be born.

The problem was that I was curious and wanted to find out [about sex]. Unfortunately, there was always a fear that sex would lead to pregnancy when you were not in love or old enough.

Jason: I had a girlfriend in kindergarten, which was an interesting experience because we played together and got dirty in the mud—all that good stuff. And basically, she was a friend, an intimate friend, but because she was a girl, people cast us in this little premarriage, "breeder couple" scenario. And it freaked the hell out of me. I still remember that feeling of fear because I thought that I would have to marry her and that meant we would have to have sex, and that scared me.

It's funny too, because sex was definitely just vaginal intercourse at that young an age. In fact, I don't think I could have imagined it any other way. I just remember people—really other kids—hassling me and asking questions like, "Are you going to marry her? Are you guys having sex?" And that brought up all these thoughts and feelings that I couldn't handle.

Warren: Well, I wondered if we might segue into another question, which is What have you felt women expect of men sexually in terms of performance, knowledge, responsibility, and communication. But also, what did other men seem to discourage or encourage?

Linnie: I'll stick to performance. One vivid memory I have was when I learned that women expected to orgasm. The whole idea seemed foreign to me. I guess like most men, I'd read that a woman usually didn't orgasm and I just wondered why not. At that time in my life, I thought, "Well I'm doing something right.

It feels good to me, so it must feel good to her. She's making the noises I've heard on television [chuckle]." And when I was done, I expected that she was happy too.

And then I came to realize there was more to it. One day a friend of mine told me, "Well, I'm not done." Or like, "I expected . . . ." This female friend helped me realize that there were more aspects of intercourse which led to orgasm for women. So as far as performance, I realized that women expect you to know that they have to orgasm also. Women expected me to be knowledgeable about what it takes to help them reach climax; not just vaginal intercourse, but all the extras.

Jason: How did you learn that, though? Did she actually tell you, show you, or did you guess and then she said yea or nay?

Linnie: We experimented somewhat. And I had read in the "sensitivity" books that you should ask, "Well, what do you want?" I'd always been afraid somewhat when talking with friends, because you're supposed to know what a woman wants. Originally the fear was about revealing that I wasn't well "versed" in the language of "lovemaking." Or at least as well versed as I "bragged" to friends that I was. So yeah, after experimenting and talking after sex, I began to realize what I didn't know and during sexual intercourse I would ask, "Am I doing this right?"

And one of the important things that I had always read about but never thought of was that some women require manual stimulation, and that helped a lot.

Jason: God shined a light on me the first day that I found out what a clitoris was, let me tell you. Like you said, Jeremy, I had this weird conception that somehow the vagina was located a little below the belly button or something. I had no idea how female sexuality worked. And I thought vaginal intercourse was the *only* thing that led to orgasm. And it can sometimes, but the clitoris is just so important, and you never learn about it in sex education classes because it's not technically associated with reproduction.

Linnie: Yeah, I never knew. After I found out what the clitoris was, I figured, "That's the G spot! That's it! [laughter.] That's what everyone is raving about."

Jeremy: Well, there's this mysterious ideology built up around the clitoris. People speak of it, and they say that's the way to please a woman, but you never know exactly where it is, what's going on with it, how to get there. I remember that the first thing I heard about it was that it was hidden under folds of skin. And that you had to kind of—

Jason: A needle in a haystack kind of thing?

Jeremy: Yeah, exactly. You had to feel around until you could find it. You had to go through—it was really kind of odd.

Jason: Where exactly do you get these kinds of messages? I can't even remember where I got all of mine.

Warren: I don't know when I first heard about the clitoris, but when I started sleeping with women, I thought, "Okay, I better find out about this clitoris thing." There were a couple of good sources of information. One was stuff written for women like *Our Bodies, OurSelves.* I thought, "Okay, *they'll* know."

Also, I had a roommate in college who was much more sexually experienced than I. He was pre-med and he'd find textbooks and things and try to show me where to find the clitoris.

I remember, too, that when I got really motivated, I thought, "Okay, what's this feel like on the receiving end? Because this is intimidating to me. I want to know how to do this right. There's this mysterious thing that's supposed to happen and she's supposed to be satisfied. And I want to know what it feels like to her." So I started looking through women's literature, like Alice Walker. I remember in *The Color Purple,* where she's talking about what that feels like. And I said, "Okay."

Jason: One other thing I was thinking about was the kind of tension I felt when learning about sexuality, especially without any sex education in school that talked about sexual emotions or pleasure. We had to learn this for ourselves. A lot of guys I've talked to have said that they actually learned most of their information through personal experience. You know, trial and error, or they've only been able to learn it from the women they've been with. There wasn't much public discussion about the reality of sex. I remember in locker rooms, guys would only talk in metaphors and stories and ridiculous things about "Oh, I fucked this. I screwed that." Nothing helpful whatsoever.

And so there was a discovery process that guys seemed to go through. All the information that I got about sex education or reproductive health was very negative and prohibitory. It said, "Oh, you don't want to mess with this. This is really serious stuff. This is *adult* stuff." So either you did it in marriage, or you did it later. But it really discouraged me from asking anybody for information when I was young.

Warren: It's like, "Here's how to prevent pregnancy, but we want to be sure you don't enjoy sex. Because if you enjoy sex, you might have a lot of it. So we're not going to tell you about pleasure. We're just going to tell you the bare minimum about how to prevent conception."

Jason: Exactly. If the only kind of sex you talk about is reproductive sex, then why does it surprise anyone that there are so many teenage pregnancies and unwanted children out there? We don't talk about any other way to be sexual. Some of that comes from religious and cultural biases, but I think there's a part that also comes from a societal fear of homosexuality. It's like saying, "As long as you're trying to have children, you couldn't possibly be queer."

Linnie: That's funny that you mention homosexuality. I think the subject of homosexuality is something that my elders didn't want to bring up because they didn't want me to know what it really was. Because you hear stories and you hear names called. "Yeah, well, so-and-so, he's a faggot. And faggots sleep with other men, and that's bad." Or "She's a bull dagger" or whatever.

But they did talk about masturbation. You would often hear, "Hey, if you do that, you'll go blind."

Jason: But the two are associated. They're always talked about as that "perverted" kind of sex.

Linnie: Right, instead of getting information about it, I was told it was perverse. And I was always afraid, because I wore glasses. I thought, "Oh my god, I'm already going blind!" It scared the shit out of me. I had a cousin tell me once, "If you have big hands, that means you've been masturbating. So let's see your hands." And I was afraid to show him. So instead of homosexuality, masturbation was fearful for me.

Andy: I think it relates back to discouraging young kids from wanting to enjoy sex. If you say that masturbation may lead to sex, then enjoying masturbation might encourage kids to enjoy sex.

Jason: I also think there's a tension between age and sexuality. The first time I masturbated was when I was thirteen. It was actually the night before I went in to see the doctor for my yearly physical, and I was scared to death that he was going to find out what I had done. I had this fear that somehow my doctor, my pediatrician who had been my physician for years, was going to know that I had jacked off the night before.

I panicked the whole night. I think part of that had to do with not wanting him to know because I didn't want to take on the responsibility of being sexually active. I had associated sex with being an adult, or at least being an older teenager in a way that I didn't want to take responsibility for being yet; I still wanted to be a kid. And yet I was still feeling horny and wanting to get off. I also remember feeling that tension in my sex education class because they talked about sex as something older people did, or responsible older people. And there I was, not wanting to take on that responsibility, and yet still wanting to be sexual.

Joe (to Warren): You had a question that was really good, and I wanted to jump back to that—what other men come to expect about your sexual activity with women. For me, anyway, now as well as when I was growing up, I was never particularly big and muscular. I was never particularly tall nor particularly good in sports. But unlike the other kids, in fourth grade, I knew where male and female body parts were and how they connected. And in middle school, I was the one who could get the girl I didn't know to dance with me at the Catholic Youth Organization dance and kiss her. In a high school religion class, of all places, I was voted the most romantic guy, the one who would know how to please a woman (I went to an all boys school). I'm not even sure why that happened.

This sexual knowledge became associated with my self-value and it made me feel important with other men. And I came to value myself as someone who knew things about women and could please a woman. And then, even in my adult life when I became sexually active with women, it became a matter of prowess that I could satisfy a woman; I could satisfy them better than other men could, because I knew how to do things. But thinking back about it now, that all stemmed from wanting to be valued in a male society.

Warren: Did similar issues come up for other people in terms of men and status?

Andy: Yeah, definitely. It's funny too how attractiveness alters the situation. I remember a lot of friends initially put pressure on me because I had a girlfriend for a long time, and she was just definitely opposed to sex. I wasn't, but I was going to respect her wishes on it. But because she was really good-looking, guys reacted much differently than I saw them treating other guys.

If she was a "mediocre" looking woman, and you said, "She doesn't want to have sex," then people would ask, "Why are you with her?" Whereas if the woman was more attractive, there was less pressure or emphasis placed on having sex with her. It's like, "Oh, well, you're not having sex, but she's really good-looking," so she's this sort of status symbol, and it's more appropriate for you to be with her rather than if she's a less attractive woman, where it's assumed you should be having sex, because then at least you're getting that from her.

Joe: So an ordinary or less attractive woman would have to provide you with sex in order . . . if you weren't getting sex off an ordinary woman, then you were wasting your time?

Andy: That was some of the attitude, yeah, especially in high school. There would be the guy who may decide for himself that he liked this woman, and without that sort of pressure, he may have stayed with her. But oftentimes, that sort of pressure from other guys would . . .

Joe: But what is it about the beautiful woman that means she doesn't have to provide sex? What did she give you in place of sex that made other guys think it was worth your while?

Andy: I think so many of your choices in high school, especially in terms of girlfriends, are about status.

Joe: Like a showpiece?

Andy: Yeah, or that this is a valued person. You're with this person so you're doing things right. You're at the place that you want to be in high school. Everyone is so conscious of their image, you know. And so she either does nothing to your image or takes away from it. If they're mediocre or unattractive, but you're having sex, then that'll boost your image. Guys will perceive you in the sexually active, stud category.

Jason: If the best-looking guy and best-looking girl in high school were going out together, we joked that they were this premier couple who would probably get married. Especially if it was the jock and the cheerleader. And this wasn't just about, as a guy, having a high-status woman, it was about, "Well, here's a good match." It was like, "Oh, look, he's already found a good match. And he's only this young."

Joe: So there are status levels, and if you find someone on the same level, then it's balanced. But if there's an imbalance, the lower person has to make up for it.

Jason: Well, I know in my high school it was very white and very upper class. And there were definitely a few good-looking black, Asian, and Latino girls in high school, but when white guys would go out with them, even though they were really good-looking, there was still more of this sexual expectation of them and less of an expectation that this was going to be a relationship that might lead to marriage. It was very much the white-bread debutante upper-class cheerleader girl who was valued. The expectation was that it's okay if you're not having sex with her because you might get to marry her and then have sex with her later and have kids with her.

Warren: I think that was true in my high school too, the sense that you wouldn't have sex with someone you might marry. You don't want a woman you might marry to know anything about sex! Because then she might want to have it with someone other than you. But if you're the one who knows about sex and she doesn't, and she's virginal with all the stuff that's supposed to mean, well, wow, she'll think she has the best guy on the planet. I think that concept was certainly floating around.

Another thing I've been thinking about is how I was not very sexually active in high school, and it raised a lot of eyebrows. There was an assumption . . . well, I was in a conservative town and I don't know if people would broadcast too much if they were having sex, but there was an assumption that if you're not with women, you might be queer.

When I look at some of the men who made a big deal about being with women in high school, I think that's one of the things it was important to them to prove, that "I'm not queer."

Jason: I want to go back to some of the stuff we talked about in terms of information about sexuality. Was there any mention at all about condoms, disease, or reproduction? I mean, I remember guys clearly talking about sex and the pressure to have sex, and a lot of these themes ring true for me. But no one ever said, "Hey man, yeah, go get her. And here's a condom." That was an afterthought. At best, it was, "Have sex with her, but make sure you don't get her pregnant."

Linnie: When I was in the seventh grade, it seemed like condoms were the fad. Guys would walk around showing how many they had. Everyone associated, "They have condoms, they must be having sex." So all the guys wanted to have condoms so they could prove, "Yeah, we're having sex."

And I remember this one guy in the neighborhood, Freckles, he'd sell them for seventy-five cents each. And I'd be sullen because I'd always forget and spend my money, and I couldn't buy a condom.

Jason: Did people talk about using them? Or did they just own them?

Linnie: No, they didn't talk about them.

Andy: You'd just see the ring in their wallet [laughter].

Linnie: They are an implication: "Well, *you* know what we're doing with them, therefore *we* must know how to use them." So guys would say, "You know what these are, right?" And you would say, "Sure, they're condoms." But I never really knew how to use one or put one on.

I developed a great appreciation for condoms in the sixth grade when I had my first sexual experience, and I literally got sick wondering if this girl, my next-door neighbor, was pregnant. So, it seems really funny after all that, by seventh grade, condoms were a fad. It's something you had to have. So I got my bag full of condoms from my uncle, who got them from the clinic—they were free. And I felt I was a man. I could go around school and show all my friends. I'd go and warn them to get a condom, just so they could put it on and claim they were having sex. As if it would facilitate having sex.

Joe: I also remember condoms being about status and about avoiding pregnancy but not really having anything to do with diseases. My brother's a teenager now, and he's bombarded with, "Be careful about what sex you're going to have. You could get AIDS." I think we're almost a half generation past that. I mean, that really wasn't an issue for us—at least until later in high school, or early in college. In grade school, when I first started thinking about sex, it wasn't really a scary idea; no one really knew about AIDS at that time.

Jason: It's interesting. I remember talking about contraception in my driver/health education class in my sophomore year of high school—it's always interesting that you got to talk about sex and cars at the same time—anyway, they ran through all the sexually transmitted diseases and talked about the biological experience of pregnancy, and then they went through all the methods of birth control. And I remember thinking and seeing all these methods that women could use, but only one besides abstinence and withdrawal that men could use—condoms. But people wanted to have sex, and no one trusted withdrawal. It was like, "Yeah, right, you're going to pull out." So there was just condoms. So I thought, "Well, chances are that she's probably going to use one of those other methods, and I won't have to use a condom."

But I had no understanding of what the real consequences of unprotected sex were. There was just this big dark fear of what happens if the condom breaks or if I didn't use one. That fear was pregnancy and fatherhood, but I didn't know what fatherhood was. I mean, I always knew what my father did, but at the time I had no idea what it would be like for me to be a parent. So I was afraid of pregnancy and fatherhood. But these were scare tactics which weren't connected to concrete experiences. I think adults didn't want us to know, like with what we were saying earlier about sex. Their idea was that if you know what sex is, you might try to do it. But this approach only partially worked, because at that time, I was resigned to, "Oh, I hope she takes care of it."

Warren: That really struck me when you were talking about that fear, because my first real girlfriend, the first person I slept with, was really big on condoms. So I was like, "Oh, condoms are great." I think I also liked them because I was worried about premature ejaculation, and I thought, "Well, there'll be less stimulation with a condom. So I'll be hard longer. And I feel really safe with my condom on."

Linnie: It's funny, I never really thought of it in terms of pregnancy. Like you said, Warren, I was always caught in performance. And I was always afraid that without condoms, that I would cum too early—you know, premature ejaculation. I was always afraid of that, so I started reading. And somewhere I learned that you're supposed to grab the base of the penis, so I tried that. And that's really uncomfortable. It was hell. It would get cold, and I would lose the erection. So I would have to stay with a condom. Not for pregnancy purposes, but for performance. And that meant a lot to me.

Joe: That's funny. I would have the opposite problem, where I would lose sensitivity with condoms. And it became this big psychological thing where—I don't know if it was the condom or just in my mind—but I just couldn't feel anything with a condom. It would be harder for me to maintain an erection. And I'd lose interest. So consequently, I would just avoid or pass up opportunities to have intercourse if the person wasn't on the pill because I didn't want to have to deal with condoms.

Even though I knew it wasn't a good idea, it got to the point where I was being manipulative. I would try to convince girlfriends to agree to have sex without a condom, knowing the repercussions.

Andy: Yeah, I think so much of that stuff is very psychological. You can read whatever, but the information about sex you consider most vital is your experience. And deviating from that or doing other things throws you off psychologically. Whether or not there is a physical sensitivity, I think there's a lot more psychologically.

Warren: I'm thinking about when Linnie was talking about finding out you're supposed to give a woman an orgasm. And I was thinking about the way condoms were presented to me before I actually started using them—like this is the moment when sex is real. When you put on a condom, that's what counts. That's when you're really having sex. This didn't encourage a lot of creativity about how to get a woman off.

Jason: What other kinds of expectations do people feel were placed on them?

Jeremy: One thing I wanted to get off my chest is about sleep. My girlfriend and I have a queen-sized bed—a huge mattress—and I think she's a victim of a media portrayal of how people should sleep. You know, once a couple has finished having sex, the man puts his arm around the woman, and the woman sleeps with her head on his shoulder, and they don't move for the rest of the night! And they wake up the next morning in the movies with, "Oh darling, what a wonderful sleep I had." Not like my arm isn't paralyzed or anything! But everything is fine, everything is fine. [Sarcastic look.]

So she has this preconception of how we should sleep. And she gets mad when I roll over and "give her my butt." I tried to talk to her about the difference between sexual relations and sleep. When you're having sex, you're awake and you're thinking, but when you're asleep, it's a whole different world. But she expects me to hold her and to wake up holding her with a smile on my face. That expectation is something that I would like to shatter.

Andy: After many uncomfortable nights, I found out another technique that's much better. Have you ever heard of the concept of "spooning"? That works really well. Just cuddle in the fetal position, with the other person in the same position.

Linnie: Also, if you face each other and intertwine your legs and just hold each other like that.

Jeremy: All right, this is the next Men Acting for Change project. We're going to change women's expectations of how we should sleep.

Linnie: Well, I don't want to change it. I think it would be great to have her sleep and you hold her.

Joe: Yeah, I want to do that. Even if only until you fall asleep. And afterwards, you probably end up moving apart.

Jeremy: Oh, I mean, in theory it's a beautiful idea, but the arm goes numb, you can't move, you can't breathe—

Linnie: See, it's part of being a man [half-joking]. You have to take being numb. You hold her. It doesn't matter. You've enjoyed the night, now you suffer a little.

Andy: Well, it seems like the larger expectation that's going on is a stylized romantic ideal that after sex you're going to hold this person all night. And the real issue which doesn't come through is communication—just saying, "I feel like doing this right now," rather than automatically assuming that it's supposed to happen, and then violating that ideal.

Jason: Well, I think there are a lot of mythical messages that we get about sex and relationships, especially gendered messages. There's this idea that sex is equated with vaginal intercourse between men and women, and that it's built around the male orgasm, which directly relates to the whole reproductive idea. It's like a symbol—"Okay, we can have a kid because I came."

Warren: It's like saying, "If you planted that seed, you better incubate it."

Jason: And if you cum as the man into a woman, then it's as if her pleasure or reward is the comfort afterwards.

Joe: And if you provide that comfort, that means you just made love. And if you don't provide it, and send her on her way, that means . . .

Jason: That she's just a fuck. There are all these messages attached to these gestures. It's like, when I turn over after a one-night stand, it seems like it's just a fuck. And it may be that, or it may be something different. And that's why I have to explain what I'm doing.

Joe: I just recently became involved with someone, and it's the healthiest relationship I've had in four years. And the second night that she stayed over, she started to put on her clothes after lovemaking. And I got upset. I asked, "Well, what's going on?" And she said, "I want to leave." And we ended up having this conversation, which was really good because we hadn't been communicating.

She wanted to leave because after the first night she stayed, she had to walk back to her room and was basically ashamed; what people thought of her was very significant to her. She had only been in one long-term relationship before, and didn't want to be seen as someone who slept around easily. For me, on the other hand, for someone to leave after lovemaking implies you were just fucking. That's what I would do if I didn't really want to be with the person. I'd want to leave, or I'd hope that they'd leave and I'd make some excuse about how I had to study or get up early so that they would leave. I coded it one way and she coded it another way; there were underlying motivations and factors that we hadn't communicated.

Jason: I think that's something that's been really tricky for me to communicate, especially when you have to talk about physical as well as emotional consequences. I've been in situations where I'd talk with my partner before having sex with her consistently. But sometimes in a one-night stand, it's hard to ask, "Well, if you get pregnant, what are you going to do?" Because I want the woman to be in charge of that choice about her own body and decide if she wants to see the pregnancy through or have it terminated.

And yet, I want to be very clear what my role is and what her expectations may be so I can make my choice of whether or not to have sex with her. It's the whole issue of "Am I ready to be a father?" And how do you deal with that? Because I feel sometimes that if we have that talk, it can't just be a fuck. You know? It can't just be casual sex if we have that talk. What do other people think? Do you feel that for it to be just less-serious sex or for it to be some kind of temporary relationship, you can't think about parenthood or the chance that something might go wrong with birth control?

Jeremy: I've never had that talk. I mean, I'm still in my teens. So it's just something that I've totally set aside for a later date. I mean, I'll be a junior in college, and it's just not something that's in the immediate conceptual future.

Jason: Why don't you talk about it?

Jeremy: It's just not something I can *conceive* of. Being a father? I mean, come on, my dad's my father. I can't be a father. And I know for a fact that my partner feels the same way, that there's a whole lot more to experience before it's time to be parents. And if there's some accidental pregnancy, though it's not outrightly communicated, it's implicit in our relationship that we wouldn't see it through. I think neither of us is in any position to do so practically, financially, mentally, and—there's no way.

Andy: Especially if it was a one-night stand, I've never had that discussion because you pray to God it does not come to that. Because if it's just going to be a one-night stand, then you're not very interested in that person anyway. And it's motivated by pure lust and you're hoping to spend as little time with them as possible.

I have never thought in terms of "Would I have that discussion?" because I'm so rarely in one-night stands. I think if I did on a more regular basis, it would loom larger in my life than it does.

Jason: Well, let's try to move on to something more concrete. Keep thinking about these ideas of responsibility, risk taking, and fatherhood. And with those in mind, let me throw out a few scenarios to get your feedback.

The first—does everyone know what NORPLANT® is? It's the birth control hormone that you can put in your arm. If a male version of NORPLANT® came out, was free, and had no side effects, would you use it?

Joe: No.

Linnie: Naa.

Andy: Nope.

Jeremy: No.

Jason: Why or why not?

Andy: It's definitely a control issue, just in terms of the options that you have. You know, you may want different things at different times. Especially at this age, I don't know where I'm going to be in . . . let's say four years. I don't want to have something that would limit my ability if I decide I want to have children at a particular time.

Jason: You can always take it out.

Andy: Yeah, I know, but I'm just saying—a surgical procedure? I just don't know.

Joe: You could tell me that NORPLANT® was free, there were no potential side effects, and it would make my penis grow an inch and I still wouldn't do it.

Jason: Why not?

Joe: I don't know. The thought of some chemical—I mean, I don't know. It's just a real instinctual reaction, not wanting some synthetic thing in my body.

Andy: To control something as personal as sexuality? I'm nervous enough about most drugs anyway. I usually don't take many at all—cold medicines, any of that stuff. I just think my own body can take care of it more easily. I don't want some medical thing to psychologically distance me from my sexuality. In terms of putting on a condom, it's something I decide at that moment.

Jeremy: Also, condoms are kind of catch-as-catch-can. If you're going to have sex, a condom is pretty much always available. But if you go through the procedure to get this thing, and you don't have sex for five years, then, "Wow, I went through this surgical procedure for nothing." But if you don't have the surgical procedure and don't have sex for five years, you just don't get any condoms. I just think it's a risky thing to go through.

Linnie: I'd also like to know what it does exactly. Will NOR-PLANT® make you sterile for five years?

Jason: Well, say while it's in, your sperm are not capable of penetrating the egg.

Linnie: Well, I still think I would not do it for psychological reasons.

Andy: Yeah, there would still be psychological reasons for me, even if everything worked out medically.

Joe: I know it's a double standard, but I'm all for a girlfriend deciding to go on birth control, even though there are associated serious health risks. I guess it's selfish on some level. I mean, I know it's selfish on some level.

Jason: Okay, the second scenario is very similar. Say a new study shows that vasectomies are 95 percent reversible. Would you consider this procedure as a means of contraception?
    Ninety-five percent, that means that you could have the procedure and you would have no chance of getting anyone pregnant, and then there's a 95 percent chance that you could get it reversed and you could be able to have kids again.

Joe: No.

Linnie: No.

Andy: No.

Jeremy: No.

Joe: Even if I was married and had two kids and didn't want any more kids. You could get divorced and want to remarry and have kids again. Why take away part of yourself? It's sort of like taking away your manhood if you can't produce viable sperm, or at least it's perceived that way.

Andy: Yeah, that's true. I am very distrustful of surgical procedures like that and don't care to have a knife anywhere on me, much less in my genitals.

Linnie: Why fix it if it isn't broke?

Warren: I really like the idea of total security. You know, that there is just no way I could get anybody pregnant. But the thought that a vasectomy might be irrevocable holds me back. I have an image that I'm going to be forty and see people playing with their children—and I mean, I *hate* kids; I really don't like kids at all. But just the thought that I'm going to see people playing with their children and I'm going to be all alone is enough to hold me back.

It's ironic, because I was willing to accept those odds with a condom. You know, reversibility and condom breakage, it's about the same percentage.

Jason: So I guess it means you'd rather have the potential result of getting someone pregnant than losing your own virility.

Andy: Yeah.

Linnie: Yeah.

Joe: On some level, when you get someone pregnant, you can dismiss this as "not my problem." I mean, it might be my fault or my responsibility, but not my problem.

Linnie: And pregnancy is not always a bad thing. Even if you don't want it, it could turn out for the best. My sister got pregnant at a young age, and I thought, "Oh my God, she should get an abortion. She's too young." But my niece is wonderful. If my sister had an abortion, I would probably have similarly positive feelings about the outcome, but I'm so much happier knowing I can go home and see my niece. To lose your virility in order to not get someone pregnant, that's so final. As bad as it sounds, I'd rather get women pregnant than permanently rule something out.

Joe (to Jason): How about you? You didn't give us your answer to those two questions.

Jason: I'd probably do both of them. I feel very strongly about taking mutual responsibility for birth control and knowing that many women, if they have the choice, have to make these choices on a very serious level. An old girlfriend was on the pill and every month we had this deal where I would take the placebos, every day at the exact same time. It was only one-fourth or one-fifth of what she took, but for one week every month, I would have to take them at the exact same time every day. And if I forgot, we couldn't have sex.

Jeremy: The deal I have with my girlfriend is that I pay for half the pill.

Jason: Yeah, that's a good thing to do too. But for me it's just realizing the responsibility that goes into it and the thought and just the constant awareness. I've been with women who won't go on the pill because of health reasons, and I can totally respect that. These are real issues in my life.

The funny thing is, a lot of women don't expect that of me because I'm a man. They really don't expect me to think about responsibility. They just assume they can't trust me, which is true on a certain level because they can't. If they get pregnant, I can jump ship if I want. But many women also think they have to take care of it. Either they're going to take the pill or whatever. And for me, it's about gender equality really coming down to this personal, physical level and what kind of physical risks people are willing to take. I think the fact that condoms don't affect you physically makes them an attractive compromise for many straight men—incorporating responsibility without threatening one's physical ability or condition.

But the fact is that if you put on a condom, you're going to be the same exact physical person afterwards. It will have absolutely no negative effect on your health, unless you're allergic to latex or something. It will not change your body chemistry, your hormones—no surgical procedure.

And it's the same thing in some ways with abortion. I mean, if the woman chooses it as an option, she's the one undergoing a physical procedure. And you may be paying for half of it or all of it, but still, on some level, I feel a great security. No matter how much I try to participate, I'm still not undergoing the procedure.

Joe: Responsibility is a big issue for men, though. When I had sex with a woman, I used to think, "Wow, I'm a man now. And I'm sensitive to women." And I thought that was being responsible. But when I was a junior in college, I did get someone pregnant, basically because I convinced her that it would be okay this one time to have sex without a condom. And I realized then how much of a man I was not and I panicked. I mean, ultimately, she made the decision to have an abortion, but prior to her decision, I was afraid she might not. I still regret to this day not being able to be equally supportive of her in either decision. Basically I panicked and made it very clear that I was hoping she would choose to have an abortion.

Jason: And yet, to commit to that level of responsibility is tough. Even though I know most of the risks I'm taking when I have intercourse with someone, I'm not willing to commit to the responsibility of being a parent every time. I don't feel like I can do that, and yet I have vaginal intercourse with women anyway.

Joe: If it happened now—if I was in a relationship and the person became pregnant—I believe that I would feel and express that I would stand by her in either decision. But I couldn't do that then.

Andy: At some point, I think it's important to be honest. I mean, you can be mutually supportive of either decision and at the same time tell someone how you honestly feel. If someone I was having sex with became pregnant, I would not feel good about saying, "This is your choice completely. I will support you in either decision," and leave it at that. I would definitely feel a responsibility to be honest and say what I felt about it: "I'll support you either way, but this is how I feel."

Just stating your own opinion might be seen as pushing her, which you're not supposed to do, but I don't agree with saying nothing. That's not taking on any responsibility. That's simply deferring to someone else—a semblance of giving them control, when in all actuality, by not being honest and open about how you feel, you're withholding important information.

Warren: I know with Liz, when we stopped using condoms and wanted to try something else, I felt strongly enough about it to say, "Look, you need to know this is how I feel. I don't want to be a father, and I feel strongly enough about this to stop having sex."

That really got her attention. When she did get pregnant, even though I was afraid she might change her mind, the fact that we'd discussed things made getting an abortion easier. But that was also a unique situation in my life. I felt pretty sure that this was someone I wanted to spend my life with. And we'd been intimate long enough that we could have that kind of conversation. There's no way, if the relationship were a week or two old or less, that a discussion like that could happen.

Then again, I did once. A woman wanted to go ahead and do something without protection, and I didn't feel comfortable, so I said, "Well, what are your views on abortion?" [laughter]. And it totally—the light came on and that was the end of that. She was out of the bed *real* fast.

Linnie: Yeah, that's the impression I got from Jason when he said he'd ask. I'd never had that encounter. I guess I always asked afterwards—like, "What age would you like to be married? What do you think about kids?" But right before, it's difficult, because for me sex is usually spontaneous.

Jason: Well, I think even if you do plan to have sex, you still want to live part of the fantasy. And your fantasy doesn't usually include fatherhood, especially when you're young. After you start having sex with her consistently and maybe have a relationship with her, that's when reality starts setting back in and pregnancy becomes more of a possibility. It's real tough, especially if you don't know someone very well, to talk about consequences, especially negative ones. It challenges the fantasy. You don't know how she's going to react. And a lot of women really don't know how to react to a guy who thinks about consequences. They don't expect it at all. So here I am, this straight guy who basically has no intention of having children, asking a woman I've just met and intend to sleep with about pregnancy and parenthood [laughter]. Go figure.

*Researchers
on Researching
Sexuality*

What Can We Learn From Sexual Behavior Surveys?

The U.S. Example

Julia A. Ericksen and Sally A. Steffen

Since 1992, we have been engaged in writing a history of sexual behavior surveys in the United States (Ericksen and Steffen forthcoming). We analyzed over 450 surveys taken between 1892 and 1992; interviewed researchers, government funders, legislative aides, and lobbyists; and read much of the contemporary literature, including newspapers that reported the survey findings. We are interested in the reasons the surveys were undertaken, the questions asked in them, the methodological issues involved, and the uses to which findings were put.

We became interested in the research after learning about a political battle in the early 1990s indicating that undertaking such research in the United States remains highly sensitive and political. On April 22, 1992, the U.S. Senate voted to prohibit the secretary of health and human services from funding two national surveys of sexual behavior previously approved by the National Institute of Child Health and Human Development. These surveys were intended to obtain epidemiological data considered essential to track the progress of AIDS. Senator Jesse Helms of North Carolina introduced the amendment prohibiting the surveys and argued that they were being pushed by the "sexual liberation crowd" in order to "cook the scientific facts to legitimize homosexual and other sexually promiscuous life styles" (*Cong. Rec.* 1992).

How did this happen, and what are the implications for others who are interested in undertaking sex research in the United States and elsewhere? In order to answer these questions, we analyzed the rationales and concerns of sexual behavior surveys since the end of the nineteenth century. The brief history of the surveys that follows shows the extent to which concerns changed over time and the ways in which researchers managed the research process in response to both their own fears about undertaking such risky research and their own preconceptions about what was important. Although the specific issues may vary from country to country, we believe that the risks in doing this kind of research—being subjected to professional vilification, misinterpreting or politicizing results by focusing on some figures and ignoring others, questioning personal motives, subjecting data to a heightened level of scrutiny—exist in many countries.

Sex is not just another research topic. Many researchers told us that they paid both a professional and a personal price for concentrating on sex. Anyone undertaking such research must assume that it is going to be politicized. Results will be used by others both friendly and unfriendly to the intent of the research. It is therefore important to take special care to manage the research process—including the presentation of results—to ensure that an accurate and intended message is conveyed, and that one's findings can hold up under scrutiny.

Our Hypotheses

The questions asked and the findings generated through this research are historically and spatially specific. But researchers frequently make claims about their results that do not acknowledge the difficulties of data collection and interpretation and that overstate the certainty of their knowledge. Instead, they seek measurable truths and frequently do not see themselves as contributing to a historically changing body of research. The frequent failure to provide the date of data collection reflects this ahistoricism. And yet there is no absolute knowledge about sexual behavior that remains true across time and space. Not only will the results vary, so will the questions, the type of respondents, and so on. This means that researchers must have a deep understanding of the culture in which they are operating in order to create and understand their findings.

Sex drives are not biologically based. Americans tend to assume that the sexual identity and interest of a person are immutable and in conflict with society. In the twentieth century, the mission of sexologists (people who believe that they have a professional expertise in issues of sexuality) has been to liberate innate sexuality from a repressive social system (Weeks 1985), and most sexual behavior surveys subscribe to this viewpoint. Many researchers create a taxonomy of human sexual behavior, break sexual acts into component parts, and document the frequencies of different types of behavior. Others judge the appropriateness of behaviors and are concerned with their control, but they do not question the existence of a sex drive.

Similarly, the surveys we reviewed reflect dominant constructions of gender differences in male and female sex drive and behavior. For example, they assume that women are aroused slowly through love, whereas men are easily aroused and consumed by an uncontrollable sex drive. These beliefs are so powerful that researchers did not always know how to handle contrary findings. Women who reported being multiorgasmic and easily aroused were sometimes characterized as incapable of sexual satisfaction and having low self-esteem. Men who were not sexually active were either omitted from the analysis or explained as adapting to their wives' needs.

These assumptions were also reflected in questions *not* asked. For example, when researchers interviewed women about their sexual experience, they assumed that all sexual acts were consensual; in 120 studies of premarital sexual intercourse, researchers ignored decision making about sexual activity. When the National Survey of Children added questions about whether adolescents had ever had intercourse voluntarily, it found that although 7 percent of fourteen-year-olds reported having had intercourse, only 2 percent reported having had *voluntary* intercourse. (Moore et al. 1989).

We maintain that sexuality is socially constructed and that these constructions change over time. While recognizing the biological bases of reproduction, our approach emphasizes the mediating influence of human agency. Drawing on Foucault (1978) and Weeks (1985), we see notions about sexuality being used as a way to self-police an increasingly complex, anonymous, and fragmented society such as the United States, where we can no longer police one another. Thus, establishing a baseline of "normality" through the findings of sex surveys becomes a way of maintaining social order. Individuals look to society for ways to monitor and reduce anxiety over sex. They develop an obsession with measuring how their sexual behavior or experience compares with the social standard.

Surveys of sexual behavior contribute to an ongoing discussion of sex as new results that provide evidence of variety and fluidity in the sexual behavior of the population challenge accepted beliefs. This is both liberating and dangerous, because it creates new opportunities for individuals and for those who monitor individual behavior.

The History of Sexual Behavior Surveys in the United States

The reasons for undertaking sex surveys in the United States have changed over time. The underlying assumptions of the research influence the questions, the collection methods, and the data analysis. This section presents a chronology of sexual behavior surveys and explores some of the methodological issues raised within different survey types.

The Early Surveys

Surveys started at the end of the Victorian era, near the turn of the century, and their emergence can be viewed as part of a general liberalization of sexual behavior and attitudes. Although this may be an accurate interpretation, the early sex surveys were narrow in their interests. Their underlying argument was that sex education was needed to protect the family and to help young people repress their sexual urges until marriage. Reformers wanted a society in which the sanctity of the family would be protected by high standards for men's sexual behavior, like those for middle-class women (abstention from sex before marriage and faithfulness within marriage). Since researchers were concerned with marriages like their own, their research concentrated almost solely on the middle class.

One of the goals of the early sex education movement was to preserve marriage by ensuring that young people selected appropriate mates. By the 1920s, with a marked rise in divorce showing no sign of abating, a concern for the quality of marriage itself began to appear in the surveys. Sex surveys were designed to document that sex was indeed important to marriage (Kerkhoff 1964). In these surveys, the successful marriage was eroticized. The research showed an increasing tendency to pressure women to be sexually aroused and to blame them for not being interested in sex. Studies were still directed entirely at bourgeois marriages; the working class was viewed as incapable of "companionate" marriages.

It was during this period that concerns about methodology surfaced in survey design and data analysis. For example, as a result of the realization that individuals might be embarrassed to appear in a sex survey, researchers went to great lengths to ensure respondents' confidentiality and, usually, anonymity. In addition, the first findings—reporting that husbands and wives did not always give the same responses to questions about their sexual relations—raised concerns about relying on retrospective data in sex research (Clark and Wallin 1964). This problem persists to the present day.

The Kinsey Survey

The man whose name is synonymous with the sex survey in the United States, Alfred Kinsey, started doing sex research as a result of teaching a marriage course, but he quickly moved beyond a strict focus on sex within marriage. It is hard now to imagine the passions ignited by the publication of the first Kinsey volume, *Sexual Behavior in the Human Male* (Kinsey, Pomeroy, and Martin 1948). Prudery was so much the fabric of everyday life in America that the *New York Times* refused to accept advertising for the book (Pomeroy 1982). But with the publication of Kinsey's data, discussions about sex became daily media fare. Although he was not the first sex researcher to make controversial statements, the response to Kinsey's research and the seemingly all-encompassing nature of his findings created the concept of "sex researcher" as an expert in the minds of the American public. Although this did a lot to legitimize sex research, it also opened findings and discussion to the scrutiny of the general public, not just experts.

Kinsey's blind commitment to scientific neutrality and his refusal to make negative moral judgments about sexual behavior troubled many. He wanted to collect "data about sex which would represent an accumulation of scientific fact completely divorced from moral value and social custom." Furthermore, he always assumed that "everyone is engaged in every type of activity" (Kinsey, Pomeroy, and Martin 1948, 53). Reviewers found many of his findings bothersome, especially his data on women. He presented evidence that women were multiorgasmic and implied that premarital sex led to improved sexual adjustment for married women.

Despite Kinsey's recognition of women's capacity for sexual pleasure, he followed a male model, emphasizing orgasm at the expense of other sexual pleasures. He talked in terms of "outlets" (orgasm), with all outlets created equal. This focus on outlets is one reason that Kinsey's data on homosexuality (which he declared to be "normal" and, indeed, biologically present in all of us) remain controversial. His finding that 10 percent of American men are homosexual has since become a powerful political tool for both the gay community and the religious right.

The most serious problem with Kinsey's data was the use of volunteers rather than a probability sample, and obtaining respondents for sex surveys continues to be a heavily debated topic. Kinsey did not use volunteers in the conventional sense; he and his associates recruited from a wide range of groups and exerted a lot of pressure to convince all group members to be interviewed.[1] His goal was to accumulate as many cases as possible, so he insisted that sampling could not be used. He was particularly incensed when prominent statistician John Tukey told him that he would exchange a thousand of Kinsey's existing interviews for a hundred done with probability sampling.[2]

Kinsey was a great believer in the use of face-to-face interviews, and he disapproved of most previous sex surveys on the grounds that the data were obtained through self-administered questionnaires. He argued that it was more difficult for individuals to refuse to answer an interviewer and that he could always tell whether a respondent was lying. Others disagreed, saying that it was easier to get individuals to admit to embarrassing behavior in the anonymity of a questionnaire than in a face-to-face interview.

These issues were not resolved by Kinsey and, in fact, still puzzle researchers.

Demographic Fertility Studies

By the 1950s, American society was increasingly prosperous and focused on the family. The high fertility rates, which demographers had assumed to be a temporary postwar effect, continued. This mistaken assumption led demographers to miss the baby boom and was one reason that Ronald Freedman and his colleagues at the University of Michigan undertook the first national fertility study in 1955. They asked about contraceptive behavior rather than sexual intercourse, but even this timid attempt to address sexual behavior made demographers nervous and affected demographic research for years (Freedman, Whelpton, and Campbell 1959).

For example, Freedman was interested in subfecundity and infertility but was told by many that he should not ask about abortion, because to do so would involve asking about crimes women had committed and would jeopardize survey results. (Even today, ambiguity about abortion means that there is little attention to obtaining accurate information.) Demographers' nervousness was also reflected in inadequate questions. In 1965, in the first national sample to do so, Ryder and Westoff (1965) asked *one* question about the frequency of intercourse. However, rather than asking about frequency in the previous week (because they assumed that one-quarter of women would be menstruating), they asked about frequency in the last month. Even so, they worried that young wives having lots of sex would not remember accurately. Indeed, it appears that most respondents multiplied from a weekly average.

In this era, only married women were interviewed at first. But as marital fertility declined, attention turned to teenage girls. (Although this eventually paved the way to interviewing adolescent boys, for a decade, the assumption was that adolescent girls made independent decisions about engaging in sex.) These teen fertility studies eventually led to government funding of research about adolescent sexual behavior. (Some speculate that the willingness to ask adolescents questions not asked of adults reflects the belief that teens may be denied privacy rights.) This set a precedent, and since that time, sexual behavior insofar as it relates to fertility has been the subject of numerous government studies.

Demographers thus legitimated sex research to the U.S. government. The first survey was funded by the Rockefeller Foundation, but increasingly the National Institutes of Health (NIH) and other government agencies became involved in sex research. Poking into citizens' bedrooms was justified predominantly by the rationale that making forecasts about family size was necessary in order to determine needs for housing, education, the labor force, and so forth. For example, Freedman, Whelpton and Campbell (1959, 8) stated that "many long range plans depend on population forecasts, and these data from personal interviews can improve our understanding of the current baby boom and the outlook for population growth."

Returning to surveys on adolescent sexual behavior, the results of the first of several studies undertaken in the 1970s by Melvin Zelnik and John Kantner showed much higher rates of sexual intercourse among unmarried American teens than had previously been estimated and caused immense concerns both in and out of the government (Zelnick, Kantner, and Ford 1981). Anxiety about the young was also exacerbated by an increase in sexually transmitted diseases (STDs) and teenage births. (Although the teen fertility rate fell, the number of teen births increased, since teens were an increasing percentage of the total population.)

Concerns about the sexual behavior of youth also resulted from changes that were occurring in society. With the civil rights movement, the antiwar movement, and the second wave of feminism, the national press focused on the "youth rebellion." The increasingly independent behavior of youth created an almost obsessive interest in studies of premarital sexual intercourse among young women, starting in the late 1960s. In 1968, the Center for Population Research was established in the NIH with an explicit research agenda focused on adolescent sexuality and pregnancy. The central questions motivating researchers concerned the existence of a sexual revolution and its impact on marriage and the family, for example, does premarital sex positively or negatively influence men's and women's experiences of sex within marriage?

Studies of the sexual behavior of unmarried college students represent over 25 percent of all sexual behavior surveys, and these surveys can be grouped by the researcher's position on premarital intercourse. Some researchers categorized it as a problem behavior, along with drug use and political activism; others were more tolerant and suggested that premarital intercourse was not necessarily deleterious to marriage. Few argued that it could have a positive impact, or they simply said that they wanted to understand sexual decision making among the young. Most researchers included no questions about contraceptive behavior, apparently fearing that to do so would be tantamount to condoning premarital intercourse.

Although most of the studies in this section were small, inexpensive, and focused on college—because of both their availability and the continued concern with the sexuality of middle-class women—a few raised methodological issues. There were studies of the bias inherent in using volunteers, of the differences between the use of questionnaires and face-to-face interviews, and of recall problems in self-reported data (finger 1947; Clark and Tifft 1966; DeLameter 1974; Wolchik, Spencer, and Lisi 1983; Catania, McDermott, and Pollack 1986; Morokoff 1986). None of these issues was resolved, but the existence of such studies was an indication that sex research was finally coming of age.

Post-AIDS Studies

In the 1980s, several factors combined to fuel controversies over sexual behavior research. In 1976, the teenage population peaked at 21.4 million, feeding images of rampant teenage sex. By the 1980s, data showing that most unmarried adolescents would engage in sexual intercourse before age twenty further fueled concerns among liberals, conservatives, and feminists over sexual liberation. When AIDS appeared, the religious right condemned homosexuals for their "repugnant," "aberrant" lifestyles and the fragile beginnings of sexual tolerance toward gays quickly crumbled. These concerns, combined with a national politically conservative backlash, had a profound impact on the public discussion of sex—in determining both what would be discussed and in what context. For example, researchers who were interested in documenting changes in gay men's sexual behavior as a result of AIDS were explicit about their intent to lessen "promiscuity," and in 1984, the first San Francisco AIDS Foundation study had as its explicit goal "to answer questions about how to go about promoting safe sex among gay and bi-sexual men in the city and county of San Francisco" (Research and Decisions Corp. 1984).

By the mid-1980s, policymakers began to realize that AIDS might infect "normal" people and that existing data on sexual behavior were inadequate to estimate the likelihood of this happening. Calls for data on sexual behavior were made by the American Association for the Advancement of Science, the National Research Council, the Surgeon General's 1986 Report on AIDS, and the 1988 Report of the Presidential Commission on the Human Immunodeficiency Virus. In 1987, the NIH released two requests for contracts to design national samples of sexual behavior: a study of teen fertility that would include questions related to AIDS and STDs (known as the American Teenage Survey), and an adult survey of risky sexual practices focusing on AIDS (known as the Survey of Health and Risky Practices, or SHARP).[3] These were to be the first national probability samples with detailed accounts of sexual behavior.

What the researchers and funders for these studies did not realize is that rationales for doing sex research have been necessary since the start of sex research and are as important as any results to be obtained. They made the mistake of assuming that AIDS was such a serious problem that the usual cautions in doing sex research could be set aside. But they miscalculated, and both surveys were halted. In the case of the American Teenage Survey—a capstone study of adolescent sexual and contraceptive behavior—the grant awardees saw themselves as neutral, apolitical scientists and were outraged when their work became the target of conservative attacks, particularly at a time when few individuals questioned the existence of a problem or argued that teenagers had a right to a sex life.

Lessons

What can we conclude from this history? Researchers should not forget that it is difficult to do this type of sex research. Most people are uncomfortable talking about their sex lives. They will not necessarily answer questions accurately, either because they cannot remember or because they are uncomfortable with the truth. We should recognize the limits of self-recall. In general, it is difficult to recall behavior that occurred some time ago. The more recent the event, the easier the recall. Individuals consistently overreport socially approved behavior and underreport socially disapproved behavior. In sex research, this can cut both ways. In some instances, individuals are as likely to exaggerate the extent of their sexual performance as they are to underestimate it.

Another key lesson is the importance of knowing just what you are interested in measuring and why, so that unnecessary or misleading questions can be eliminated.

Researchers have a bias toward wording questions identically for all respondents on the grounds that this makes the data comparable across interviews. This downplays the fact that there are not necessarily terms for sexual behavior that everyone knows and is comfortable with. For example, many Americans do not know what "masturbation" means because they use a variety of slang terms. Others would be offended if they were asked whether they ever "jerk off."

Researchers must be sensitive to the race, gender, and ethnicity of interviewers. Alfred Kinsey believed that white married men made the best interviewers, regardless of the respondent. This is no longer believed. Now, female interviewers of the same ethnicity as the respondent are usually used, but the issue is still being debated. There is general agreement that most interviewers can be trained to overcome their own sensitivities about sex, at least in the United States.

Issues of confidentiality can easily bedevil sex research. Short of shredding all documents that identify the respondent, it is not clear that confidentiality can be assured; respondents are right to be nervous.[4] This concern was cited in the congressional debates over the national samples and was a contributing factor to their demise.

The history of sexual behavior research has smaller lessons. Because the research is likely to be attacked, it is important that it be as defensible as possible. There is a great deal of reason to be suspicious of volunteer respondents, so resources need to be devoted to obtaining the best possible sample and to minimizing nonresponse rates. This means paying attention to item nonresponse as well as survey nonresponse, since in sex surveys, there are often quite high levels of the former, usually on particularly sensitive questions (Bradburn and Sudman 1979). When there are inadequate resources to undertake a high-quality survey, other kinds of data collection may be preferable. Unless there is a need to obtain behavioral parameters, a small number of open-ended, in-depth interviews or focus groups may be the best use of resources.

Like many worthwhile undertakings, sex research is scary for the researcher. However, in spite of our misgivings, we believe, like other researchers, that sex research helps liberate issues of sexuality and brings light to areas that were formerly dark. We need to understand sexual behavior if we want to understand how it interacts with other issues, such as women's health. Doing sex research, particularly if one understands the context of the research, can be a powerful political act. It is no accident that much of the best research on the sexual behavior of gay men, essential to delineating the exact mode of AIDS transmission in the United States, was done by gay men with survey research or social science training.

Notes

1. Interview with Paul Gebhard, February 18, 1994. He described the technique they used to obtain "100 percent samples" of the groups they interviewed as so coercive at times that he doubted whether today they would pass a human subjects review.
2. Interview with Wardell Pomeroy, May 20, 1993.
3. The SHARP survey subsequently became the "National Health and Social Life Survey" (Laumann et al. 1994).
4. Recent advice by University of Chicago lawyers indicates that even sending documents to another country is no guarantee that an angry, suspicious spouse will not be able to persuade the courts to obtain their return and release.

References

Bradburn, Norman M., and Seymour Sudman, with the assistance of Edward Blair, William Locander, Carrie Miles, Eleanor Singer, and Carol Stocking. 1979. *Improving interview method and questionnaire design.* San Francisco: Jossey-Bass.

Catania, Joseph A., Lois McDermott, and Lance Pollack. 1986. Questionnaire response bias and face-to-face interview sample bias in sexuality research. *Journal of Sex Research* 22:52–72.

Clark, Alexander, and Paul Wallin. 1964. The accuracy of husbands' and wives' reports of the frequency of marital coitus. *Population Studies* 18:165–71.

Clark, John P., and Larry L. Tifft. 1966. Polygraph and interview validation of self-reported deviant behavior. *American Sociological Review* 34: 516–23.

Congressional Record. 1992. S4737. April 22.

DeLameter, John D. 1974. Methodological issues on the study of premarital sexuality. *Sociological Methods and Research* 3:30–61.

Ericksen, Julia A., and Sally A. Steffen. Forthcoming. *Kiss and Tell: Revelations of sexual behavior surveys.* Boston: Harvard University Press.

finger, Frank W. 1947. Sex beliefs and practices among male college students. *Journal of Abnormal Psychology* 42:57–67.

Foucault, Michel. 1978. *History of sexuality: The use of pleasure.* New York: Random House.

Freedman, Ronald, Pascal K. Whelpton, and Arthur A. Campbell. 1959. *Family planning, sterility and population growth.* New York: McGraw-Hill.

Kerkhoff, Richard K. 1964. Family life education in America. In *Handbook of marriage and the family,* edited by Harold T. Christensen. Chicago: Rand McNally.

Kinsey, Alfred, Wardell B. Pomeroy, and Clyde Martin. 1948. *Sexual behavior in the human male.* Philadelphia: W. B. Saunders.

Laumann, Edward O., John H. Gagnon, Robert T. Michael, and Stuart Michaels. 1994. *The social organization of sexuality: Sexual practices in the U.S.* Chicago: University of Chicago Press.

Moore, Kristen, et al. 1989. Nonvoluntary sexual activity among adolescents. *Family Planning Perspectives* 21:110–14.

Morokoff, Patricia. 1986. Volunteer bias in the psychophysiological study of female sexuality. *Journal of Sex Research* 22:35–51.

Pomeroy, Wardell B. 1982. *Dr. Kinsey and the Institute for Sex Research.* New Haven, Conn.: Yale University Press.

Research and Decisions Corporation. 1984. A report on: Designing effective AIDS prevention campaign strategy for San Francisco: Results from the first probability sample of an urban gay male community. Prepared for the San Francisco AIDS Foundation.

Ryder, Norman B., and Charles F. Westoff. 1965. *Reproduction in the United States: 1965.* Princeton, N.J.: Princeton University Press.

Weeks, Jeffrey. 1985. *Sexuality and its discontents.* New York: Routledge.

Wolchik, S. A., S. Lee Spencer, and Iris S. Lisi. 1983. Volunteer bias in research employing vaginal measures of sexual arousal. *Archives of Sexual Behavior* 15:399–408.

Zelnik, Melvin, John F. Kantner, and Kathleen Ford. 1981. *Sex and pregnancy in adolescence.* Beverly Hills: Sage.

Researcher Bias in the Field of Sexuality and Reproductive Health

Ana Amuchástegui

Conducting research on the sensitive and private topic of sexual behavior and its meanings in different cultures presents many problems, including how to maintain confidentiality, elicit meaningful responses, put the interviewee at ease, establish trust, and interpret responses or nonresponses. These difficulties are confounded by the researcher's own biases about "appropriate" sexual values and behavior, his or her presumptions about a society's dominant sexual norms, the potential for the researcher and the study participants to influence each other, and issues such as who determines the research agenda and how the findings will be used. This chapter reviews some of the ethical dilemmas and personal biases that I confronted in a recent study.

Research Project and Objectives

My research project was entitled Hybrid Cultures: The Coexistence of Traditional and Modern Meanings of Virginity and Sexual Initiation for Mexican Youth (Amuchástegui Herrera 1994). This study attempted to illuminate and describe the cultural forms and meanings that young people in three Mexican communities attached to virginity and to their first sexual relationships. It also sought to examine the place of gender and power issues in sexual initiation.

My research goals were to (1) study sexual attitudes and practices within specific Mexican communities, focusing particularly on the sexual initiation among young people and their notions about virginity; (2) examine the differences between these communities in the meaning attached to sexuality and reproduction; and (3) to explore the ways in which the collective norms of the traditional cultures shape and interact with modern ideas about individual choice. In doing this research, I wanted to use a qualitative methodology so that in-depth interviews with community members would form the backbone of my fieldwork. The objectives of the Population Council (the organization under which this research was conducted) also had to be taken into consideration. Fortunately, there was strong overlap between my interests and those of the Population Council, which sought to produce a series of comprehensive, qualitative studies on the cultural aspects of sexual practice.

In addition to these specific research goals, my work addressed the need for more information on sexual meanings,[1] particularly in light of the risk of HIV infection. At the same time, "gender" has been legitimized as a research issue for the population and family planning fields thanks to long-standing efforts by feminist organizations to incorporate their agenda into mainstream social research. Indeed, many are coming to recognize the importance of strengthening women's position in intimate partnerships when it comes to discussions and decisions regarding sexual and reproductive behavior. In this way, my project was probably reflective of a broad shift in reproductive health and family planning research toward a more multidisciplinary and qualitative approach to research.

Fieldwork was conducted in three communities with geographic, economic, cultural, and ethnic characteristics that illustrate Mexico's highly unequal process of industrial development and modernization. The three communities included a Zapotec Indian community, a rural community in Guanajuato (central Mexico), and a working-class urban community in Mexico City.

The Zapotec community, in the Valley of Oaxaca, was chosen because Mexico has been shaped as much by native cultures as by the Spanish one, and because a great many Mexicans continue to live in traditional native ways. At the same time, a large proportion of the local men travel periodically to the United States to work as temporary laborers, and many young Zapotec girls migrate to Mexico City to work in domestic households as maids, where they are exposed to modernization. In the rural community in Guanajuato, as well, many people seek work in nearby cities or travel to the United States. However, the Catholic Church and religion form an important part of daily community life and play a considerable role in shaping local sexual values and practices. Finally, the young people from Mexico City are the children or grandchildren of manual laborers or salaried employees, and they have better access to education than youths from the other two sites.

I began by holding an initial group meeting in each community to discuss several aspects of sexuality—mainly, the concerns of young people regarding sexual initiation, reproduction, and formation of couples—to introduce possible informants to the research, and to recruit volunteer interviewees. Potential interviewees were primarily recruited through nongovernmental organizations (NGOs) that had already involved them in some kind of reproductive health project. Some subjects, however, were referred spontaneously by other interviewees and had not participated in any previous projects. This distinction was important, since the informants' prior "training" in reproductive health issues and their earlier experience in discussing such topics made a difference in the kind of information they provided, in terms of traditional and modern frameworks of meaning.

Among those who were introduced to the project, twenty-five men and women between fifteen and thirty-two years of age asked to be interviewed. After the meeting, in order to address any doubts or queries they might have about the issues raised, I made myself available to the volunteers. This approach allowed the great majority of the interviews to be responsive to the participants' needs.

I conducted twenty-two individual and seven group interviews with the volunteers. Some interviews were loosely structured, and others were in-depth or semistructured; they were all supplemented by conversations with key sources such as municipal workers, doctors, midwives, and health promoters to provide a better context for the interpretation of my discussions with young people. Initially, I was responsible for interviewing the female volunteers and a male colleague was responsible for talking to the male volunteers. However, in reviewing the data from the first two interviews with men, I was frustrated by the interviewer's inability to draw out more information about the men's first encounters with sexual intercourse. So I decided to try to talk to the men myself. I found that my being a woman did not inhibit the men's responses to my questions. My status as a bearer of scientific, specialized knowledge and as someone from outside the community had a greater impact on the interviews than whether I was the same sex as the person being interviewed.

Researcher Bias and Its Consequences

Choosing the Research Topic

The very act of choosing a subject and determining that it merits investigation already implies a particular interpretation of reality—a particular bias. Consequently, I did not pretend to discover any particular "reality" with this research project or try to discover some sort of "truth" about the possible meanings of the first sexual experience. Rather, I attempted to build an approximation of what such meanings might be.

I selected my research focus on the basis of several considerations. In a wide range of cultures and societies, sexual initiation is among the most central and significant events on the road to adulthood. The meanings a person gives to his or her sexual practices (or the range of sexual behaviors in which he or she engages) are the most intimate links to the values of a particular society and reveal the complex nexus between individual experience and community norms. Since each culture produces a set of norms—including sexual norms—to which its members are expected to conform, studying sexual initiation can open windows on the process by which identity is formed.

In addition, as a therapist, I had seen the tremendous pressures that traditional gender role ideologies create for both boys and girls, and I observed the strong relationship between gender values and an individual's assumptions about his or her own sexuality. For example, I saw demands on boys to start their sexual activity at a very young age. These were as strong as the command that girls should not engage in sexual activity until they get married. I decided to focus on the first sexual experience because, for both boys and girls, the dominant cultural stereotypes about gender and sex are particularly acute.

My choice was also determined to a great degree by my desire to understand the transformation of sexual values that is taking place in Mexico as a consequence of the nation's cultural and material modernization. Despite holding rather rigid gender role norms, my clients—both male and female—exhibited behavior that, to me, reflected resistance to those norms. I also had a personal stake in this inquiry. I, too, am immersed in this cultural change and have struggled to come to terms with my own Catholic upbringing, in which female sexual desire and pleasure were regarded as undesirable at best. My own bias in favor of modern values and autonomous behavior, especially for women, inspired me to try to comprehend the way in which ideas about sexuality are formed and then accepted or resisted.

I began—as any researcher does—with certain theoretical and conceptual preferences and assumptions that determined my approach to the problem and the research process. For example, the project was limited by the fact that I conceived it in terms of the socially dominant model for sexual behavior: a heterosexual reproductive model. This emphasis reveals that I am a part of my culture's dominant moral prescriptions and that I have absorbed its biases. For example, a study less shaped by my own research interests might have focused on what the interviewees considered the most significant sexual experiences of their lives.

Role of the Interviewer

It is extremely important to be aware of the effect that research on sexuality can have on interviewees, especially when the interviewer urges the subjects to relate personal experiences. In many instances, individuals ask spontaneous questions that demand responses from the researcher. The attempt to remain scientifically "neutral" at such times can have negative consequences in this type of qualitative research. It can destroy the sense of trust that has been established between the interviewee and interviewer, or the interviewee might interpret a nonresponse as a sign of judgment and be unwilling to reveal anything else. Therefore, it is essential that researchers be prepared to respond to the needs generated by the relationship with the subject.

It is easy for us, as professionals, to forget the difficulty inherent in being interviewed about our sexual practices. We should try to imagine just how daunting such an in-depth interview might be for some of our subjects. On reflection, a good exercise in this regard would be to subject ourselves to the same types of interviews and then to register, analyze, and report on our experiences.

I typically began the interview by asking if the volunteer had any questions. Most often, they asked for help with difficulties in sexual or family relationships. For example, a fifteen-year-old male from the capital wanted to know if early sexual initiation could retard growth. Other interviewees had medical questions about, for example, stomach problems, mental deficiencies, and treatments for sexually transmitted diseases. My background as a family therapist and a psychologist often enabled me to answer such questions. However, when informants had questions that I could not answer or demands that I could not meet, such as requests for a medical consultation, they were sent to governmental institutions or NGOs that would take care of them. I attempted to answer all questions with an eye toward the interviewee's perspective and her or his cultural context.

I had only to imagine being asked the questions that I was asking my subjects to conclude that my work was an invasion of their privacy. This realization may well have interfered with my ability to explore certain subjects, especially those linked to sensuality, the erotic sensations of the interviewees, and the details of their first sexual encounters. I chose to respect the spontaneous silence of my subjects after certain questions and to record their responses as such. The following excerpt from an interview with Bertina, a thirty-year-old woman from Guanajuato, illustrates this situation:

Bertina: No, that's all, it [her first sexual encounter] was just sudden.

Interviewer: All of a sudden? And you weren't afraid? Were you pleased, did it give you pleasure or were you afraid?

Bertina: Well, when I felt sick, yes, I was afraid.

Interviewer: Afterwards?

Bertina: Right, afterwards, not at the moment. But afterwards, yes, because I got very sick, yes, I got very sick.

Interviewer: You got very sick afterwards?

Bertina: I threw up, I had diarrhea.

Even though I asked about her actual sensations, feelings, and experience the first time she had sexual intercourse, Bertina chose to tell me about her reactions to it *afterwards*, which I believe indicated that her responses during intercourse were too intimate to talk about.

However, there were other occasions during the interviews when I felt compelled to intervene. For example, Sául, a youth from a rural community in central Mexico, expressed great anger over the fact that his young bride had not become pregnant in the two months since their wedding. The manner in which he was blaming her seemed to portend a violent incident in the near future, and I felt compelled to intervene:

Sául: Here I am, you know, two months married, practically two and a half months, and my wife keeps telling me that she doesn't feel any symptoms of pregnancy, so I tell her, "Listen! I'm working away as hard as I can, I can feel myself wasting away, but no, you're still empty, so to speak, and you have the gall to tell me that I seem to have a hard time coming up with [sperm]." Is it true what they say that a man has to give up part of his life in order to give life?

Interviewer: It is too early for you to be worrying that your wife isn't pregnant, way too early. You have to keep in mind that there is only a period of a few days each month when she could get pregnant. It can't happen every day.

Sául: You can't do it every day?

Interviewer: No, there is only one opportunity per month. Keep in mind that you've only had a few chances so far.

Sául: In two months? And what if in those two months I've had ten ejaculations, or more than ten?

Interviewer: But if they haven't taken place on fertile days . . .
Sául: And what if I am wasting away each time I give it?
Interviewer: Don't worry, you are not going to run out of that.

Finally, just asking the questions that opened these discussions was a form of intervention. It seemed that most of the informants, especially the young and the less educated ones, were unaccustomed to talking about themselves and their experiences, as if it was unusual to find someone who would listen to them. I discussed this observation with the groups in Guanajuato and Oaxaca, and they confirmed it. They explained that some of them enjoyed my interviews because they could tell their stories without fear of being judged or punished. In many cases, the subjects of this study seemed pleased merely to have a chance to relate their stories, their experiences, and their doubts to someone outside their community, someone who had the added prestige of possessing specialized knowledge. I often heard the phrase, "I've never told that to anyone but you."

Confronting Researcher Bias

Although it is important to recognize the impact of this kind of research on the interviewees, it is equally important to recognize that the subject of sexual behavior and sexual norms also affects researchers. Through each stage of the research process, from conceptualization to analysis, the social scientist's own subjectivity interacts with the study participants and with the data encountered. Whether we acknowledge it openly or not, we tend to identify with our interviewees or to judge them and condemn their conduct or their decisions, or we are surprised by their opinions about sexuality.

Hearing about the meaning of sexual experiences in other people's lives inevitably leads one to question one's personal positions and how they affect one's research and interpretations of the research findings. As I worked with the transcripts of my interviews, I often found myself identifying with elements in the stories, especially with those narrated by women, so that I was continually forced to remind myself of our differences in order to analyze the material from the subject's perspective instead of from my own.

My identification with some of the experiences related by the interviewees forced me to confront my own biases. For example, some of the volunteers were struggling to reconcile their feelings of desire and eroticism with their concomitant sense of sinfulness or transgression—not to mention real punishment if they were "caught." In these instances, I sympathized with their individual and more modern feelings. For example, in the interview with Bertina, I asked if I could be of any help to her, in return for her time and her generous telling of her story.

> *Interviewer:* Listen, Bertina, tell me, what doubts or questions do you have? Do any of the things we've discussed worry you. . . . could I possibly answer a question about any of them?
>
> *Bertina:* Well, no . . . just that one thing . . . whether having [sexual] relations is a sin.
>
> *Interviewer:* Look, that is something that comes from the Church, and it depends on how much of a believer you are, doesn't it? If you are a devout believer and are very close to the Church, then for you it is going to be a sin. But now, you know that, well, young people are changing . . . there are many people that no longer put so much stock in religion and they don't consider it a sin, right? So really this all depends on how you feel, it depends on you. Maybe . . . you think that God can't frown on something that gave you so much pleasure and so much joy, right? So this depends on you . . . very much so. The Church says it is a sin, but many people no longer feel that way, right? That depends on you.

I responded to Bertina's question about collective and institutional norms and values (with which she might be trying to comply) from my individualistic, modern, and democratic standpoint, emphasizing her right to choose. I am not sure if such an option is available to her, but my response was intended to support her resistance of a cultural or community mandate that constrained and judged some parts of her experience.

My bias also became evident to me when my findings failed to confirm my preconceived notions about the communities under study. This conflict first surfaced when I observed the degree of vigilance that rural communities, and especially indigenous ones, were exercising over their women, to the extent that women's very freedom of movement was being controlled and governed by their neighbors. My romantic vision of native peoples as "our cultural heritage" was shattered by this graphic evidence of how power was exercised in daily community life. Having always thought of exploitation in terms of class struggle, I was now forced to see it played out within the community and among family units. As a consequence, any attempt to understand whole Indian communities solely in terms of "victimization" by another social group became entirely inadequate. I was forced to see that power is exercised in the smallest social spaces, and though I had known this in theory, it was difficult to accept it at such close range.

The most difficult discovery for me, however, was that sexual norms in the three communities turned out to be largely the same. I had expected these constructions of sexual meanings to be qualitatively differentiated and divided by communities, but instead I found that sexuality had homogeneous meanings across the three communities. Therefore, my original idea that traditional societies are somehow isolated from the social transformation process taking place around them was challenged with the recognition that all cultures participate in the modernizing process by incorporating within their own systems of values and norms various ideas from dominant social groups. Eventually, the concept of "hybrid culture"—the idea that traditional cultures can absorb the characteristics of a modern society, so that the values of both coexist in one community (García Canclini 1990)—helped explain such uniformity.

Research Dilemmas

My experience in conducting these interviews and my confrontations with my own personal biases made me aware of several dilemmas both in undertaking this type of research and in interpreting and presenting findings. Acknowledging these conflicts does not render this study invalid, since even within these limits, it ultimately yielded a great deal of useful information. Nevertheless, it is essential to recognize and account for these biases and contradictions if researchers are to properly comprehend, contextualize, and evaluate the results of research on sexuality and reproductive health.

Even when one wants to conduct meaningful research, a tension exists between the goals and objectives of the research and the real needs of the community. Researchers must acknowledge these conflicts and, when possible, adjust their research design accordingly or account for the conflict in reporting their findings. One possibility might be to work with community groups in order to negotiate the needs of both the informants and the research, and to discuss with them the findings and report their opinions. The following suggestions are not offered as definitive solutions; my purpose is merely to propose that these issues need to be incorporated into the broader discussion of how research in sexuality and reproductive health is carried out.

First, although my motivation included a desire to improve the conditions of the people who were interviewed, it cannot be said that the subjects themselves desired or demanded this research project. In fact, they might have identified different priorities for research. Nevertheless, I was able to make the process useful to them by offering information or referrals to services at their request.

Second, I had some politically founded concerns about how the study results, once they were published and in the public domain, might be used to justify interventions that show little respect for the cultures on which the study was based. Policymakers or others might design programs and services based on these findings with only their own agenda in mind, without consulting the persons and communities involved in the study, thus imposing goals, values, and practices that are alien to the community's own needs and culture. For example, family planning services could use information on sexual meanings and behavior in a community to achieve the goals of controlling population growth rather than considering the reproductive goals of a particular individual or couple. Although such a risk is never completely avoidable, researchers can try to prevent it by, for example, including in the recommendations of their research a statement that the active participation of the communities should be sought *before* any intervention based on the findings of studies is designed.

Finally, it is difficult—if not impossible—to present research findings as "the truth" on the elusive and sensitive subject of sexuality, because of the complexities involved in talking about it and the researcher's personal biases in interpreting the findings.

These issues and questions require further reflection and discussion among researchers, donors, and policymakers on the subject of sexual behavior. As work in this field continues, researchers, program managers, and donors must make a commitment to analyze the element of bias in their work in order to make the agenda underlying any study explicit and to make sure that future work in sexuality and reproductive health is as open and transparent as possible.

Notes

1. As explained by Dixon-Mueller(1993, 275), sexual meanings refer to "the social construction of sexuality . . . the process by which sexual thoughts, behaviors, and conditions (for instance, virginity) are interpreted and ascribed by cultural meanings. This incorporates collective and individual beliefs about the nature of the body; about what is considered erotic or offensive; and about what and with whom it is appropriate or inappropriate for men and women (according to their age and other characteristics) to do or to talk about sexually."

References

Amuchástegui Herrera, Ana. 1994. *Culturas híbridas. El significado de la virginidad y la iniciacíon sexual para jóvenes mexicanos. Finale report de investigación*. Mexico City: Population Council.

Dixon-Mueller, Ruth. 1993. The sexuality connection in reproductive health. *Studies in Family Planning* 24(5):269–82.

García Canclini, Néstor. 1990. *Culturas híbridas. Estrategias para entrar y salir de la modernidad*. Grijalbo/CNA, Col. Los Noventa. N° 50, México, 1990.

Notes on Rethinking Masculinities

An Egyptian Case

Kamran Asdar Ali

*I*n 1993–94, I undertook fifteen months of fieldwork for my doctoral dissertation in anthropology. I researched contraceptive decision-making processes among poor urban and rural households in Egypt.[1] I investigated how poor women and men, informed by their notions of sexuality, fertility, body, and health, reach decisions on fertility control in extremely insecure social and economic conditions. Concurrently, I looked at the construction of femininity and masculinity in Egypt, not as idealized, fixed categories but as processes that are linked with people's experiences as gendered beings in contested, changing, and unstable terrain.

In the Middle East, as in most cultures, fertility control is not an individual woman's decision. Although the influence of male partners and of other household members has been amply documented, male understandings of sexuality, the body, and fertility control have not received comparable scrutiny. Several recent surveys conducted in developing countries to study male beliefs and practices related to fertility control have aided in the understanding of male behavior in fertility regulation and identified trends for future family planning policy initiatives (see Mustafa 1982; Mott and Mott 1985; Makat 1987; Mbizvo and Adamchak 1991;

Jejeebhoy and Kulkarni 1989; Khalifa 1988; Abdel-Aziz, Hussein, and Cross 1992). Yet these studies give us minimal information about the constraints of daily life on the choices people make. Especially in relation to the Middle East, they take the inequality in gender relations as a given of society and culture, never questioning how it is maintained, perpetuated, or changed. They also exaggerate the separation of the male and female spheres. Inequalities do exist between the genders, but missing is an understanding of how these differences are maintained and undermined within the social context. Moreover, cooperation and sharing between the genders often coexist with practices and rhetoric that generate male power and authority.

Seeking to give some depth to the homogeneous representation of male behavior and notions of masculinity, Kandiyotti (1994) discusses the notion of dominant ("hegemonic") and subordinate ("subaltern") masculinities in the Muslim Middle East. She places the production of masculine identities in generational and institutional terms and shows how masculinities are produced and change as men move through their life cycles and different occupations. Through a reading of life histories and literary texts, she illustrates how young boys become gendered in relation to older men in the household. When the older men of the household are absent, a young man's mother and sisters may jokingly treat him as the man of the house. However, in the presence of his father and older brothers, a young man retains a position inferior to the older women of the family. Kandiyotti gives examples of how men negotiate their masculinity in all-male institutions such as the army. The humiliations that subordinate men suffer at the hands of their superiors and the homosexual relationships common in these surroundings complicate the construction of masculinity. By providing such examples, Kandiyotti argues that for most men in the Middle East, masculinity is related to the arena of power and its negotiation.

Although this analysis shows how masculinity varies within a particular culture, culture itself is dynamic. In the Middle East, as elsewhere, gender roles are transformed in response to a number of influences. The changing socioeconomic conditions in Arab countries have created economic disparities and, at the same time, have meant an increased participation of women in the labor force. These changes, along with the increase in female education, have threatened the more "traditional" organization of households and have redefined female space and boundaries. The undermining of male authority brought about by unemployment and subsistence on one's wife's pay is another crucial window to understanding male behavior.

Although I spoke with many women during the course of my work, for the purposes of this chapter, I focus on my conversations with men. Although almost all the men I spoke with upheld the standard of a patriarchal Middle Eastern man, I perceived that, individually, their actions and motivations were not as rigorous and were sometimes in contradiction to this standard, suggesting a range of Middle Eastern masculinities. After innumerable in-depth and often private conversations with men, I began to develop an understanding of male notions of self and body that could not be easily grasped by questions commonly asked in survey methodology, such as, Would you like your wife to use contraception? or Who makes the decision on contraception in the household? A more nuanced picture of male decisions and behavior began to emerge.

In this chapter, I present this picture as a series of observations and, in some instances, hypotheses rather than as a comprehensive framework for understanding men's fertility decisions and behavior. Despite its tentativeness, I believe that this information illuminates some of the complexities of gender relations in the Middle East, particularly as they affect fertility decisions. Finally, because of the personal and sensitive nature of this work, I also share some of my own experiences as a researcher and reflect on the ways in which I was forced to reconsider this role.

My Evolution as a Researcher

I spoke primarily with men from lower-income families in a poor neighborhood of Cairo and in a village in the governorate of Sharquiya, two hours northeast of Cairo. In both communities, I presented myself as a physician (I have a medical degree) doing research on family planning. In the village, with the help of a locally respected physician, I conducted several focus group sessions with men and women from different social and generational backgrounds. At both sites, I gathered further information by a small sample survey. As the study continued, I participated in the daily lives of these communities and spent considerable time talking to men informally about their occupational and personal histories, issues of fertility and infertility, marriage, domestic and sexual relations, and changing socioeconomic patterns in the community.

Most of my information came from a free exchange of views between myself and my informant-friends. In the urban area, a group of us would meet every Thursday evening (Friday being the weekly holiday) and talk into the late hours of the night on any number of topics ranging from the country's current politics to marriage rituals in Pakistan (my native country). My friends were industrial workers, and almost all of them were married. At the rural site, I followed similar patterns. During the day, I spent most afternoons in the agricultural fields talking to farmers about their crops, helping them with minor chores, listening to village gossip, and being questioned endlessly about my personal life.

Focus Groups

In the village, I was introduced to the community through a reproductive health clinic linked to a medical university in Cairo. To ease my introduction, the senior medical doctor in the clinic suggested that he and I conduct focus groups with different subsets of the local population on issues of birth control and fertility. The participants were randomly selected through the network of other clinic staff members who lived nearby. Most were organized with young men, community leaders, *dayas* (midwives), religious leaders, or women who lived in the surrounding villages and hamlets. As the participants were more familiar with my doctor friend, he moderated most of the sessions, and I participated as his assistant. The discussion below centers on three focus group sessions that we conducted with young men whose ages ranged from early twenties to mid-thirties (all of whom were married, some for the second time).

The focus groups proved helpful in enabling us to establish links with the communities and to ascertain certain general ideas about people's attitudes toward gender relations and contraception. However, they were less helpful in eliciting honest responses regarding domestic decision-making processes and relationships. In part, this is because these are highly dynamic and complex interactions that are difficult to grasp through a simple question-and-answer format.

Based on our stereotypical reading of gender relations, we initially assumed a model of male-dominant rural households. To understand the links between gender roles and fertility decision making, we asked such questions as: Would you allow your daughters to study? Do you allow your wives to visit other households without your permission? What kind of contraceptives would you allow your spouse to use and why? Do you think it is acceptable to beat your spouse? In response to these questions, men would often articulate standards of male authority. The answers were important in showing the manner in which men chose to represent their private lives in public.

Men's responses to the issue of domestic violence proved particularly illuminating. All agreed that it was necessary to beat one's spouse under certain circumstances, such as suspicion of infidelity or disobedience of orders. And yet almost all the men denied ever being violent with their wives. This unanimity may be explained in part because these men lived in nearby villages and therefore knew one another; in some cases, they were related through marriage. Another explanation may be their hesitancy to talk about their spouses in a public forum. In a society in which modesty and shame, honor and respectability, play major symbolic roles, probing, personal questions such as those on domestic violence were always resisted.

It was also difficult to get men to respond to questions that were perceived as being too personal; questions about individual behavior or attitudes were resisted. For example, we encountered a certain level of hesitancy among informants when we asked about choice of contraception in some detail. Most men preferred the IUD because it has fewer medical complications for women. When asked how the problem of breakthrough bleeding was handled, some men whose spouses were using IUDs responded that it did not matter because they treated it like part of the menstrual cycle and did not have sex with their wives on such days. When we asked whether they indulged in foreplay on such occasions, a primary school teacher shot back, "Do you have foreplay with your wife before having sex or on days she menstruates?" This question caught us off guard, but made us aware of the boundaries between acceptable questions and those that would be resisted. This and similar responses somewhat subverted our authority. As researchers and doctors, we had assumed a right to probe the "private" lives of these men while at the same time assuming that we were beyond the realm of such questions. In order to break through these barriers, I realized that it was important for me to move to a level of participant-observer by living in the village.

Beyond Focus Groups

After a month of working through the clinic, I moved to a nearby village. A coworker in the clinic, Atef, introduced me into the community as a member of his family, and I was graciously accepted. By taking this step, my "authority" as a researcher and doctor was lessened. Although I was still looked upon as an outsider and a university graduate, I was dependent on the people for my day-to-day living, and my vulnerability was evident to my informants. I was also exposed to similar kinds of questioning that I was forcing on them.

After I had been in the village for a few days, Atef's brother-in-law, Ismael, invited me to see his *feddans*,[2] which were ready with the cotton crop. While walking toward his fields, Ismael casually asked, "Ya doktor, how many times should I have sex in a day?" I was caught unawares. I had never been asked such a direct question before. What could I say? Any number of times. I do not know. Ask your wife? I wanted to present myself as a knowledgeable doctor, so I gave the best answer I could think of and told him "Any number of times, as long as you both agree."[3] Then I asked him what had prompted him to ask me such a question. He answered that he worried about the health of his wife and did not want to burden her with excessive sex.

As our conversation developed, he told me that he had always opposed any kind of contraception for his wife on religious grounds, but now that he had six children, further childbirth might affect his wife's health, youth, and fullness. Therefore, he had given her permission to use the IUD. He had resolved the apparent contradiction in his beliefs by asserting that if Allah really wanted him to have a child, no contraceptive could prevent it.

Moreover, he drew a distinction between *tanzeem* (spacing) and *tahdeed* (complete cessation) and did not disagree as forcefully with *tanzeem* which was necessary so that women could recuperate their health after delivery of a child and also during the breast-feeding months.[4]

It was through informal and honest exchanges such as these, in which I participated as an equal partner and shared my thoughts and experiences, that I began to develop a more contextualized understanding of men's decisions regarding contraceptive use. In the following section, I discuss some of the factors that influence men's decisions.

Findings

Recent studies in Egypt have shown that many men leave the choice of a specific contraceptive method to their wives after the initial decision to limit or space births has been made (Abdel-Aziz, Hussein, and Cross 1992; Johns Hopkins University, unpublished focus group results, 1988). In my work, however, I came across men who systematically influenced these decisions. For example, they often opposed oral contraceptives and IUDs because, besides other symptoms, they may produce breakthrough bleeding or spotting. As Muslim women cannot pray when they are menstruating, this is a particularly undesirable side effect. Furthermore, sex during menstruation is not permissible in the popular belief system.

Men also influenced these decisions through their received notions and knowledge (albeit usually from their wives) of health problems caused by certain contraceptives. They frequently invoked folk body imagery to explain their decisions. For example, according to my informants, the obesity associated with oral contraceptives was due to the retention of fluids (bad blood); these fluids were then stored under the skin, creating swelling with no concomitant gain in strength. My informants told me that in these situations, the woman is always tired and listless and can be cured only with a proper and balanced diet.[5]

My informants also shared the notion of an open and fluid body in which objects and fluids may travel to different parts, which is quite prevalent in Egyptian folk constructions of the body (see Early 1988, 1993). They conceive different parts of the body to be in dynamic interconnectedness. During sexual activity, the body is considered to be hot and more open than usual. I was constantly told not to drink cold water after a sex act because water could gravitate to the knee and ankle joints, causing excruciating pain. Similarly, according to some, the IUD could travel up into the heart and cause serious problems. It could also penetrate the head of the fetus if there was an accidental pregnancy—everyone knows that contraceptives cannot compete with the will of Allah.

The imagery of an open and fluid body also played a part in explaining the nonuse of condoms by almost all my male informants. I interviewed a number of men who complained of pain in their inguinal regions after using condoms. This they attributed to their fear that sperm may travel back into the urethral orifice, lodging in muscles or joints and causing pain or arthritis. Similarly, men dreaded having intercourse with women who were menstruating, as menstrual blood could enter into them and lodge in their joints.

However, the main reason that the men gave for not using condoms was that, with condoms, they did not receive and were incapable of giving sexual pleasure. Both rural and urban men insisted that women received heightened sexual pleasure when they felt the male ejaculate passing through the vagina into the uterus. (Of course women have different constructions of pleasure that may or may not overlap with those mentioned by men.) This pleasure was linked with the gradual cooling down of the female body from a hot, sexually excited state.

In my discussions with men, there was often a preoccupation with their spouses' orgasmic pleasure, and several men reported using certain medicines to maintain erections so that they could help their wives reach sexual climax. This is not surprising, given that the popular Islamic belief system encourages sexual relations not only as a procreative act but also as something to be enjoyed by both sexes. However, I began to understand this theme of being able to sexually "satisfy" their wives as an important element in the construction of masculinity.

For example, the focus on female orgasm may work as a subtle form of social control over women, who, in popular imagery, are seen as oversexed and unfaithful.[6] In a context of competing masculinities, it may also reveal the fear that an unsatisfied woman will seek others to fulfill her needs; men with more erect penises are potential rivals. In this context, impotence becomes the most extreme insult. In the communities in which I worked, impotence was periodically blamed on curses and black magic by rival men. An erect penis and its power to satisfy a woman is directly linked to the rhetoric and practice of power and control over both women and other men. Condom use, therefore, may not only reduce pleasure for both men and women but also destabilize certain constructions of gender linked to the practice of power.

Finally, the attainment of sexual pleasure was, according to my informants, linked to various social and economic aspects of life. Many men spoke of the inability to have pleasure in life, including in their sexual relationships, if they could not provide a "decent" living for their families. The Egyptian poor have been tremendously affected by the structural adjustment program, which, under the advice of the International Monetary Fund and the World Bank, has resulted in the devaluation of the Egyptian pound; increases in transportation costs; elimination of long-term subsidies on bread, flour, tea, sugar, and other items of daily use; and an increase in indirect taxes (Korayem 1993). Similarly, shrinking employment opportunities, both in urban areas and in neighboring Gulf countries and Iraq, have taken a heavy toll on men's sense of well-being.

Some of my luckier informants held two or three jobs—a civil servant in the morning, taxi driver in the afternoon, and seller of home-cooked *tamiya* (falafel) at night. However, they too complained of not having enough money to feed their families. These money shortages had a direct impact on their sexual lives, since certain energy-giving foods, popularly combined for *proteinate* (proteins), which are thought necessary for a healthy sexual life, consist mostly of different kinds of increasingly inaccessible meat products. As one man said, "Without meat and with all these worries, I ejaculate in a few minutes, whereas the rich man can keep his erection for half an hour and satisfy his spouse."[7]

Thus, the notions of hegemonic masculinity to which these men aspired were undercut by their socioeconomic conditions: poverty demasculinized them. School fees, transportation costs, expenditures for clothing, house rent, union dues, monthly installments for the stove—all these and more have made life frustrating and tense for the poor. Their sexual performance suffers and simultaneously, their own standing as men suffers.

———————

My claims are modest. I have tried to suggest the continuously negotiated nature of masculinity in Egyptian society. I have sought to show glimpses of male experiences in Egypt and to confront the stereotypical representations of masculinity in the Middle East. I have placed the construction of the masculine ideals of my informants in their relationship to power. Although a part of this power is related to their ability to control women in "public" and "private" domains, masculinities thus created are on unstable terrain. Moreover, notions of masculinity that rely on sexual performance and relations between genders are further challenged by the changing social and economic circumstances. Such description and analysis of different levels of male experience force us to comprehend decision making about contraception as a complex process. To grasp this complexity, which is embedded in symbolic and socioeconomic structures, social research needs to pay attention to people's lived experiences.

Notes

1. This research was supported by a Population Council Fellowship in the Social Sciences. Dr. Barbara Ibrahim and the staff of the Cairo office provided patience and support. In Egypt, the American University in Cairo provided institutional affiliation. The research would not have been possible without the support and intellectual stimulation of my friends and field assistants Dahlia Abul Hadi, Sameh Saeed, and Mustafa Abdur Rahman. Special thanks to Dr. Gamal Suroor and Dr. Ahmed Ragai of the International Islamic Center for Population Studies and Research, Al-Azhar University. I am most indebted to my informants, who tolerated my queries and who always accepted me with open arms. Finally, thanks to Syema for everything.
2. A *feddan* is a unit of land in Egypt, equal to approximately 1.035 acres.
3. My liberal, politically correct answer was also meant to show my disdain for these oversexed peasant men who, as I had been told by my upper-class Cairene friends, had no respect for women. Who said anthropologists do not carry biases?

4. Many informants couched their reluctant acceptance of contraception in terms of caring for their wives' health. Paradoxically, although the men spoke to me about the dangers of different female contraceptives, they encouraged and tolerated their use if periodic pregnancies were affecting the health of their spouses, even recommending them, as in the case of my friend Ismael, to help their wives space their pregnancies.

5. Poverty and lack of resources in poor households complicate the situation, making a healthy diet out of reach for most of these women.

6. Social constructions of women as wives, mothers, and daughters, which carry definite ideological underpinnings and systems of prestige, are balanced against a competing construction of the essential woman who is chaotic and represents disorder (*fitna*) (see Mernissi 1975), particularly in relation to her overwhelming sexuality. In my interviews, the construct of a sexually charged woman was also used as an argument for the need to physically restrain and circumcise women (circumcision is believed to cool a woman down sexually).

7. This may also point to an unstable relationship between husbands and wives in poorer communities, where husbands cannot satisfy their wives and hence do not have sexual control over them. Such explanations may be in the realm of the ideal and symbolic, but the construction of gender roles in the communities I worked in were often reflected through this kind of narrative.

References

Abdel-Aziz, Sayed, Fatma Hasan El-Zanaty Hussein, and Anne R. Cross. 1992. *Egypt male survey 1991.* Calverton, Md.: Demographic and Health Surveys/Macro International.

Abdel-Aziz, Sayed, Fatma Hasan El-Zanaty Hussein, Hasan Zaki, and Ann A. Way. 1993. *Egypt demographic and health survey 1992.* Cairo: National Population Council; Calverton, Md.: Macro International.

Capmas. 1991. *Role of Egyptian women in the family.* Cairo: Capmas.

Early, E. 1988. The Baladi curative system of Cairo. *Culture, Medicine and Psychiatry* 12(1):65–83.

———. 1993. *Baladi women of Cairo: Playing with an egg and a stone.* Boulder, Colo.: Lynne Reinner.

Jejeebhoy, Shireen J., and Sumati Kulkarni. 1989. Reproductive motivation: A comparison of wives and husbands in Maharashtra, India. *Studies in Family Planning* 20(5):264–72.

Kandiyotti, Deniz. 1994. The paradoxes of masculinity: Some thoughts on segregated societies. In *Dislocating masculinity: Comparative ethnographies,* edited by A. Cornwall and N. Lindisfarlane. New York: Routledge.

Khalifa, Mona A. 1988. Attitudes of urban Sudanese men towards family planning. *Studies in Family Planning* 19(4):236–43.

Korayem, Karima. 1993. *Structural adjustment and reform policies in Egypt: Economic and social implications.* Amman, Jordan: United Nations Economic and Social Council, Economic and Social Commission for Western Asia.

Lindisfarlane, Nancy. 1994. Variant masculinities, variant virginities. In *Dislocating masculinities,* edited by A. Cornwall and N. Lindsfarlane. New York: Routledge.

Makat, J. F. 1987. *Child spacing in Lesotho.* Working paper in demography no. 9. Lesotho: National University of Lesotho.

Mbizvo, Michael T., and Donald J. Adamchak. 1991. Family planning knowledge, attitudes, and practices of men in Zimbabwe. *Studies in Family Planning* 22(1):31–38.

Mernissi, Fatma. 1987. *Beyond the veil.* Bloomington, Ind.: Indiana University Press.

Mott, Frank L., and Susan H. Mott. 1985. Household fertility decisions in West Africa: A comparison of male and female survey results. *Studies in Family Planning* 16(2):88–99.

Mustafa, M. A. 1982. *Male attitudes towards family planning in Sudan.* Khartoum, Sudan: Sudan Fertility Control Association.

Naguib, Nora Guhl, and Cynthia Lloyd. 1994. *Gender inequalities and demographic behavior: The case of Egypt.* New York: Population Council.

Rugh, A. 1984. *Family in contemporary Egypt.* Syracuse, N.Y.: Syracuse University Press.

*T*alking to Men and Women about their Sexual Relationships

Insights from a Thai Study

Napaporn Havanon

I conducted a research project, Sexual Networking in Provincial Thailand, during 1991–92, when the spread of AIDS in Thailand was beginning to become a cause for alarm.[1] High-risk groups in danger of becoming infected with HIV were (and remain) intravenous drug abusers who shared hypodermic needles, hemophiliacs who were treated with infected blood products, promiscuous people, and sexually active homosexual males. Although policymakers and the general public were beginning to understand that these were not the only groups at risk for HIV infection, it was believed that prostitution was the chief cause of the spread of AIDS among a wider population. Men patronizing entertainment establishments and sleeping with service girls were deemed to be at high risk for infection. It was also widely believed that foreign tourists played a major role in the prevalence of the flesh trade in Thailand and were carriers of HIV, transmitting it to prostitutes whose services they used.

I took issue with this perception and argued that the rapid spread of AIDS in Thai society probably did not stem chiefly from the development of the tourism industry and the inflow of foreign tourists. I reasoned that the culture of the indigenous people and their sexual behavior played an equal, if not more important, role in the promotion of the flesh trade in the country. I believed this to be the case because, even though Thai society is monogamous according to the law, in practice it is not considered a major taboo for a married or single man to have sexual relations with several different women, including service girls. Thus, the main objective of this research was to learn more about the sexual behavior of people with multiple sexual partners. A secondary objective was to explore the extent to which Thai women who are not commercial sex workers become linked to the commercial sex network through their partners' behavior.

The study's primary focus was a cross section of married and single men working in white-collar and blue-collar jobs as well as some students, all of whom had had more than one sexual partner in the previous twelve months. We also interviewed women who were likely to have had multiple sexual partners, such as singers, waitresses in restaurants with music, masseuses at traditional massage parlors, and score markers at snooker halls, as well as women who occasionally engaged in commercial sex arrangements. Additionally, we interviewed students and unemployed teenagers who frequented nightclubs and pubs, and women who were wives of clients with sexually transmitted diseases (STDs).

Before the fieldwork began, the principal investigators on the project (Anthony Bennett, John Knodel, and I)[2] held numerous in-depth discussions to select locations and research methods. We decided to carry out the research in a central province not far from Bangkok. The province had moderate industrial development and several educational institutions. Moreover, the province was not famous for tourism. Although it had many places of entertainment, such as restaurants with music, bars, pubs, nightclubs, snooker halls, and traditional massage parlors, these entertainment spots were intended more for local people and Thais visiting from other provinces.

A total of 181 men and 50 women were interviewed, employing an in-depth interview method with flexible, open-ended questions. All the interviews were conducted in a relaxed and informal atmosphere, and questions were asked in a conversational style. Only male researchers contacted and interviewed men, and only female researchers contacted and interviewed women. Both men and women were asked similar questions, including their perceptions and attitudes about premarital sex, extramarital sex, and men's sexual relationships with commercial sex workers; the number of sex partners in the past year and their partners' occupations;[3] and details about their own sexual behavior, such as coital frequency, use of condoms, and reasons for use or nonuse.

I present my experience in conducting this research in two main sections: a discussion of my experiences and difficulties in conducting the research—including recruiting and educating personnel to collect data and attempting to solve problems that arose during the data collection process; and a reflection on how my experiences strengthened my knowledge of the sexual behavior of men and women and deepened my understanding of the gulf between men's and women's sexual experiences and perceptions. As a Thai woman, I was particularly affected by meeting and interviewing other Thai women and talking with them about subjects that they had never discussed with their spouses, parents, relatives, or colleagues.

Overcoming Obstacles to Research

I was apprehensive when the research began, partly because I had no experience studying sexual behavior and knew this to be a sensitive issue that could not be discussed openly. Consequently, I was uncertain whether the field research would provide enough knowledge to paint a clear picture of the sexual behavior of men and women. I also doubted whether I would have access to the female respondents targeted in the study, as I would have to go through provincial or district public health officials; operators of restaurants, bars, pubs, traditional massage parlors, and snooker halls; and owners of factories, banks, and other establishments to reach them.

To overcome some of these obstacles, I met with public health officials in the selected province. The public health chief of the province was very cooperative and introduced me to four officials (one male and three female) whose daily work brought them into contact with owners and employees of entertainment places. I explained the objectives of the study and the main topics to be discussed and reviewed sample questions for the interviews. Three out of the four gave pessimistic responses, saying that it would be difficult to gain access to female respondents, get their coopera- tion, or obtain truthful responses. The remaining official said that it would be possible with some effort and a tactful approach, but added that she foresaw some difficulties. I was impressed by her attitude and felt some encouragement; I asked for her assistance. She had a colleague who was also interested in participating in this research and they both joined our research team, which remained together until the field research was complete.

Both officials played an important role in making the data collection among women respondents a success. They provided me with access to various entertainment places by letting me join a work team that distributed condoms and visited service girls. They also helped me identify places where potential respondents could be located—restaurants, pubs, public parks, local schools. They helped me find an intermediary who could introduce me or my research assistant to the owner of the establishment or a friend of the people gathered at the site. They also introduced me to various people who arranged interviews with other mem- bers of the community. Generally, all contacts with female respondents were made through at least one intermediary. If necessary, a second intermediary was contacted by me or my research assistant.

The health officials' cooperation in arranging these introduc- tions anonymously was essential, as I did not want the respon- dents to know that I knew the officials. If they had known, potential respondents might have been suspicious of the confidentiality of the study. The officials respected the need for confidentiality and never asked me for any information from the interviews, restrict- ing themselves to an intermediary role.

Yet both were very interested in this work, as their only research experiences to date had been with structured question- naires in which the researcher is not required to probe for details about people's behavior and attitudes. They enjoyed working with researchers who chose respondents carefully, allowed the respon- dents to choose an appropriate time to be interviewed, and allowed for open-ended responses. They appreciated our patience with respondents who were reluctant to give either time or infor- mation. For the first time, they felt that research work could be exciting and challenging.

As mentioned earlier, the interviewer in this study was always the same sex as the respondent. I chose former or current graduate students in the social science field as male interviewers. The interviews with women were conducted by me and my research assistant. She had done data collection with me in the past, and she also had prior experience gathering data on sexual behavior and family planning.

The students I invited to join the research team had analytical minds, were interested in and had an understanding of social problems, and were friendly and self-confident. They were keen to participate, as they recognized the value of this research experience. I spent a lot of time with them before the research began to discuss the overall study objectives as well as the objectives for each question. Their knowledge of AIDS and how it is transmitted also had to be developed. I learned later that this time spent in preparation was beneficial for another reason. The male students told me that they had been apprehensive about me—their teacher and a woman—talking with them in detail about sexual behavior. They needed some time, which was provided by our discussions, to become accustomed to me and to this work.

The data collection process was slow. I assigned researchers to interviewees, instructing them to make brief notes during the course of the interview from which they would make complete field notes later. This process proved challenging for the researchers, as many had little experience taking detailed notes of their interviews. Earlier, I had asked them to make field reports immediately after the interviews; I would then review the reports and ask them to provide more details, if necessary. So now, to help them with their difficulty, I suggested that they make extended notes during the interviews (like the responses they gave to my requests for additional information) as a way of taking down more accurate information.

Because earlier studies had indicated that condoms were unpopular and perceived as unnatural, I thought that it was important to explore the issue of condom use or nonuse in greater detail. However, many of the researchers thought that questions such as "Did you use a condom when having sexual relations with this person? If not, why not?" were too personal. At first, they did not try to persuade respondents to elaborate on their reluctance to use condoms because they were concerned about offending them and creating a situation in which a respondent would refuse to answer additional questions. I encouraged the interviewers to approach sensitive or personal questions gradually, for example, by asking the respondents' opinions on condom use first, and *then* asking whether they used condoms. I also encouraged the interviewers to introduce such topics in a light-hearted way by sharing a story of something that had actually occurred, either to them or to an acquaintance. Finally, I explained that if respondents refused to answer questions, the researcher could terminate the interview.

This approach probably allowed the researchers to relax and enabled respondents to talk more freely about their sexual experiences and behavior. In fact, some people voluntarily and unexpectedly told researchers private stories. For example, a male interviewee said that he had had a sexual experience with another man because he was drunk, but he insisted that he was not gay and did not like that kind of sexual behavior. He considered the event an accident.

Talking to women presented a different kind of problem. There is a perception in Thai society, particularly among the middle class, that it is an impropriety for women to discuss sexual behavior or anything to do with sex openly. A woman who introduces a subject such as condoms in conversation is considered unladylike, lacking finesse. We thought that this cultural bias would create barriers when we tried to talk to women. However, we learned that when we introduced our questions in a semiformal manner, explaining that we sought the information for a better understanding of sexual behavior in the general population, the respondents felt that they were making a contribution and were willing to talk about their sexual lives, behaviors, and relationships with their partners quite openly.

Personal Insights

My experience of interviewing female respondents and reading the male researchers' field notes greatly changed my understanding of relations between women and men in Thai society. I once believed that the social status of Thai women was quite good in comparison with that in other Asian countries. My belief was based on my observation of Thai society. Although men do not traditionally take a role in domestic chores and child care, they do participate in raising families by farming, gardening, and animal raising. Women are responsible for managing the budget and have a say in other issues such as family planning, the number of children, and the children's education. Thai women also enjoy the freedom to travel within their own country without restriction and to maintain relationships with both female and male relatives.

However, my research experience demonstrated to me that the status of Thai women in intimate relationships is very low. I already knew that, in Thai culture, women face many restrictions regarding premarital and extramarital sexual activity. For women, premarital sex is strongly discouraged, and extramarital sex is forbidden. Men have more freedom to have premarital and extramarital sex, including sexual relations with commercial sex workers. In fact, one way to be a "good woman" in Thai society is to allow men the privilege of a double standard by accepting their sexual relationships with other women. Now, as I heard more about men's and women's attitudes and experiences regarding sexual behavior, I began to appreciate that the differences in their viewpoints created a potential health risk for women. Both the women and the men interviewed in this study thought that having sex with commercial sex workers was acceptable behavior for both single and married men.

"Whoring is normal for men. Even if some of us have girlfriends, we can't always have sex with them. So when we feel the urge, we have to go to a prostitute." —Male student

"Visiting prostitutes is normal for men because men have to go whoring. If you don't, you might as well go to the monkhood." —Married white-collar male

"Visiting prostitutes is normal for both single and married men. It is their right. If they like to go, they can go. Service girls are, by definition, available to provide sex services for men." —Waitress, single

"Visiting prostitutes is not unusual; it's normal. Men get tired of having sex with just their wife. Once in a while, it's okay to go out and have fun, and the young prostitutes really know how to make you feel good." —Married white-collar male

Women, however, are expected to be "naive" and "passive" in sexual matters. This standard of a passive female role in sexual relations creates a profound lack of awareness about women's risk status, because women do not understand or even know about their partners' sexual behavior. Women do not question their husbands or boyfriends about their affairs with other women or service girls or discuss their concerns or suspicions about contracting STDs. They tend to assume that their partners are not the type who have affairs or that they have enough sense to use condoms with other women.

The women interviewed in this study thought that it was solely their partners' responsibility to protect themselves from catching diseases. It was also clear from the interviews that women perceived condom use to be a man's prerogative—they thought it inappropriate to suggest that their partner use a condom.

"We never use a condom because he doesn't want to." —Female pool hall scorekeeper

"I don't use condoms with this guy because he has high education and should know how to protect himself." —Unemployed female teenager

"I never use condoms because my boyfriend knows what is good and what is bad and he should know to protect himself if he sleeps with another girl." —Female singer

No woman mentioned asking her husband to use a condom.

As I am also a Thai woman whose attitudes and behavior have been shaped by my culture, the findings of this study caused me to look at myself. Believing that one has a right to be "safe" in a sexual relationship, I began to understand that a relationship with a member of the opposite sex must be based on *real* equality. The findings from this research underscored for me the importance of providing women and men with an accurate picture of the risks they face in sexual relationships, particularly of acquiring HIV. I hope that Thai women, given the opportunity to learn and understand the facts as I did, will rethink their roles in relationships with men and immunize themselves against the dangers created by their passive role in sexual matters.

Notes

1. For further information on this study, see Havanon, Bennett, and Knodel (1993).
2. Anthony Bennett is a resident advisor for the AIDS Control and Prevention Project, Family Health International, in Bangkok; and John Knodel is a professor of sociology at the University of Michigan.
3. This information was collected in an attempt to develop a better understanding of how sexual networks are created; for example, if a woman worked in an entertainment spot, she was likely to have more than one sexual partner.

Reference

Havanon, Napaporn, Anthony Bennett, and John Knodel. 1993. Sexual networking in provincial Thailand. *Studies in Family Planning* 24(1): 1–17.

*W*hat's Love Got to Do with It?

The Influence of Romantic Love on Sexual Risk Taking

Dooley Worth

Currently, the number of new AIDS cases is growing fastest among women. The life experiences of the women with whom I have had the privilege of working suggest that women are more at risk of contracting HIV and AIDS than men not *just* because of their physiological makeup or their social or economic status but because they engage in sexual risk taking in the pursuit of love. For these women, sexual behavior is not necessarily driven by a need for sexual fulfillment but rather by the need to be "loved" by a man in order to feel whole. To attract romantic love, women suppress their own sexual needs; they take sexual risks that work against their own health, against their physical survival.

Although I have done research primarily among poor minority women living in inner cities ravaged by drug use, I believe that many women in all social and economic circumstances are influenced by the belief that romantic love will bring them fulfillment, and that they engage in sexual risk taking to obtain such love. This chapter discusses my experience discovering and attempting to understand the links between childhood experiences, women's search for romantic love, and sexual risk taking.

Background

I was trained in New York City as a researcher, a medical anthropologist. My doctoral work focused on the impact of colonialism and, subsequently, nationalism on health care in developing countries such as Vietnam. After obtaining my doctorate, however, I chose to work closer to home, on Manhattan's Lower East Side, where the social and economic problems are severe.

In 1986, I noticed an increasing number of women coming to the community clinic where I worked for treatment of HIV or AIDS. At the time, there was almost no talk of women and AIDS, except among a handful of medical care providers. Working in cooperation with the New York City Department of Health and the medical director of the Stuyvesant Clinic, I helped set up the first women-specific HIV testing and counseling services in the city. Heterosexual, bisexual, and lesbian, the women included heroin addicts, sex partners of injection drug users and bisexual men, prostitutes, housewives, students, artists, businesswomen, public employees, and medical professionals. In a facilitated weekly group, they shared their fears, problems, courage, and treatment experiences. The women were grappling with extremely complex decisions due to their roles as caretakers of men and children—decisions men did not face. In order to help design programs for women, I felt that I needed to have a greater understanding of the interaction of drug use and sexual risk taking in women's and their partners' lives.

In 1987, I was offered an opportunity to help set up a similar program funded by the U.S. Centers for Disease Control at Montefiore Medical Center, also in New York City. As part of my research, I made weekly observations of the behavior of heroin-addicted women in one of Montefiore's methadone clinics in the South Bronx—another community characterized by severe social and economic problems. As details of the women's lives emerged, so did evidence of a specific set of risk-taking behaviors related to HIV and AIDS.

During the second year of the ethnographic study of HIV-related behaviors in women in methadone treatment, I continued to observe the women's behavior in the group but devoted most of my time to individually interviewing a representative sample of the women. The interviewing took place in a small medical examination room where we had complete privacy. Employing an open-ended interviewing style (I simply asked the women to tell me about their lives and touch on what was most important to them), I documented their life histories and thoughts about their behavior, in their own words.

The women's accounts left little doubt that, contrary to the opinion of many health professionals, their risk-taking behaviors had a rational basis, given the crises-ridden context of their lives. The majority of these women were still actively using drugs despite being on methadone maintenance. As a result, they were frequently faced with eviction, family and health crises, arrest, and confrontations with social welfare authorities. Their triage system for decision making was firmly rooted in dealing with the most pressing present need (for drugs and the money to obtain them) or crisis (losing welfare benefits, homes, custody of their children). They did not have the luxury of addressing possible health needs or crises that might take place in the future. In many cases, the women were not sure that they would have a future. The environment they lived in supported this belief. Some had family members who had died prematurely due to the affects of alcoholism or drugs, several had been widowed more than once before the age of thirty-five, and all had been exposed to drug-related violence.

As I analyzed the women's life histories, specific risk factors emerged that appeared to contribute to behaviors that culminated in HIV or AIDS. Many of the women had been born into families with histories of addiction to alcohol and drug abuse (*"I was raised in an alcoholic home . . . watching my mother and father fight a lot and everything was bad, growing up seeing that . . . I was depressed a lot."*) or families with histories of mental illness (*"My mother was an alcoholic and she is a mental case. . . . I had two uncles that killed themselves."*). One-third of the women I interviewed privately spontaneously disclosed that they had been victims of incest or childhood sexual abuse (*"All my brothers raped me. . . . They didn't penetrate me completely . . . [this from] . . . the time I was about seven, eight years old."*). Others had been physically abused as children (*"She [mother] just beat the shit out of me. . . . I remember the beatings, they were like very severe. Sometimes it seemed like she wasn't going to stop."*) or they had grown up watching their mothers or siblings being physically abused. Women spoke of a connection between these events and the initiation of risk taking later in their lives.

Comparing the Montefiore interviews, I calculated that the majority of the women had progressed along what appeared to me to be an identifiable lifelong continuum of risk. For about half the women in the program, such risk taking had already led to HIV or AIDS. The continuum of risk taking usually began as the women approached adolescence and began acting out: staying out of school, running away from home, and getting into trouble with the police or juvenile justice system. AIDS was just one of a number of possible end points for such risk taking. Others were multiple unwanted pregnancies (*"I had a relationship with this guy . . . I was pregnant three times by him and they were all aborted."*) or involvement in repeatedly abusive relationships (*"My husband used to beat me up all the time . . . he ended up hurting me really bad . . . I was in the hospital . . . I had a concussion . . . I had . . . a blow-out eye."*).

Concerned that these women's childhood experiences might be atypical of those of other women with HIV and AIDS, I decided to explore whether a similar continuum of risk existed in a group of heroin-addicted women who were not in drug treatment. I returned to the Lower East Side and interviewed a small sample of women who were actively injecting drugs, matching my study participants for age and ethnicity with the women in the South Bronx. Again I employed a nondirective, open-ended interviewing technique. The small sampling of women, interviewed in a neighborhood storefront, disclosed an even higher rate of sexual and physical abuse in childhood than the women in treatment at Montefiore, although they were not asked if they had been abused (Worth et al. 1990). Comparing their life histories, I found a similar pattern of risk taking.

The data from both studies indicated that there were links between women's adult risk taking and their childhood experiences. At this point, I had to wonder whether such a linkage was limited to women who were heroin addicts. What about women who had used other noninjected drugs? What about the increasing number of women who had not used drugs at all but were at risk of HIV infection through sex?

Wanting to explore this question, I agreed to participate in a five-site study of female sex partners of male injection drug users funded by the Community Research Branch of the National Institute on Drug Abuse (NIDA) in 1992. The women recruited included non-drug users, former drug injectors, and non-injection drug users. The interviewers were asked to try to recruit non-drug-using women, but in the inner cities it was difficult to find women partnered with male injectors who had not used drugs themselves. Over two hundred women were interviewed in five cities (Boston, San Juan, Juarez, San Diego, and Los Angeles). One hundred eighty-nine interviews were accepted for analysis. The interviews were open-ended and explored the women's experiences with risk-taking behaviors over a lifetime. The semistructured questionnaire included nondirective questions about the women's family history, childhood, sexual history, health history, and history of drug use. The study focused on women's relationships with men (it was targeted at heterosexual women). Relationships were probed through questions exploring the women's concepts of ideal relationships, love, and marriage. Their actual relationships—how they began, why they were attracted to their partners, sexual decision-making roles, and sexual behavior and risk taking within (and outside) the relationship—were also documented.

The experience raised important questions regarding what type of training and background is most appropriate when conducting research in sensitive areas such as sexual behavior and personal relationships. The questionnaires were administered in the field by trained, experienced ethnographers in three sites and by community outreach workers in two sites where there were no ethnographers available. The ethnographers and the outreach workers were brought together for one day of training on the use of the questionnaire. Back in the field, the ethnographers were able to collect indepth material on the women's sexual decision making and behavior over time, working under difficult conditions (such as working on the street) and in a short period of time. The community workers, who matched the women interviewed in ethnicity and age, were far less successful in eliciting sensitive sexual information from their informants, although they had much better access to them. It must be noted that there were cultural differences in the two sites where the community workers conducted the interviews, which appeared to influence women's ability to talk openly about sexual desire or behavior. Even taking this into account, the outcomes of the interviews suggest that the quality and depth of information obtained are more dependent on the training and skill of the interviewer than on their ethnicity or ability to "culturally bond" with the informant (Worth 1993).

The data collected in the NIDA study, which employed a more structured instrument, confirmed the previous findings, that is, risk taking appeared to be linked to and grow out of childhood trauma or neglect and the behaviors adapted to survive those experiences. Over half the women in the NIDA study said that they came from homes where there had been abuse (*"He [father] physically beat her [mother], he was killin' her. He was beatin' her, choking her, and he had dragged her to a window and tried to throw her out."*). Thirty-seven percent of the women in the five-site study said that they had been sexually abused as children (*"I was ten years old. He [mother's boyfriend] used to come by my mother's house . . . he forced me to have sex with him and he told me if I didn't he was going to beat me or he'll kill me."*). Forty-one percent said that they had been physically abused as children (*"My father gave us Apache-style punishments. He knelt us on grates with pieces of glass . . . he would leave us tied down like this."*). A few women experienced both sexual and physical abuse, but most were exposed to one or the other.

The women also described another childhood experience that they said had an impact on their later risk taking: 40 percent referred to an experience they called a "loss of childhood" (*"I played the mother in my family . . . I did the cleaning, the cooking, the discipline; I was just a mother in my childhood."*). Women who had experienced a loss of childhood said that they engaged in risk taking as adolescents to escape these responsibilities and to get the attention they missed as children (*"I need attention . . . I was desperate so I started skipping school."*).

Another group of women who felt robbed of their childhood said that they turned their disappointment and rage into acting out (*"[I] was angry because as a child I never really was a child."*). As adolescents, their anger led them into using drugs, staying away from home, hanging out with "street kids," and entering sexual relationships with men who they thought would take care of them. These were predominantly older men or drug dealers, often the most affluent men in their neighborhoods (*"This man was like Sugar Daddy to me, so I didn't have to work, I didn't pay no rent, I didn't have to do nothing. I was drunk seven days a week."*).

Examining the data across the study sites, women seemed to cope with experiences of sexual abuse by adopting consistent, specifically identifiable coping patterns. They tried to distance themselves from what had happened to them by blocking out all their feelings (*"I was molested as a kid . . . it's just a part that's blocked out."*). They felt that they had lost control of their bodies and lives (*"After that happened to me, I would not go outside . . . I would just sit like in a shell, wouldn't do nothing, talk to nobody . . . I wouldn't even go to school."*). They sought to bring control back into their lives—often through drugs or sex (*"All this stuff [the effects of abuse] [was] coming through my drug addiction."*). And they confused love with having sex (*"Ever since that happened I felt that the only way you show love is by having sex with men . . . I felt this is the only way you showed affection."*).

Girls who were physically abused also tried to distance themselves from their experience by running away from home (*"I was picked up by juvenile authorities."*) and by becoming pregnant (*"I had a baby . . . I gave the baby up for adoption . . . I ran away."*). They had trouble distinguishing love from abuse; many told the interviewers that they had been physically abused by a partner (*"He ran me off the freeway in my car . . . he beat me up, left me bloody . . . pulled so much hair out of my head."*). five percent of the women said that they had been sexually abused by a partner (*"He tried to rape me . . . I did not want to have sex with him . . . he locked me in the bathroom and I cut all my back because the bathroom has mirrors and they broke."*) and over 50 percent described emotionally abusive relationships (*"Being called names, puttin' you down . . . sayin' that I was no good, I was a whore . . . you know, I started believing that."*).

Girls who had been neglected as children often bought into "rescue" fantasies, running away from home with men they didn't know (*"I met a boy and I ran away with him without knowing him well . . . I had known him for a week."*); experimenting with drugs, sex, or both (*"I was runnin' the streets . . . getting picked up by men."*); and entering into inappropriate, often abusive relationships with men who expected them to assume the very caretaking role they were fleeing (*"When I went off with my husband I thought this was going to be different and well everything was a little worse."*).

As adults, all the women in the NIDA study had male partners who put them at risk for HIV and AIDS through their use of injected drugs. Some of the women clearly did not know about their risk for HIV and AIDS because they were unaware of, or in denial about, their partners' drug injection. *However, the majority of women told the interviewers that they did know about their partners' drug injection and about the risk of HIV and AIDS and other sexually transmitted diseases. Yet more than 80 percent did not protect themselves from repeated sexual exposure to HIV.*

Women's Search for Romantic Love

Believing that the women were making rational decisions, given the context of their lives, I felt compelled to understand what was going on. Why did they continue to put themselves at risk sexually? Some clearly did it out of economic necessity. Others took risks because of cultural or family pressures. Fear (over 60 percent of the women in the NIDA study were physically abused by their partners) also played a role in sexual compliance. But women's decisions to stay in their relationships and expose themselves to risk did not appear to be based solely on socioeconomic, cultural, or fear factors. In fact, some women left relationships because of physical abuse or the threat of it. And women stayed in relationships that they were not economically dependent on. For example, in San Juan, most of the women were not dependent on their male partners for financial support; they were on welfare that they received directly.

Something else, something less obvious than socioeconomic, cultural, or fear factors seemed to be motivating at least some of the women to stay in relationships that placed their lives in jeopardy. The majority of the women interviewed in the NIDA study told the interviewers that they were very disillusioned and unhappy with their relationships and with their partners' sexual behavior, but they insisted that they really "loved" their partners and therefore remained sexually available to them. Studying individual women's accounts of why they made the sexual and relationship decisions they did, I began to see another factor emerge: what I would call their belief in, search for, and vulnerability to romantic love.

I had first encountered this issue in my discussions with the women in the Montefiore methadone program. From their conversations, it appeared that many of the women had mothers who were alcoholics. The women were asked to discuss why they thought their mothers drank. Several talked about how their mothers had been brought up with an idealized notion of romantic love, of how they would be loved and cherished by their husbands. They said that the reality of their mothers' relationships (*"[My father] wasn't faithful to my mother . . . when we were growing up*

. . . there were periods when he would leave for up to a year." "He was a chronic woman chaser.") had left them massively disappointed, and they had started drinking to cope with the disparity between what they wanted and expected from love and what they had gotten in their actual relationships.

The issue of disappointed love appeared again in the NIDA study when such expectations were specifically probed. Many of the women's lives were unconsciously focused on a search for love to replace the love and care they had not received as children (*"[I] felt nobody loved me and nobody cared about me . . . I really felt like I wanted to die."*). The lack of love in childhood was graphically described and linked to later risk taking (*"When you feel that nobody loves you . . . you're looking for a certain kind of attention in other areas which are not good for you—that's when you turn to drugs and stuff like that."*). The women said that a lack of parental love also left them vulnerable in their adolescent and adult relationships (*"I was looking for love, I didn't get love at home. . . . No attention, no one caring. . . . Until this man came into my life . . . caressing and touching. . . . I didn't get it from my mother, no kisses no hugs no nothing."*).

Such experiences played into the "white knight" syndrome that one of the ethnographers in the NIDA study noted. The women she interviewed were, she thought, clinging to a romantic childhood fantasy that a man (knight) would come along and make their lives all right, even when their experiences indicated that this was not likely to happen. The women's ideal mate was a nondrug-using, nonabusive male who worked, was faithful, spent time with his partner, and was good to their children. Ideal situations included a husband, a single-family house, and children. The Latina women specifically mentioned that they also wanted a husband who was affectionate. Affection for them connoted intimacy, as traditional Latino cultural norms support a nonsexual ideal for women (women respond to men's sexual needs rather than their own) (Worth and Rodriguez 1987).

Few women in the NIDA study had found such a partner or romantic love or affection in their adult relationships with men. Men often played into women's fantasies of "romantic love." In fact, some of the women in the NIDA study said that they were attracted to heroin-addicted men precisely because they were more "romantic" than other men, more sensitive.[1] In spite of their disappointment, many women upheld their part of what they perceived to be the relationship contract; that is, they provided their male partners with sex, usually when the men wanted it and how the men wanted it—often without condoms.

Dangers of the Ideal of Romantic Love

Although gender roles have been slowly changing, the ideal of romantic love remains a powerful icon for most women. This ideal is dangerous because it obscures the need for individual women to develop a strong sexual identity. Traditionally, it has portrayed women as empty vessels whose emotional and sexual fulfillment comes through reflecting their male lovers' passion rather than their own. It is the male lover who is in control of sexual desire and choices in the romantic love scenario. He chooses her, and in doing so, gives life to her sexual desires—desires that are hidden from her.[2]

The discouragement of strong sexual identities in women has served men's desire to control women's sexuality. The lack of awareness of their own sexual selves has rendered women powerless to express their deepest sense of themselves, one that is simultaneously spiritual, emotional, and physical. Unable to express who they are sexually, women are not in control of the form their sexual responses take. They lack sexual parity. In the absence of sexual parity, asking women to demand sexual protection can place them at heightened risk of being abused.

Although many of the women in the studies were not in touch with their own sexual needs, they were very aware of their need for love. It was this need that appeared to me to unconsciously drive the women to take sexual risks. Their sexual decisions were driven not by the conscious need to know or please themselves but by an unrecognized yet deeply felt need not to feel alone. Sex was described by the majority of women in rather stark terms, primarily as penetration or coupling, for example, vaginal, "normal," or "straight up [missionary position]" sex. Sexual pleasure, fantasy, foreplay, and other types of sexual activity were seldom mentioned, except in the context of their absence. Women were penetrated without foreplay (as though the goal of sex was merely to fill a void). Women's acceptance of such penetration (which some described as "use," as in "he used me") seemed to be linked to their need to be loved, not to be alone.

Women also participated in unsatisfying and unsafe sex because they had difficulty conceiving of a successful life or socioeconomic future without a male partner. As one woman said, she put up with an unsatisfying sex life because *"I see a future with him."* Condom use interfered with the belief in such a future, with its implied need to protect against past encounters with others. Many women said that they had not even asked their partners to use condoms because they thought that condom use would signify a lack of fidelity—a lack of future. Furthermore, the women thought that introducing condoms into a relationship was unromantic; it destroyed the illusion of what they were searching for—romantic love.

Not all the women interviewed in the studies continued to buy into the notion that romantic love would fulfill their need for love and nurturance. Some women in the NIDA study said that they had become disillusioned with men and with sex lives that did not address *their* needs (*"I've been hurt and manipulated so much I can't trust men."*). Often these women were in recovery and had been forced to get in touch with their own feelings, to take a good look at their lives. Many said that they had given up on the search for love or sex. Some of them attempted to obtain a feeling of self-worth, of completeness, by immersing themselves in their children's lives (*"Without them I would be nobody."*). Such immersion, however, is dangerous, because it has adverse effects on children; they are, in effect, being asked to parent or partner their parent. When children have to parent or partner their mothers, they are robbed of the love *they* need to develop a healthy sense of themselves. When mothers turn away from romance and, in some cases, sexual satisfaction, they expect their children to fill the gap in their lives. This creates a vicious intergenerational cycle of need; feelings of emotional abandonment and neglect create a new generation of risk takers searching for love, as was observed in this study.

Reflections

My experience suggests to me that only when we ask what love has to do with sexual choices and behavior—when we approach behavior change with a new sense of awareness of the full complexity of womens' lives—will we understand sexual risk taking. But before we can do this, we as researchers and program staff have to become comfortable with our own sexuality and our feelings about these issues of love and nurturance. The experiences of childhood sexual and physical abuse, incest, and neglect are not limited to clients. Many professionals have had similar experiences, and they will not be able to deal openly with clients' problems if they have not faced and dealt with their own problems first. Training (and possibly counseling) is often necessary before asking staff to work with clients on issues related to sexuality, relationships, abuse, and neglect. Other professionals—whether researchers or clinicians, male or female—are simply not comfortable with issues of sexuality and find it difficult to bring up or discuss the subject with clients. In far too many cases, they also lack the social and cultural sensitivity to engage women in such discussion. The result is that very few researchers or clinicians have ever engaged their clients in discussions of sexuality and the effect of abuse or neglect, even though all these issues have an impact on women seeking their services.

The pervasiveness of the avoidance of such discussions was brought home to me by the surprise expressed by many of the study participants upon being asked to talk about their sexuality, their sexual desires and needs. Over and over in the NIDA study, women told the interviewers that they had never thought about or been asked about their own sexuality (*"You [are] giving me questions I ain't think about . . . sex."*).

One of the ethnographers in the NIDA study asked a client if she minded being questioned about her sexuality. The woman said no. The same woman later said of the experience, *"The woman who interviewed me, she was good . . . she got deep . . . she left a lump in my throat, she reminded me of a lot of stuff I did."* This lack of questioning about their sexual experiences is astonishing if you reflect that these women have been interacting with myriad social service and health care providers for years and have participated in numerous research projects.

To effectively intervene with women engaging in risk taking that makes them vulnerable to HIV and AIDS and other sexually transmitted diseases, we have to examine the role of love in sexual risk taking. More researchers have to become aware of, and seek the means to understand, how different women define themselves and *their* most profound needs. We have to explore how women's sexual behavior is related to those needs within the context of their specific cultural or ethnic values. *We have to recognize that the definition and recognition of women's sexual needs have traditionally been related to and stem from male needs and fears.* We need to adopt new ways of framing and asking questions about the links between love, sexual desire, relationships, and sexual behavior. We have to listen to the experiences of the women we work with.

We will not be able to assess women's potential to bring about change in their lives and relationships and reduce their sexual risk-taking behavior until we can initiate comfortable conversations with women about their sexuality and place it in the context of their entire lives. To do this, we need to develop methods of studying the "ecology" of sexuality for different groups of women (the context that influences their individual sexual decisions).

An ecological understanding is, however, just a first step. As program planners and administrators, we have to adapt new models that can deliver services in a broader context, models that are multi- rather than monosystemic. We have to learn how to work with entire families, with different generations of the same family, with couples, with mothers and daughters, with fathers and sons to address the context of risk-taking behavior (which is intergenerational). We have to find better ways to address the abuse and neglect that result in lack of self-esteem in both men and women and lead to risk-taking behavior. We have to become strong advocates for change in traditional gender socialization, which has promoted the idea that women's ultimate fulfillment results from attracting romantic love. We have to encourage women to develop the ability to identify and address their own needs rather than expecting their male lovers to set the tone and the terms for sexual exchanges—exchanges that often require women to sacrifice their sexual possibilities to fulfill those of their "sexually undeveloped" male partners.

Our goal should be to see that women no longer have to trade their own sexual and emotional needs for the gauzy hope that they will be "loved" and protected by a male partner, that the void they feel within themselves will be filled by the resection of his sexual desire. This Faustian exchange leads women to take risks that threaten their lives.

Notes

The research described in this chapter was funded by a number of sources, including the Stuyvesant Polyclinic, the New York City Department of Health, Montefiore Medical Center, the U.S. Centers for Disease Control, the HIV Center for Clinical and Behavioral Studies of the New York State Psychiatric Institute, the National Institute on Drug Abuse, the Human Resources Services Administration, and the Community Consultation Center of the Henry Street Settlement.

1. Unfortunately, the men who tended to respond to the women's needs had similar needs themselves, having also been abused and neglected as children. Their needs had already resulted in many of them becoming involved in drug use or were played out in the exploitation of women.
2. Western literature abounds in such situations—from Cinderella, whose true goodness and beauty come to light only through the prince's love, to Jane Eyre, whose passion is brought to life by Rochester's dark love. In romantic stories, women are not in control of either their own passion or their own destiny. They are also more likely to be subjected to humbling or dangerous situations from which they are saved by men.

References

Worth, D. 1989. Sexual decision-making and AIDS: Why condom promotion among vulnerable women is likely to fail. *Studies in Family Planning* 20(6):297–307.

———. 1993. Cross-site qualitative research report for NIDA. Unpublished.

Worth, D., E. Drucker, K. Eric, and A. Pivnick, 1990. Sexual and physical abuse as factors in continued risk behavior of women IV drug users in a South Bronx methadone clinic. Poster presented at the Sixth International Conference on AIDS, San Francisco, June 20–24.

Worth, D., and R. Rodriguez. 1987. Latina women and AIDS, *Siecus Report* (January–February):5–7.

PART TWO

Understanding and Acting on the Links among Sexuality, Contraception, and Reproductive Health

*Bringing Sexuality
into Family Planning
Services*

*T*he Sexuality
Connection in
Reproductive Health

Ruth Dixon-Mueller

*A*ttitudes and behaviors surrounding sexuality and gen-
der carry profound meanings for women and men in every
society and affect the quality of life in fundamental ways.
Knowledge of sexual attitudes and behaviors is important to family planning researchers, policymakers, and service providers,
because such attitudes and behaviors underlie virtually all the
conditions that their programs address. Yet little is known about
how family planning clients interpret their sexual lives or what
providers can do to help women gain more effective control over
their sexuality and reproduction.

This chapter identifies some of the linkages between sexuality
and reproductive health that are relevant to family planning professionals. Women's and men's sexual attitudes and behaviors
influence contraceptive adoption, choice, and use effectiveness,
for example, and the use of particular methods can affect the way
people experience their own and their partners' sexuality in positive or negative ways (see, for example, Bruce 1987). More generally, sexual relationships often incorporate power disparities
based on age, class, race, and patronage (for example, employer-
employee, teacher-student, landowner-laborer relationships) as

well as gender. They incorporate disparities in physical strength and in access to material and social resources. Girls and women often have little control over what happens to them sexually, that is, over men's sexual access to their bodies and the conditions under which sexual encounters take place. Yet the extent to which a woman is able to negotiate the "terms of trade" of a particular sexual act or relationship defines her capacity to protect herself against unwanted sexual acts, unwanted pregnancy, or a sexually transmitted disease (STD). More positively, it defines her ability to enjoy sex and to seek family planning advice and health care. From the most intimate to the most public level, then, interpersonal power relations affect sexual and reproductive health outcomes.

Sexuality and Gender in Family Planning Literature

A visitor from another planet would be mystified about sexual behavior if she/he/it were to depend on demographic and family planning journals for information. A review of articles, commentaries, and reports in five journals[1] over twelve years of publication reveals that sexuality and male-female power dynamics are discussed (or at least mentioned) in three contexts: (1) how "coital frequency" within marital or consensual unions—and/or how men's and women's attitudes about sexuality, reproduction, and gender roles—influences contraceptive use, method choice, and use effectiveness, and vice versa (forty-one articles); (2) how adolescent sexual activity and contraceptive use are related to the risks of out-of-wedlock pregnancy and childbearing, and how sex education might change these behaviors (twenty-four articles); and (3) how "high-risk" sexual behaviors are related to the spread of STDs, including AIDS (eleven articles).[2] Some articles report quantitative data from surveys, and others include commentary on sexual behavior and gender roles derived from in-depth interviews, focus-group sessions, or ethnographic research. What can family planning providers learn from these articles that would help them reduce the risks to girls and women of unwanted or unprotected sex and promote more mutually enjoyable and responsible sexuality? What assumptions do researchers make, and what information gaps remain?

Taken as a whole, this review tells us something about the scope and limitations of the treatment of the subjects of sexuality and gender-based power in selected demographic and family planning journals. They conclude, for example, that clients are influenced in their contraceptive choice and continuation by the frequency of their sexual activity (and vice versa) but offer little insight into how more qualitative aspects of sexual relationships are affected. They point out that adolescent gender roles can have a powerful impact on teenage sexuality and pregnancy rates but suggest little about how gender roles might be transformed. They examine patterns of sexual networking and STD transmission but typically do so within a narrow conceptual framework. The assumptions that are made and the way questions are framed tend to limit the capacity of reproductive health providers to design more effective policies and programs. An approach based on a broader understanding of the dimensions of sexual attitudes and behaviors in diverse settings, and of variations in gender power dynamics, would be more useful.

Sexuality in a Gender Framework

Sexuality has different meanings for different people in different contexts. Drawing on sociological and anthropological literature, I propose a simple framework here that identifies four dimensions of sexuality and sexual behavior that are socially organized along gender lines. Sexual behavior consists of actions that are empirically observable (in principle, at least): what people do sexually with others or with themselves, how they present themselves sexually, how they talk and act. In contrast, sexuality is a more comprehensive concept that encompasses the physical capacity for sexual arousal and pleasure (libido) as well as personalized and shared social meanings attached to both sexual behavior and the formation of sexual and gender identities. As a biological concept transposed by culture, sexuality becomes a social product, that is, a representation and interpretation of natural functions in hierarchical social relationships (Grupo Ceres 1981).

The framework presented here is an expanded version of a working definition drawn from a review of sexual behavior in sub-Saharan Africa (Standing and Kisekka 1989). The first two dimensions are primarily behavioral and objective; the last two are physiological or cultural and subjective. Each dimension of sexuality intersects with and is shaped by the experience of gender; thus, gender differences (and commonalities) in sexual behaviors, meanings, and drives can be analyzed systematically for particular social groups. All four aspects of sexuality are relevant to the design of reproductive health programs and policies.

Sexual Partnerships

The first element of the sexuality-gender framework addresses the number of sexual partners, current and past; the timing and duration of sexual partnerships throughout a person's lifetime; the identity of partners (socioeconomic characteristics, relationship); the conditions of choice under which each partner is selected or imposed; and the rate and conditions of change of partners. Numbers and identities of partners are commonly incorporated into models of sexual networking and disease transmission (Dyson 1992). Equally important from a policy perspective, however, are the factors that influence how partners are chosen and changed and the terms of the sexual relationship.

Patterns of partner selection can change dramatically over the course of a lifetime, from childhood and adolescence through adulthood to old age. Conditions surrounding sexual initiation appear to be particularly important in shaping subsequent attitudes and behavior, including long-term reproductive and health outcomes. Research in three Caribbean countries, for example, suggests that girls who have experienced physical or sexual abuse as children are more likely than others to have early first intercourse and more sexual partners as adolescents and young adults (Handwerker 1991; see also Boyer and Fine 1992 on adolescent pregnancy in the United States). The authors of the Caribbean study contend that family violence, sexual abuse, and the level of sexual activity are linked from one generation to another and have a common origin in structural features that regulate gender relations. For instance, sexual relations initiated in early arranged marriages can carry long-term implications. A study of health care clients in Ethiopia, for example, found that half of the women interviewed said that they had first had intercourse with their husbands before their first menstruation, and one-fifth were aged twelve or younger at the time (Duncan et al. 1990). In addition to the physical dangers of youthful childbearing, early onset of sexual activity was associated with a higher prevalence of STDs and cervical cancer and with a higher likelihood of divorce and subsequent partner change.[3] A simple question to clients about the timing and conditions of their first intercourse as well as about subsequent partner change could uncover important physical or emotional vulnerabilities.

Gender differences in the timing of initiation (or cessation) of sexual activity and in the identity, number, and choice of subsequent partners reveal a double standard in virtually every society. Reflecting both structural and ideological forces, power and resource imbalances are played out in ways that impinge deeply on girls' and women's ability to determine their own sexual and reproductive lives. Although reproductive health professionals have been concerned with women's ability to make contraceptive choices and to protect themselves from STDs, at the heart of these decisions lies a woman's ability to choose whether, when, and with whom to have sexual relations or to engage in a particular sexual act. The question of choice is complex. What seems on the surface to be purely voluntary sexual activity, for example, may be driven by deep economic need. In one study of a Nigerian Yoruba community, few wives who had extramarital affairs said that they did so for their personal enjoyment; instead, most traded sexual favors for some form of assistance withheld by their husbands. The husbands, in turn, commonly had relations with "friends" in town, most often divorced or separated women who themselves had children to support (Orubuloye, Caldwell, and Caldwell 1991).

Sexual Acts

The second element of the framework encompasses the nature, frequency, and conditions of choice of specific sexual practices in which individuals and couples engage. Focusing on reproduction, the conventional demographic literature makes the simplistic assumption that sex consists of voluntary heterosexual intercourse with vaginal penetration and ejaculation. Different styles of intercourse are rarely mentioned (for example, repeated encounters in quick succession), nor are oral or anal intercourse (heterosexual or homosexual), nonpenetrative forms of sexual expression (for instance, mutual or solitary masturbation), sex with animals, children's sex play, rape or "milder" forms of coerced sex, the use of pleasure-enhancing devices or techniques (some of which may be physically damaging, such as surgical alteration of the labia or the use of drying or tightening vaginal astringents), or other practices.

The frequency and forms of sexual expression in which people engage are important elements of sexual and reproductive health. Some sexual practices negate the need for contraception but not for disease prevention; others may require both. A study of first-year college students in Canada found that one-fifth of the female students had experienced anal intercourse, and one-fourth of the women with ten or more partners (among whom anal intercourse was more common) reported having had an STD (MacDonald et al. 1990). Whether the scarcity of inquiries about such practices derives more from the researchers' and service providers' embarrassment at asking such questions or from the presumed reluctance of respondents and clients to answer them is difficult to say.[4] Unless questions about specific noncoital sexual practices are asked, however, important health consequences and counseling possibilities are likely to be missed.

Homosexual (and bisexual) practices are often invisible to researchers and providers when clients are assumed to be purely heterosexual. Although the literature on North American and European societies recognizes female and male homosexuality as a specific lifestyle, most commentaries on Asian, African, and Latin American societies tend to assume it away, despite the prevalence of male prostitution in some areas. Yet transitory adolescent homosexual experimentation is probably common, especially among boys, in virtually all cultures. Moreover, as Standing and Kisekka (1989, 52–53) point out, opportunistic homosexual encounters between men where access to females is restricted—as well as longer-term relationships between older men (who are often married) and younger men or boys—are typical of many societies that deny the existence of a homosexual "class." In rural Bangladesh, for instance, researchers found that older boys often lure young boys into having anal sex with them if they "don't have access to a vagina" (Aziz, Ashraful, and Maloney 1985, 108). Family planning providers clearly need to consider the possibility that boys and men—married or unmarried—may be having penetrative sex with other men or boys as well as with girls or women, thus raising their own as well as their partners' exposure to STDs. Questions relating to same-sex partnerships should be routine elements of research on sexual networking in seemingly heterosexual populations.

Practitioners also need to be sensitized to the possibility that their adult female clients as well as adolescents and children of both sexes may be subjected to violent sexual acts such as forced oral, vaginal, or anal intercourse and physical abuse. Victims are unlikely to mention such practices, even in the face of obvious physical evidence of harm, if they are frightened or ashamed. Sometimes children are the victims: 22 percent of female clients of one STD clinic in Ibadan, Nigeria, were under ten years of age (Sogbetun, Alausa, and Osoba 1977). Spousal and child abuse appear to be endemic in many societies and across social classes (Levinson 1989). As noted earlier, physical threats or actual violence form a theme in women's complaints about their partners, even in the more conventional family planning literature. Ironically, spousal abuse is sometimes rationalized as an expression of love or concern. A researcher in one Indian village reported that wife beating was a widely prevalent custom that was justified as a way of showing regard. "It is not surprising if sometimes a man gets carried away and really hurts his wife," he wrote, expressing the village men's point of view, "but the intention is noble—to demonstrate love" (Kapur 1987, 21). This interpretation of violence relates to a third element of sexuality: the ascription of personal and cultural meaning.

Sexual Meanings

The social construction of sexuality refers to the process by which sexual thoughts, behaviors, and conditions (for instance, virginity) are interpreted and ascribed cultural meaning (Ortner and Whitehead 1981; Vance 1991). This third element incorporates collective and individual beliefs about the nature of the body, about what is considered erotic or offensive, and about what and with whom it is appropriate or inappropriate for men and women (according to their age and other characteristics) to do or to talk about sexually. In some cultures, ideologies of sexuality stress female resistance, male aggression, and mutual antagonism in the sex act; in others, they stress reciprocity and mutual pleasure (Standing and Kisekka 1989).

The social construction of sexuality is inevitably linked with cultural concepts of masculinity and femininity. They are inter-locking domains (Vance 1984). Ideas about what constitutes the essence of "maleness" and "femaleness" are expressed in sexual norms and ideologies. Cross-cultural studies reveal that, as is the case for females, the imagery of manhood in most societies is "a culturally imposed ideal to which men must conform [often at great cost to themselves and to others] whether or not they find it psychologically congenial" (Gilmore 1990, 1; see also Hearn and Morgan 1990). Being a "real man" is typically associated with viril-ity and potency as well as with bravery, honor, and responsibility. Men are vulnerable to attacks on their manhood by elders, male peers, and women who share and enforce the cultural ideals.

The contradictions of male power and sexuality are expressed in men's efforts to dominate women, which derive from male physical, material, and ideological advantage, and in their anxi-eties about failure and loss of face. Men who are sexually predatory themselves realize that their own wives and daughters are targets for other such men (see Folch-Lyon, Macorra, and Schearer 1981 on Mexico). This realization intensifies their anxiety about their own power and maleness, as well as their resentment toward women, whom they accuse of infidelity. Sexual potency is equated with men's authority over women; thus, attacks on potency threaten male power, and vice versa.

Shifts in the meaning and expression of sexuality occur throughout the life cycle for both women and men, especially in response to the changing likelihood of conception. In some culturally conservative South Asian societies, intercourse is con-sidered appropriate only through the period of married adult-hood when children are being conceived and reared. Premarital and extramarital sex as well as marital sex beyond middle age are thought to be improper (Vatuk 1985). Among the !Kung of Botswana, in contrast, child sex play is tolerated or even encouraged; adolescence is a time for experimenting with several partners; early adulthood is a time of marital pairing and sexual jealousy; and menopause marks a transition to more open and relaxed female sexuality, which may include taking younger male lovers (Lee 1985). Age- and status-graded social constructions of male and female sexuality carry important implications for service delivery and research. Clients of a certain age or status may be reluctant to admit certain sexual activities to a provider, for example; providers, acting on their own assumptions, may not even think to ask about them.

Sexual Drives and Enjoyment

Physiological and sociopsychological aspects of sexuality interact to produce varying levels of arousability and orgasmic capacity that differ generally and situationally among individuals and that change over the course of a lifetime. This element includes women's and men's knowledge of the body's sexual and reproductive capacities and the ability to obtain physical and emotional pleasure from fantasy, sexual encounters, or self-stimulation. What is the nature of the individual's sexual identity and response? Do women and men differ in their assessment of the sexual relationship as a whole—or of particular sexual practices—as pleasurable or not? In what ways are sexual relations a source of anxiety?

Individuals' perceptions of their own and others' sex drives and enjoyment are inevitably mediated by the social construction of male and female sexuality as defined above. In some studies, men insist that women are less interested in sex than men are (see Folch-Lyon, Macorra, and Schearer 1981 on Mexico). A Japanese study, noting that "female sexual repression is a strong theme throughout present-day Japanese culture," found that "with only one exception . . . wives expressed indifference or explicitly negative attitudes toward sexuality regardless of their educational level" (Coleman 1981, 35). In other settings, women are thought to have powerful sex drives that require strict controls over their physical mobility (see Sabbah 1984 on Islamic societies) or frequent sexual appeasement (see examples in Standing and Kisekka 1989 for sub-Saharan Africa). Frequent sexual intercourse for men may be thought to cause weakness and to require restorative efforts (see Brody 1981 on Jamaica; Aziz, Ashraful, and Maloney 1985 on Bangladesh), even though the same men consider intercourse important for maintaining overall health. Cultural beliefs about particular sex acts also influence subjective pleasure, especially if an act is considered deviant or dangerous. Low-income men in Jamaica interviewed by Brody (1981) believed that cunnilingus was "unmasculine" and exposed them to dangerous substances. The polluting power of menstrual blood is often mentioned in the literature.

Little is known about how much pleasure women and men obtain from their sexual relations or how much they know about sex. Men's pleasure is often assumed, yet pathbreaking work in the United States by Rainwater in 1960 and 1965 and more recent research show that this is not the case. In India, Kapur's (1987) conversations in a Himalayan Kumaoni community revealed that "very few men or women even claimed a satisfactory sex life within marriage" (53). Some men said that they felt "trapped" or "suffocated" when they were inside a woman and that quick ejaculation was the "best fun." Women, in turn, complained that men were in too much of a hurry to satisfy them sexually. "Young men are seldom any better than older men," one woman remarked of her husband, his brother, and several young men that she knew. "They are all so keen to discharge and be on their way that one is left looking at the hills with a surprised feeling" (65).

Each of the four elements of sexuality—the number, timing, choice, and social identity of sexual partners; the mode, choice, and frequency of specific practices; the cultural and subjective meanings attached to sexuality and gender; and the individual's level of sex drive and enjoyment—is related to contraceptive behavior, to the risk of STDs, and to other aspects of sexual and reproductive health (see figure). Each of the elements is also related to the others, both within and across dimensions. A married man is likely to engage in different sex acts (and think differently about pleasure, pregnancy, and disease) when he is with a commercial sex worker, for example, than when he is with his wife. Finally, each element is shaped by characteristics of the larger social system in which it is embedded: by social and economic institutions that determine power hierarchies and life choices based on gender, age, class, ethnicity, and other distinctions; and by ideologies of gender (and other differences) that

Linkages between the Sexuality-Gender Framework and Reproductive Health

Sexual health

Protection from STDs
Protection from harmful prac-
tices and violence
Control over sexual access
Sexual enjoyment
Information on sexuality

Reproductive health

Safe, effective protection from
(and termination of) unwanted
pregnancies
Protection from harmful reproductive practices
Contraceptive choice and satisfaction with method
Contraceptive and reproductive
information
Safe pregnancy and delivery
Treatment of infertility

**Social organization
of gender differences**

Sexual partnerships

Number of partners
Partnership timing, duration
Social identity of partners
Conditions of choice/coercion
Conditions and rate of change

Sexual acts

Nature of sexual acts
Frequency of sexual acts
Conditions of choice/coercion

Sexual meanings

Masculine/feminine sexuality
Perceptions of partnerships
Meaning of sex acts

Sexual drives and enjoyment

Formation of sexual identities
Socially conditioned sex drives
Perceptions of pleasure

each system elaborates. The connections between sexual behavior and these structural and ideological forces also must be better understood for the design of responsive programs.

Applications of the Sexuality-Gender Framework

Understanding the linkages among particular aspects of sexuality, gender, and reproductive health can be useful to family planning providers, policymakers, and researchers in a variety of ways.

What Can Programs Do?

When a woman complains that her husband "uses her" sexually, or when she says that she cannot risk her partner's anger by using contraceptives without his permission, what do such statements mean to the family planning provider? What could providers learn about the sexual behaviors and belief systems of the clients and communities they serve? What could clients learn about their own and their partners' sexual capacities and rights in order to make informed decisions?

Family planning practitioners deal on a day-to-day basis with fundamental questions of sexual and reproductive choice. Yet—with some important exceptions—contemporary practitioners, like their counterparts in demographic research, appear to have adopted a sanitized version of sexuality that treats intercourse as an emotionally neutral act. Sexual behavior is relevant insofar as it may create a demand for contraception or abortion, that is, for conventional birth control services. Its variations and subjective meaning to adolescent and adult women and men in different circumstances are rarely explored, however, despite the obvious impact of people's sexual experiences on their perceptions of their physical and emotional well-being.[5] Moreover, nonreproductive, noncoital, nonconsensual, and commercial sexual relations among persons of all ages (including young adolescents) do not fall under the rubric of conventional family planning programs. Indeed, many programs are still grappling with the issue of whether their moral legitimacy and clarity of purpose are compromised by treating STDs (Germain et al. 1992). Few programs offer special clinic hours or counseling for boys and men. Yet male clients have concerns of their own, such as fear of sexual inadequacy, ignorance about sexual and reproductive functioning, risk of STDs, risk of unwanted pregnancies with their partners, or misunderstandings about how male- and female-controlled contraceptive methods work.

Family planning providers can learn about their clients' sexual and reproductive concerns through intake questionnaires, physical examinations, contraceptive counseling, and clinic-based group discussions, among other avenues (Bruce 1990; Joffe 1986). For example, intake questionnaires used to collect basic demographic and health information from clients could include questions about sexual history as a guide to advising clients about contraception and as an aid in identifying other health problems. Providers need to know about the range of clients' sexual partnerships (both same- and opposite-sex partners) and practices if they are to offer appropriate advice about protection from disease, harmful practices and pregnancy. Clients could be asked whether their partners are fully cooperative in matters of contraception and disease prevention and the issues of whether, when, and how to have sexual relations. They should be asked routinely about genital discharge or sores and whether they experience pain or discomfort during intercourse or other sexual acts. Persons conducting physical examinations should look for signs of physical and sexual abuse, reproductive tract infections, and damage resulting from genital mutilation, vaginal medication, and other practices (Dixon-Mueller and Wasserheit 1991; Heise 1992). Clients exhibiting signs of harm or disease should be asked to bring in their children (both male and female) and partners for consultation, because patterns of violence and disease tend to be replicated across and within genders and generations.

Ideally, individual counseling and group discussions in clinic settings would offer a safe haven for male and female clients in segregated groups or as couples to discuss their sexual concerns. Clients and providers could identify misinformation, provide support, and articulate needs that programs could address. Discussion topics with obvious sexual components include common reproductive tract infections; transmission of STDs, including

AIDS; problems of infertility; contraceptive preferences, menstrual beliefs, and taboos; fecundity cycles in females; misconceptions about menarche and menopause; causes of unwanted pregnancy and abortion; and male responsibility for birth control and child rearing.

Just as clients' sexual attitudes and behavior affect their reproductive health, so too providers' sexual knowledge and values influence the quality of their service delivery. Providers may withhold contraception or abortion services from sexually active unmarried women, for example (indeed, many programs have formal policies of this type), or fail to deal realistically with STD prevention if a client is homosexual. Providers may have little knowledge of sexual functioning and may feel uncomfortable when clients ask for information and advice. Providers' sexual attitudes should be identified and challenged so that mutual learning takes place. Training modules could be developed for both providers and clients with basic information about sexual functioning (physiology, male and female sexual response, capacity for orgasm); about life-cycle changes in sexuality, fertility, and menstrual patterns; and about the rights of girls and women— and of vulnerable boys and men—to have control over their own bodies and to be free of sexual coercion and violence, among other topics. Based in part on locally defined concerns, these modules would be responsive to the contexts of women's and men's lives in specific situations.

Community outreach programs can address many issues of sexuality and gender-based power in the context of family planning and disease prevention. Some techniques lend themselves to entertaining as well as informative treatments: community "teach-ins" that include mock public tribunals to identify and debate folk beliefs about sex and reproduction;[6] videos tailored to particular audiences (for instance, teenage boys, men and women with many sexual partners); performances of sexual or family planning dramas involving gender role switching; rap music contests; comic books and novellas; radio talk shows; newspaper and popular magazine columns and quizzes; peer counseling centers purveying a sense of humor as well as accurate information and a point of view. The medium would inform and entertain; the message would confront misperceptions and identify and transform sexual double standards that assume male entitlement to women's bodies. Girls, women, and vulnerable boys and men need to learn how to negotiate their sexual and reproductive rights, that is, to protect themselves from STDs and unwanted partners or sexual acts, and to assert their right to sexual enjoyment within mutually caring and responsible relationships. If community members can understand how they construct and reinforce concepts of sexuality and gender, they can become active agents in the deconstruction and transformation of these same social scripts.

Notes

This chapter is excerpted from *Studies in Family Planning* 24, no. 5 (1993):269–82.

Research for this paper was supported by the International Women's Health Coalition (IWHC), New York. Members of the Working Group on Sexuality and Gender, cosponsored by IWHC and the Population Council, offered valuable insights into the issues considered here as well as useful comments on earlier drafts of the paper. A special note of appreciation goes to working group members Judith Bruce, Amparo Claro, Joan Dunlop, Chris Elias, Andrea Eschen, John Gagnon, Adrienne Germain, Sia Nowrojee, Jacqueline Pitanguy, Deborah Rogow, Nahid Toubia, and Beverly Winikoff, and to Tracy Brunette of the Department of Demography, University of California, Berkeley, for her assistance with the literature review.

1. The five journals are *Studies in Family Planning, Family Planning Perspectives, International Family Planning Perspectives, Demography,* and *Population and Development Review.* These journals were selected as examples of mainstream English-language publications with wide readership. Journals dealing with some aspects of reproductive behavior, such as *Social Biology* and *The Milbank Memorial Fund Quarterly,* were not reviewed, nor were more specialized journals on contraception or sexual behavior. Of approximately 2,100 articles included in the journals, seventy-six incorporated some mention of sexual behavior or gender relations as they relate to reproductive health.

2. Twenty-four of these articles appeared from 1980 to 1985, and fifty-two from 1986 to 1991, with *Studies in Family Planning* and *Family Planning Perspectives* accounting for fifty-one of the seventy-six. Twenty-four were based on data from the United States or Canada, twenty-two on sub-Saharan Africa (almost all since 1986), twelve on Latin America or the Caribbean, nine on Asia, two on Europe, and none on North

Africa or the Middle East; seven were cross-national comparisons. Articles summarized in the "Update" or "Commentary" sections of *Family Planning Perspectives* were included, even if they were originally published elsewhere. Excluded from this review were contributions to *Population and Development Review* that examined institutionalized family and community controls over marriage and reproductive behavior more generally in selected Asian, sub-Saharan African, and Latin American contexts.

3. Emotional aspects of early sexual initiation are equally important. Researchers in Bangladesh found that although most villagers believed that girls should be married at an early age (the preparatory seclusion of girls begins at about eight to ten years), some suggested that younger girls are too immature and may be frightened by the sexual act. "When a girl is given in marriage at a tender age, she is likely to become afraid of her husband and scream when he wants to have coitus with her," one villager said (Aziz, Ashraful, and Maloney 1985, 56).

4. According to historians, Roman Catholic missionaries conducting confessionals among indigenous peoples in Mexico in the sixteenth century were instructed to ask questions about adultery, anal intercourse, avoiding procreation, intercourse during menstruation, sex with animals, homosexual sodomy, masturbation, sex between women, incest, and other "sins" (Marcos 1991). The confessional instructions are uniquely suited to demographers because each query about whether the supposed sinner has committed a particular act is followed by another: how many times?

5. Early family planning clinics in the United States under the guidance of Margaret Sanger and her colleagues were far more likely than clinics today to define sex education as part of their mission, in part because so many women were pleading for help in overcoming their sexual ignorance and unhappiness (Chesler 1992).

6. In a community outreach campaign in Costa Rica, for example, a team of health workers used a combination of questionnaires, role playing, mock tribunals, and community counseling to find out what adolescents and adults believed about sex and birth control and to correct misinformation. "Finding the myths and taboos about sexuality and unraveling them is the task of health workers," reported one team leader, adding that health workers themselves "need to be clear about their own sexuality in order to adequately respond to the needs of adolescents" ("Health Team" 1993, 22).

References

Aziz, K., M. Ashraful, and Clarence Maloney. 1985. *Life stages, gender and fertility in Bangladesh.* Dhaka: International Centre for Diarrhoeal Disease Research.

Berelson, Bernard. 1969. Beyond family planning. *Studies in Family Planning* 1(38):1–16.

Blanc, Ann K., and Naomi Rutenberg. 1991. Coitus and contraception: The utility of data on sexual intercourse for family planning programs. *Studies in Family Planning* 22(3):162–76.

Bledsoe, Caroline. 1991. The politics of AIDS and condoms for stable heterosexual relations in Africa: Recent evidence from the local print media. *Disasters* 15(1):1–11.

Boyer, Debra, and David Fine. 1992. Sexual abuse as a factor in adolescent pregnancy and child maltreatment. *Family Planning Perspectives* 24(1): 4–11.

Brody, Eugene B. 1981. *Sex, contraception, and motherhood in Jamaica.* Cambridge: Harvard University Press.

Brown, Prudence. 1983. The Swedish approach to sex education and adolescent pregnancy. *Family Planning Perspectives* 15(2):90–95.

Bruce, Judith. 1987. User's perspectives on contraceptive technology and delivery systems: Highlighting some feminist issues. *Technology in Society* 9:359–83.

———. 1990. Fundamental elements of the quality of care: A simple framework. *Studies in Family Planning* 21(2):61–91.

Caldwell, John, Pat Caldwell, and Pat Quiggin. 1989. The social context of AIDS in sub-Saharan Africa. *Population and Development Review* 15(2): 185–234.

Caldwell, John, K. H. W. Gaminiratne, P. Caldwell, S. de Silva, B. Caldwell, N. Weeraratne, and P. Silva. 1987. The role of traditional fertility regulation in Sri Lanka. *Studies in Family Planning* 18(1):1–21.

Caldwell, John C., I. O. Orubuloye, and Pat Caldwell. 1991. The destabilization of the traditional Yoruba sexual system. *Population and Development Review* 17(2):229–62.

Chesler, Ellen. 1992. *Woman of Valor: Margaret Sanger and the Birth Control Movement in America.* New York: Simon and Schuster.

Coleman, Samuel. 1981. The cultural context of condom use in Japan. *Studies in Family Planning* 12(1):28–40.

Darney, Phil D., et al. 1990. Cited in Hormonal implants prove to be highly acceptable although nearly all users experience side effects. *Family Planning Perspectives* 22(5): 234–35.

Dixon-Mueller, Ruth. 1993. *Population policy and women's rights: Trans- form- ing reproductive choice.* New York: Praeger.

Dixon-Mueller, Ruth, and Judith Wasserheit. 1991. *The culture of silence: Reproductive tract infections among women in the third world.* New York: International Women's Health Coalition.

Duncan, M. Elizabeth, G. Tibaux, A. Pelzer, K. Reimann, J. F. Pentherer, P. Simmonds, H. Young, Y. Jamie, and S. Daroughar. 1990. First coitus before menarche and risk of sexually transmitted diseases. *Lancet* 335: 338–40.

Dyson, Tim, ed. 1992. *Sexual behaviour and networking: Anthropological and socio-cultural studies on the transmission of HIV.* Liège: Ordina Editions.

Feyistan, Bamikale, and Anne R. Pebley. 1989. Premarital sexuality in urban Nigeria. *Studies in Family Planning* 20(6):343–55.

Folch-Lyon, Evelyn, Luis de la Macorra, and S. Bruce Schearer. 1981. Focus group and survey research on family planning in Mexico. *Studies in Family Planning* 12(12):409–32.

Forrest, Jacqueline Darroch, and Jane Silverman. 1989. What public school teachers teach about preventing pregnancy, AIDS, and sexually transmitted diseases. *Family Planning Perspectives* 21(2):65–72.

Germain, Adrienne, King K. Holmes, Peter Piot, and Judith N. Wasserheit, eds. 1992. *Reproductive tract infections: Global impact and priorities for women's reproductive health.* New York: Plenum Press.

Germain, Adrienne, and Jane Ordway. 1989. *Population control and women's health: Balancing the scales.* New York: International Women's Health Coalition.

Gilmore, David D. 1990. *Manhood in the making: Cultural concepts of mas- culinity.* New Haven, Conn.: Yale University Press.

Gregersen, E., and B. Gregersen. 1990. Cited in Users approve of female condom. *Family Planning Perspectives* 23(1):5.

Grupo Ceres. 1981. *Espellode Vênus: Identidade social e sexual da Mulher.* São Paulo: Editora Brasiliense.

Handwerker, W. Penn. 1991. Power, sex, and violence: The political econ- omy of sexual behavior. Unpublished paper, Department of Sociology, Humboldt State University, Arcata, Calif.

Hardy, Ellen E., Quintina Reyes, Fernando Gomez, Ramón Portes-Carrasco, and Aníbal Faúndes. 1983. User's perceptions of the contraceptive vaginal ring: A field study in Brazil and the Dominican Republic. *Studies in Family Planning* 14(11):284–90.

Health team tries to explore reproduction myths. *Tico Times,* March 26, 1993, 22.

Hearn, Jeff, and David Morgan, eds. 1990. *Men, masculinities and social the- ory.* London: Unwin Hyman.

Heise, Lori. 1992. Violence against women: The missing agenda. In

Women's health: A global perspective, edited by M. A. Koblinsky, Judith Timyan, and Jill Gay. Boulder, Colo.: Westview Press.

Herold, Joan M., E. Monterroso, L. Morris, G. Gastellanos, A. Conde, and A. Spitz. 1988. Sexual experience and contraceptive use among young adults in Guatemala City. *International Family Planning Perspectives* 14(4):142–46.

Howard, Marion and Judith Blamey McCabe. 1990. Helping teenagers postpone sexual involvement. *Family Planning Perspectives* 22(1):21–26.

Joffe, Carole. 1986. *The regulation of sexuality: Experiences of family planning workers.* Philadelphia: Temple University Press.

Kakar, Sudhir. 1989. *Exploring Indian sexuality.* Chicago: University of Chicago Press.

Kapur, Tribhuwan. 1987. *Sexual life of the Kumaonis.* New Delhi: Vikas.

Lee, Richard B. 1985. Work, sexuality, and aging among !Kung women. In *In her prime: A new view of middle-aged women,* edited by Judith K. Brown and Virginia Kerns. South Hadley, Mass.: Bergin and Garvey.

Levinson, David. 1989. *Violence in cross-cultural perspective.* Newbury Park, Calif.: Sage Publications.

MacDonald, N. E., et al. 1990. Cited in Knowledge of HIV risks does not always prompt safer sexual behavior. *Family Planning Perspectives* 22(6): 277–78.

Marcos, Sylvia. 1991. Clergy, goddesses, and eroticism: Excerpts of an essay on Catholicism's confrontation with Meso-America. *Conscience: A Newsjournal of Prochoice Catholic Opinion* 12(5):11–15.

Moore, Kristin Anderson, Christine Winquist Nord, and James L. Peterson. 1989. Nonvoluntary sexual activity among adolescents. *Family Planning Perspectives* 21(3):110–14.

Nichols, Douglas, Oladipo A. Ladipo, John M. Paxman, and E. O. Otolorin. 1986. Sexual behavior, contraceptive practice, and reproductive health among Nigerian adolescents. *Studies in Family Planning* 17(2):100–07.

Nichols, Douglas, Emile T. Woods, Deborah S. Gates, and Joyce Sherman. 1987. Sexual behavior, contraceptive practice, and reproductive health among Liberian adolescents. *Studies in Family Planning* 18(3):169–76.

Ortner, Sherry B., and Harriet Whitehead, eds. 1981. *Sexual meanings: The cultural construction of gender and sexuality.* Cambridge: Cambridge University Press.

Orubuloye, I. O., John C. Caldwell, and Pat Caldwell. 1991. Sexual networking in the Ekiti District of Nigeria. *Studies in Family Planning* 22(2):61–73.

Pick de Weiss, Susan, Lucille C. Atkin, James N. Gribble, and Patricia Andrade-Palos. 1991. Sex, contraception, and pregnancy among adolescents in Mexico City. *Studies in Family Planning* 22(2):74–82.

Rainwater, Lee. 1960. *And the poor get children: Sex, contraception and family planning in the working class.* Chicago: Quadrangle Books.

———. 1965. *Family design: Marital sexuality, family size and contraception.* Chicago: Aldine.

Rehan, Naghma, and Audu K. Abashiya. 1981. Breastfeeding and abstinence among Hausa women. *Studies in Family Planning* 12(5): 233–37.

Roemer, Ruth, and John M. Paxman. 1985. Sex education laws and policies. *Studies in Family Planning* 16(4):219–30.

Sabbah, Fatna A. 1984. *Woman in the Muslim unconscious.* New York: Pergamon Press.

Santiso G., Roberto, Jane T. Bertrand, and Maria Antonieta Pineda. 1983. Voluntary sterilization in Guatemala: A comparison of men and women. *Studies in Family Planning* 14(3):67–73.

Sogbetun, A. O., K. O. Alausa, and A. O. Osoba. 1977. Sexually transmitted diseases in Ibadan, Nigeria. *British Journal of Venereal Disease* 53:158.

Soskolne, Y., S. Aral, L. S. Magder, D. S. Reed, and G. S. Bowen. 1991. Condom use with regular and casual partners among women attending family planning clinics. *Family Planning Perspectives* 23(5):222–25.

Standing, Hilary, and Mere N. Kisekka. 1989. *Sexual behaviour in sub-Saharan Africa: A review and annotated bibliography.* London: Overseas Development Administration.

Townsend, John W., E. Diaz de May, T. Sepúlveda, Y. Santos de Garza L., and S. Rosenhouse. 1987. Sex education and family planning services for young adults: Alternative urban strategies in Mexico. *Studies in Family Planning* 18(2):103–8.

Tsui, Amy O., S. Victor de Silva, and Ruth Marinshaw. 1991. Pregnancy avoidance and coital behavior. *Demography* 28(1):101–17.

Tucker, Gisele Maynard. 1986. Barriers to modern contraceptive use in rural Peru. *Studies in Family Planning* 17(6):308–16.

Udry, J. Richard, Luther M. Talbert, and Naomi M. Morris. 1986. Biosocial foundations for adolescent female sexuality. *Demography* 23(2):217–30.

Vance, Carole S., ed. 1984. *Pleasure and danger: Exploring female sexuality.* Boston: Routledge and Kegan Paul.

———. 1991. Anthropology rediscovers sexuality: A theoretical comment. *Social Science and Medicine* 33(8):875–84.

Van de Walle, Francine, 1991. Family planning in Bamako, Mali. *International Family Planning Perspectives* 17(3):84–90.

Van de Walle, Francine, and Narssour Ouaidou. 1985. Status and fertility among urban women in Burkina Faso. *International Family Planning Perspectives* 11(2):60–64.

Vatuk, Sylvia. 1985. South Asian cultural conceptions of sexuality. In *In her prime: A new view of middle-aged women,* edited by Judith K. Brown and

Virginia Kerns. South Hadley, Mass.: Bergin and Garvey.

Verzosa, Cecilia C., Nora Llamas, and Richard T. Mahoney. 1984. Attitudes toward the rhythm method in the Philippines. *Studies in Family Planning* 15(2):74–79.

Warren, Charles W., D. Powell, L. Morris, J. Jackson, and P. Hamilton. 1988. Fertility and family planning among young adults in Jamaica. *International Family Planning Perspectives* 14(4):137–41.

Weisman, Carol S., Stacey Plichta, Constance Nathanson, Margaret Ensminger, and J. Courtland Robinson. 1991. Consistency of condom use for disease prevention among adolescent users of oral contraceptives. *Family Planning Perspectives* 23(2):71–74.

Winter, Laraine. 1988. The role of sexual self-concept in the use of contraceptives. *Family Planning Perspectives* 20(3):123–28.

World Health Organization Task Force on Psychosocial Research in Family Planning. 1982. Hormonal contraception for men: Acceptability and effects on sexuality. *Studies in Family Planning* 13(11):328–42.

Worth, Dooley. 1989. Sexual decision-making and AIDS: Why condom promotion among vulnerable women is likely to fail. *Studies in Family Planning* 20(6):297–307.

Zabin, Laurie, Marilyn Hirsch, Edward Smith, and Janet Hardy. 1984. Adolescent sexual attitudes and behavior: Are they consistent? *Family Planning Perspectives* 16(4):181–85.

Zelnick, Melvin, and Farida K. Shah. 1983. First intercourse among young Americans. *Family Planning Perspectives* 15(2):64–70.

*L*earning about Sexuality

through Family Planning Counseling Sessions in Indonesia

Ninuk Widyantoro

*I*n Indonesia, as in all countries, there are many firmly held beliefs about sexuality and women's sexual roles. Many people (decision makers, teachers, doctors, religious leaders) have told me that it is not necessary to teach about sex, because it's a natural thing. Like a child who will be able to talk and walk, so it is with sex. Everybody will master it, when the time comes. In the national family planning program, discussion or education about sexual matters has been absent, although recently the program has begun to include information about very basic reproductive physiology, such as the process of fertilization, in its informational materials.

It is also commonly accepted that most women do not have the same sexual needs and desires as men and are not willing to discuss their intimate experiences. Based on my day-to-day experience as a family planning counselor, these assumptions are not correct. Women come to family planning clinics to get either counseling or advice about contraceptives or to obtain medical services, but in the counseling room, most discussions about contraceptives lead to discussions about sexuality.

This has been my experience not only in my urban work but

also in my work with village women. There seems to be an assumption among service providers and decision makers that poor or rural women are uneducated and incapable of logic, that they do not dare ask questions or forward their opinions and thus cannot make wise decisions. Almost all my experiences tend to show that these assumptions seriously underestimate women's capabilities. It is true that many women in Indonesia lack high levels of formal education, but that's only because they can't afford it. Talking about and sharing experiences of their own sexuality and learning from one another do not require formal education.

The experiences gathered below—which were shared during individual counseling, group sessions, formal and informal gatherings, and lectures—suggest that women do want to know about sex. They do care about it and enjoy it, and they also become worried, stressed, or depressed when they encounter sex-related problems. What follows are descriptions of such complaints or problems and the steps I took to answer them.

Contraception and Sex

A client complains that after using the injectable contraceptive for more than two years, she is not as eager to have intercourse with her husband. Her husband complains too, and she feels sorry for him. She wonders why lovemaking is not as enjoyable for her as it was before, since she still loves her husband as much as before. Suddenly she thinks that maybe the injectable, because it is a hormonal method, may be the cause. She asks me whether the hormone could affect her gairah seks *(libido). If so, she would certainly like to change methods.*

A woman in a group session in Lombok asks: "Will vasectomy decrease male libido? If yes, I won't let my husband do it!"

A client complains that she has gained so much weight while on the pill that she feels she can no longer arouse her husband with such a "fat body."

In Indonesia, one rarely hears, especially from health care providers, about effects on libido linked to contraceptive use.

Perhaps this is more a reflection of whether anyone has an opportunity to ask this question than of the real situation. Women who use contraceptives not only complain about medical or physical side effects but are also concerned about the effect of contraceptive use on their sexual lives—their psychological needs.

For the first woman, I advised that she could try another method temporarily at the end of the current cycle of injectables, to see whether it made a difference in her libido. She wanted a simple method for this purpose and decided that condoms would be best. As follow-up, her husband was taught the proper use of condoms.

In the case of vasectomy, we know that there are frequent misunderstandings about the nature of the operation and its side effects. With the help of pictures and diagrams, the process of vasectomy was explained to the second woman and her husband. It was very important for the couple to understand not only the exact location and size of the incision and the operation itself but also the process of male erection from both physiological and psychological perspectives.

Clients also link perceived side effects of contraception, such as weight gain, to their sexual lives. Women's responses to this kind of side effect differ. For example, one woman who used to be very thin responded positively to the fact that she gained five kilograms (eleven pounds) while using oral contraceptives; her body became fuller, she felt more attractive, and her self-esteem and confidence rose. This led to a better sexual relationship between her and her husband. Another woman, such as the third woman cited above, may feel ugly as a result of weight gain, particularly if her husband makes criticisms. In this case, we can encourage her to choose another contraceptive. It is important for us to explore the root of her complaint, to decide whether it is caused by psychological or physiological factors (although the two are closely intertwined).

A woman using the IUD complains that it hurts her husband's penis during intercourse.

The fact that women have very little knowledge about their own bodies can influence their perceptions of and experiences with contraception. Family planning personnel often refer to side effects as "not serious," meaning that they are not a serious health threat. However, this approach fails to take into account a wide range of side effects that can have serious social and other impacts. There are frequent requests for IUD removal based on perceived problems in the sexual relationship. It is not surprising that even urban women with higher educations don't have a clear picture of where the device is put in their bodies. Apparently it is rare for family planning providers to explain this. Some imagine that during intercourse the penis enters the womb, touching the IUD.

The placement of the IUD and the position of the sex organs during intercourse were explained to this woman using a picture from a "pop-up" book. Together we discussed any possible reasons for her husband's perceived pain, including the possibility that the IUD's string needed to be shortened. She was advised to consult the health center to have this checked.[1]

Wider Reproductive Health and Sexual Health Needs

In some discussions, clients expressed concern about common reproductive health problems, such as vaginal discharge, which they linked to decreasing sexual pleasure.

A woman is concerned because her husband complains that during intercourse her vagina is too "wet," which limits his sensation and pleasure. She has used a traditional method of drying the vagina: a plant root that has an astringent quality and is inserted into the vagina before intercourse. However, after two weeks of use, she experienced pain and burning and, on consulting a doctor, was advised to discontinue the practice. She hopes that there is another way of achieving the same result without the side effects.

In this case, we led a discussion on the function of lubrication in sex and the dangers of overusing materials that can injure the sensitive tissue. We need to find out more about this practice and the possible health effects, as there is accumulating evidence from other countries that "dry sex" practices can lead to vaginal injury and increased risk of sexually transmitted diseases, including HIV and AIDS.

A woman in Lombok asks: "Can we have intercourse during menstruation? I feel an increasing desire during that period."

This question is one that is surprisingly difficult to answer in unqualified terms. Some medical specialist colleagues advise that there is a higher risk of infection during menstruation, an issue that may be receiving greater prominence in the context of HIV and AIDS. Other doctors advise that intercourse during menstruation does not result in problems, particularly after the first day or two of strong menstrual flow. In Indonesia, religious issues are also pertinent; however, the proscription against sex during menstruation is not as strict as some others, allowing people some latitude in their decision. All these considerations need to be discussed frankly when this issue arises. Usually it leads to the advice that couples should discuss the issue and make the decision together.

Questions of sexual dysfunction, such as premature ejaculation and serious problems of sexually transmitted disease, also arise during family planning counseling sessions.

Another woman from Lombok expresses her worries: "My husband has been experiencing premature ejaculation lately. It's driving me mad and making me frustrated. I'm easily upset and on edge. Do you know how this can be cured?"

Questions about sexual satisfaction always require a discussion about potential psychological causes as well as physical causes, such as diabetes, and the need for communication and experimentation within the relationship. Since women in low-income communities often cannot afford medical examinations, they usually prefer to try to rule out nonphysical causes first—probably the opposite of the approach in industrialized countries.

Again in Lombok: "Lately I have seen sores around my husband's penis; his semen has a yellowish color and sometimes it smells bad. His condition has made me reluctant to have sex with him. Is that a sign of infection or sexually transmitted disease [penyakit kotor]?

We must address this kind of question with great sensitivity. Women need to be advised that all unusual symptoms require medical attention for both partners. However, this is a particularly difficult issue. Through observation and direct communication with health care providers,[2] we have learned that most are reluctant to conduct partner notification. They don't want to disturb or possibly destroy the husband-wife relationship. Because women lack knowledge about symptoms of reproductive tract infections and sexually transmitted diseases, and because health care providers have been limited in their response to clients' need for more information and counseling on these subjects, some nongovernmental organizations and counselors have become aware that informational materials that can help women and their partners deal with such problems must be developed.

General Reproductive Health Knowledge

Women in rural and urban areas alike have the same curiosity about their bodies and reproductive systems. A frequently asked question is: "What does the hymen *[selaput dara]* look like? Where is it located in the body?"

A book of illustrations is essential to describe not only the location of the hymen but also its nature, as it is frequently perceived as an impermeable, inflexible barrier. Looking at a picture often leads to a discussion of the fact that intercourse is not the only cause of perforation of the hymen among virgins. This is particularly relevant, because proof of virginity at marriage is still demanded among some families in Indonesia, and reclosing or stitching of the hymen is sometimes requested of physicians.

Sexual Relations

We need to question the frequent assumption that Indonesian women take only a passive role in intercourse. In group discussions about family planning or related matters, some women have expressed concern when they no longer feel like taking an active role in sex. Other women have shared stories about the ways they initiate intercourse:

"I and my husband are the same age. Now I'm forty-one; our three children are grown up; I feel old and it doesn't seem right to be having sex as often as when we were young, but my husband is as eager as before and complains about my passive behavior lately. Do you have any medicines or herbs [obat/jamu] *to arouse me?"*

One woman in Jakarta said, "My husband is a very quiet person, he does not talk much if not necessary. His routine schedule is when he comes home from work, he sits with us for dinner, takes a bath, and goes to bed after reading for a bit. So if I feel I want to have sex with him, what I do is to show us a blue movie. That seems to work, because he then follows what we see on the film . . . and does it with me."

Other women tell of a more subtle approach: they bathe; put on sheer nightgowns; dab perfume behind each ear, on their necks, in between their breasts, and around their intimate areas; and then snuggle up to their husbands in bed—perhaps also dimming the lights and putting on sweet music. But one woman said, "Well, why do you have to go round and round like that? In my case, I just go straight to my husband and tell him what I feel, and we do it!"

The most fundamental concerns and questions about sexuality among rural women differ very little from those of urban women, who have more opportunity for higher education and contact with the outside world. What differs are mainly the trappings of sex, which in the city can include such things as "blue films," "sheer nightgowns," or "soft and romantic music." The basic commonality is the eagerness and need to please and to be pleased in their sexual relationships with their spouses.

A client, married for a long time, is concerned because lately her husband has begun to demand oral sex. At first she was shocked, and worried that he may have learned this practice from someone else. But after discussing it with him, she thought she would be willing to engage in the practice except for two questions: one, does the Muslim religion forbid it? and two, will there be health implications of swallowing the sperm?

Other clients have raised questions about anal sex that mirror these concerns. Discussion about such questions needs to emphasize communication—thinking and talking through the doubts people may feel—and the challenges of trying something new. As information about HIV becomes more available, counselors in Indonesia have to add this issue to the discussion: the risks involved and protection needed. With regard to Muslim religious teachings, there is no universal prohibition on these practices.

There is also a darker side to sexual relations, which can relate to instances of abuse.

A client complains that her husband often slaps her, beats her head against the wall, and otherwise abuses her, but later expects her to have sex with him as though nothing had happened. She has begun to fear sex and has become frigid. She cannot respond physically to him under such conditions yet somehow feels that it is her duty to yield to his needs. Her husband cannot understand why she is no longer fully responsive.

As a counselor, in cases like this, I need to give both knowledge and support. Issues that should be covered range from basic physiology to helping couples communicate better; ideally, both husband and wife are invited to counseling sessions. Over and above the need for sensitive counseling are broader issues of legal protection and support networks such as shelters for abused women—issues that are still not widely debated in Indonesia.

The Need for Sex Education

It may be of interest to Indonesian service providers, who are often reluctant to discuss sexual matters with clients, that many of the above questions (including the question from the woman who feared that her husband had a sexually transmitted disease) came from group sessions with women that included me, the local doctor, and the community health worker. The other professionals were not only surprised at the openness of the women, particularly in a strict Muslim community, but also had to admit that they were not equipped to answer many of the questions. Even if they knew some of the physiological aspects of the issues raised by the women, their attempts at explanation often involved medical terms and technical information that the women could not understand.

Most women are not knowledgeable about sexually related reproductive functions and processes. Lack of knowledge about sexuality can lead women, both married and unmarried, to the tragedy of an unwanted pregnancy. In addition, mothers can't effectively educate their children about these matters. Female adolescents, lacking clear knowledge, are thus at risk of unwanted pregnancy and sexually transmitted diseases. Among young adolescents, the following examples illustrate how naive they are about the risks of pregnancy:

> *"I thought that a single act of intercourse could not cause pregnancy."*

> *"My boyfriend suggested that if we made love in a standing position, it would prevent us from risk of pregnancy."*

> *"I never took off my panties during intercourse (that is, they thought that panties would function similarly to a condom), and now my boyfriend is so mad at me because I am pregnant."*

All these cases reflect the need for very basic factual knowledge before adolescents become sexually active.

In the family planning clinic where I worked for thirteen years, many women came for abortion (*induksi haid* or menstrual regulation) services. However, because the legal status of this service is still unclear in Indonesia, many women try other methods—drinking herbal mixtures, undergoing rough abdominal massage by traditional midwives, or other means of abortion. When these efforts are unsuccessful, women sometimes come for counseling for how to best manage the burdens of their unplanned pregnancies—burdens that include husband-wife conflict, economic stress, cessation of schooling, influences on their health, and psychological pressures that manifest themselves in a variety of ways. This suffering, which could also affect the quality of the child's life, made me even more resolved to try to assist people in this situation—through not only "curative" but also "preventive" strategies, such as sex education for the young.

And yet today, most Indonesian decision makers and religious leaders do not approve of explicit or direct sex education—for example, through schools. The family planning program, however, has strong support from the government and informal leaders throughout the country, as well as a large infrastructure of both clinic and field-based personnel.[3] As we have seen, information exchange on family planning can and does lead to related sexual matters. If a sympathetic, practical sex education information package and approach were developed for use by selected family planning personnel, it would make a major contribution to family health and welfare.

A Practical Approach

My day-to-day experiences dealing with women—urban, rural, young, old, with and without education—have led me to take a more proactive stance in providing information that will help women. My job as a counselor has led to ongoing involvement with research, contacts with experts from Indonesia and internationally, and the preparation of material that can be used in intervention projects. For example, I have tried to formulate a simple information and education packet that can be given solely as sex education—where the context is supportive—or linked to information about family planning, either in the clinic setting or in the field.

The main ingredients of the packet are fairly basic:

1. *The approach (the key determinant).* The person who is going to give the information or education (a counselor, clinic worker, or field-worker) has to have a warm and caring attitude, be a good listener, and create a situation or atmosphere in which women will not hesitate to ask any question. She should adopt a two-way communication or client-oriented approach that reflects a willingness to learn from the questions asked by the women. Sometimes it is more helpful to assist women to find their own answers from among a range of possibilities; sexuality counseling is a mixture of factual information, exploration of feelings, and effective efforts to overcome the problems women experience.

If Indonesia were to involve family planning workers in the task of counseling or educating peers, during recruitment, attention would have to be given to candidates' attitudes and interpersonal skills. In my experience, there are many such people within the system who have this potential and who need only minimal training and support to bring out their natural skills. Ideally, attention would also need to be given to other health care providers throughout the system so that they too would have at least basic insights into client-oriented approaches.

2. *Content.* Discussion can begin with a specific question, but in a group session, it could begin by a review of the human reproductive process, including descriptions of:

- The reproductive system (female and male), using words that are familiar to each group, trying to avoid difficult medical or scientific terms.

- The process of human reproduction (menstruation; ovulation; pregnancy, including the development of the fetus; and the delivery process).

- Fertility regulation.

- Physiological problems, disease, or infections that could affect the normal process, such as reproductive tract infections and infertility.

This review should always be accompanied by open discussion, with participants encouraged to ask questions (an average of one-quarter lecture time and three-quarters discussion time is ideal). If there is a difficult question, we should be frank and seek help in answering the question. One of the most rewarding aspects of group discussions occurs when they take on a life of their own, with the counselor playing only a facilitating role and the participants themselves putting forward their suggestions and experiences.

3. *Teaching Aids.* For my first five years of counseling, I used a diagram of the female reproductive system in counseling sessions to explain the process of human reproduction, where we put an IUD, how to use jelly as a contraceptive, where ectopic pregnancy takes place, and so on. One day a good friend of

mine gave me a three-dimensional book entitled *The Facts of Life* (Miller and Pelham 1984), which has pop-up pictures of male and female reproductive organs, the development of the fetus in the uterus, a sperm, an ovum, and others. After I started using the book, the counseling sessions became more lively and enjoyable both for me and especially for the clients.

In the city, it's easy to use transparencies, slides, or even short films; however, in the field, I use the pop-up book or a very simple book I developed from the Facts of Life principles. In Lombok, more than 100 tutors (health communicators trained in reproductive health counseling skills) now own this book, and even in a restricted Muslim community, the people and the Muslim leaders accept the use of the book and seem to appreciate it.

4. *Process.* Once we become experienced in this kind of work (as counselor or tutor), we do not need more than ten to fifteen minutes to explain the content—the basic process of human reproduction—using the necessary materials to give a clear picture to clients, either on a one-to-one basis or in a small group consisting of no more than ten people. What we need the most time for is discussion and questions.

This process is not limited to the clinic setting. For example, I have had many invitations to give lectures about family planning. I show the audience a film about reproduction or simply bring the Facts of Life book. I always find that discussions become wider when issues of abortion and sexuality are included. These discussions turn out to be very open and frank.

Information and education on sexuality are basic and important. They increase not only knowledge but also the capacity of women in all stages of life to be familiar with their own bodies and their own needs, to take care of their own health, and to understand when to seek outside help. A knowledgeable woman will then share her knowledge with her friends, helping others to dispel myths and misinformation and—if the time comes—to pass on honest and full information to their children and the future generation.

A woman concerned with her inability to achieve orgasm is especially distressed by her husband's humiliating comments about her "frigidity." After fairly long-term counseling, which involved discussion of her self-

esteem, the need for communication with her husband, as well as guid-
ance on physiology involving clitoral stimulation and other forms of
achieving sexual satisfaction, she proclaimed herself to be "like a reborn
person." "Ninuk, I am not only pleased for myself, but I have been able to
share what I have learned with my sisters and my daughter. I'm so proud
to be able to help others."

Notes

I would like to thank Valerie Hull of the Population Council, Jakarta, for
her assistance with this chapter.

1. It was this experience that led to the development of a local version
   of a detailed book of illustrations that could enrich the explanation
   of such issues and reach a broad audience who would not have access
   to physiological models or imported books.
2. "Women's Perspectives of RTI and STD," conducted by Women's
   Study Center, University of Indonesia.
3. Although the family planning movement in Indonesia has been
   broadened to emphasize family resilience and family welfare, the
   central importance of sexual relations to family harmony is often
   overlooked because of the pervasive fear of female sexuality and the
   tendency to associate sex with negative connotations.

Reference

Miller, Jonathan, and David Pelham. 1984. *The facts of life.* London:
Jonathan Cape.

Bringing Men and Women Together in Family Planning Clinics

María Isabel Plata

Asociacion Pro-Bienestar de la Familia Colombiana, PRO-FAMILIA, an affiliate since 1965 of the International Planned Parenthood Federation (IPPF), is the leading private, nonprofit family planning association in Colombia. Today it provides more than 65 percent of all family planning services delivered in the country. It runs forty-eight clinics located in all regions and directly markets contraceptives in pharmacies and small shops throughout the nation. The role of the association is "to promote and defend the basic human right of family planning in Colombia and work toward achieving better sexual and reproductive health by offering information and other services."

PROFAMILIA began to incorporate reproductive health and rights into its programs in the mid-1980s as the result of a number of coinciding forces. Most notably, by the late 1980s, there was a growing awareness among staff of how women's roles in their families and in society affect their reproductive health and their ability to make and implement decisions regarding fertility and contraceptive use. The success of the women's movement in Colombia in putting reproductive rights on the government's agenda also created some external pressure for PROFAMILIA to

171

reexamine its mandate and service delivery structure so that it no longer focused solely on family planning. The following is an overview of various initiatives undertaken by PROFAMILIA so that its services would contribute to an effort to support noncoercive sexual relationships between men and women.

Recognizing Gender Issues

The first opportunity to address power relations between men and women arose in the main family planning clinic in Bogotá in 1986. Our administrative and medical staff were often confronted in their day-to-day work by women's low power status in intimate relationships. For example, a doctor or nurse would notice bruises on a woman who had come to the clinic for contraceptive services. Upon questioning, she would admit to living in an environment of perpetual fear at the hands of a violent and abusive husband. Or a patient would reveal that she was fighting with her common-law partner for custody of a child or for child support. In such instances, the clinic staff would listen sympathetically and try to offer comforting words of encouragement or advice, but apart from human kindness, they could provide little assistance of any practical value.

In November of that year, PROFAMILIA began a pilot project, initially funded by Population Concern (based in London) and subsequently by the Ford Foundation, to offer legal advice, negotiation, and services, including litigation in the area of domestic and family law, to both women and men. Women who came to the family planning clinic and who had observable legal problems were referred to the legal services clinic. Men came to the legal clinic because they heard of it through brochures and posters distributed through both women's and men's clinics. Often, women and men came with similar problems, particularly in the area of child support. This has proved to be a successful component of our services, and six legal services clinics have since been established.

As time went on, however, we became aware of other problems faced by women that could not be as easily detected or solved by legal assistance. These problems often manifested themselves in conflicts between clients and staff. For example, a patient who had a vaginal infection had a terrible argument with one of our doctors because the clinical procedure she required could not be done at the clinic and she had to go to a nearby hospital. She felt that we had not treated her well and demanded her money back. After talking to her, we learned that she feared that her husband would find out that she had to go to the hospital for treatment of the infection. Whereas the doctor saw the infection as a medical problem, the woman saw it as a sexual problem that she could not talk about with her husband.

Our staff were not aware of or could not easily understand how the imbalance of power between men and women, particularly in intimate relationships, impaired women's ability to successfully use contraception or protect themselves from disease or unwanted pregnancy. Nurses and doctors assumed that female clients were engaged in sexual relations as equal partners; they did not consider the fact that men are usually in control in sexual relationships and that women are often not in a position to demand specific practices. Thus, staff would counsel a woman that, for medical reasons, she should use vaginal tablets and have her partner use a condom, not appreciating the social or cultural context that would interfere with her ability to do so. It became increasingly apparent that staff needed to understand how gender issues manifested themselves in clients' needs and in their responses to those needs. This meant that PROFAMILIA as an institution would need to examine whether the structure of its staff and services contributed to gender biases or imbalances.

A History of PROFAMILIA's Experience

Our first challenge was to learn what terms like "reproductive health," "reproductive rights," and "women's human rights" meant or could mean within a family planning clinic. We decided to build on the contacts and good rapport we had established with local and regional women's groups when setting up the legal services clinic. This was a valuable experience because, in overcoming the initial skepticism of women's groups toward family planning and toward PROFAMILIA, which receives funds from the U. S. government, doctors from our clinics and feminists came to know and respect one another.

Recognizing the expertise and experience that women's groups had in the area of reproductive and women's rights, we thought it important to continue to work with them. So in order to give our staff an opportunity to internalize these new concepts, we organized a meeting for medical staff, feminists, and lawyers from Colombia and other Latin American countries. This meeting, which took place in 1991 with funding from the IPPF/Western Hemisphere Region, proved very congenial and has led to many subsequent joint activities and mutual support.

Staff from the main clinic in Bogotá then began to work with some of the smaller PROFAMILIA clinics in other cities to establish similar workshops (financed by a grant from the Planned Parenthood Federation of Canada). With the help of three Colombian women's groups, we organized sessions in twelve clinics. The first workshops, which were organized for executives and administrators, focused on gender issues and discrimination against women and how these affect women's health in the context of their day-to-day lives. The content included basic issues concerning reproductive rights, women's rights, and the 1991 Colombian Constitution, which had incorporated new concepts around the issue of individual rights and women's rights. In these workshops, we also started to look into issues of self-esteem and empowerment of women. Again, the purpose was to help managers and providers understand the reality of women's lives and some of the conflicts women may experience when they come to a clinic. Some participants liked the experience, but others were critical. One of our directors, for example, could not see why issues of self-esteem and related workshop exercises were valid in a family planning clinic. These mixed results showed us that if we wanted to advance discussion of these issues, we had to work at two levels: with our clinic directors at annual meetings and more directly with local staff.

While we continued to work with senior staff in a number of different, and often specially convened, venues, we also began organizing workshops for counselors so that they could integrate these ideas into their sessions with clients. The objective for these workshops was to enable staff to look at services from a client's perspective and make more appropriate decisions about how to provide services and how to respond to particular clinical situations. We also encouraged providers to think about how they could take proactive measures to educate clients about their legal rights and their rights to health services. Again with the help of the Planned Parenthood Federation of Canada, we recently developed a series of workshops for our paramedical staff of men and women who do counseling in our clinics and provide community-based information and education. The purpose is to advance together in the search for equality and to change the traditional language of sexuality.

Family Planning Counseling from a Gender Perspective

The initial results of our work with service providers and counselors have been promising; our counselors have started to question their own attitudes. For example, one counselor always felt frustrated when dealing with women who wanted their tubal ligations reversed. She began to understand for the first time why a woman with four or five children would request the reversal. She had come to realize that women do not always act as free agents, particularly when they do not have a sexual identity independent of their husbands or partners. She could now come to terms with these kinds of requests. We have learned that the analysis of men's and women's different perspectives allows us to understand our clients better.

Our interest in contributing toward noncoercive sexual and reproductive relationships between men and women—relationships that are based on mutual respect and personal responsibility—has had a direct impact on the way we organize counseling and services. For example, we have developed special counseling around those contraceptive methods that are provider controlled (IUDs, NORPLANT®, and tubal ligations) rather than client controlled in order to ensure that our women clients are making fully informed decisions that they are comfortable with. With long-acting methods, we extend the initial consultation, the medical examination and counseling, and the actual procedure over several days, both to give the woman time to think about her decision and to provide various stages at which she can involve her partner, if she chooses to do so.

If a woman comes alone seeking a sterilization, she is asked in the initial counseling session whether she wants to come back with her partner so that they can both receive counseling and reach a joint decision. She is asked if she knows that tubal ligation is irreversible and if she knows about vasectomy. Her partner's role in the question of reproductive responsibility is explored. Unfortunately, a vast majority of our women clients still consider family planning their responsibility and are reluctant to involve their male partners.

PROFAMILIA also has several male-only clinics, and these have proved to be ideal places to educate men about their participation in family planning activities and safer sex. When a couple comes in for a sterilization, they are sent to a male-only clinic, where they receive joint counseling. A typical interview starts with the man announcing that *he* has decided to bring his wife for a tubal ligation. After asking how many children they have, our counselor begins to explore "his" decision by asking if the woman wants the procedure. The counselor asks the woman questions like Who impregnated you? Who is also responsible for those pregnancies? Who should be doing the family planning? and eventually, Would you like him to participate in the family planning? If the answer to this last question is yes, our counselor asks the man if he knows about vasectomy. Since he usually does not, the counselor explains how it is done and uses a chart to compare the two surgical procedures. At this point, the couple commonly asks questions like Does it hurt? How far away is the clinic from the workplace? Will it affect our sexual life? When can normal sexual activity resume? The counselor refers to both procedures when answering these questions. Often this leads to a discussion among the couple and the counselor of the stereotypes surrounding male and female sterilization that result in wives having the procedure because this is what "traditionally is done." At this point, the counselor points out that more and more Colombian men have decided to get vasectomies.

Another significant change is that when a couple arrives for the first time and asks for information concerning fertility control methods, our counselor offers them the opportunity to participate in a group counseling session with other women, and perhaps other men. This is always cleared with other members of the group ahead of time. If a participant in the group objects, the couple is asked to wait and is counseled individually.

The dynamics of mixed groups are quite interesting. We have found that men lack basic information concerning contraceptive methods and that they often ask some of the same questions and express some of the same concerns that women had ten years ago. For example, men ask if the IUD produces cancer. Men also tend to focus on "scientific" questions like How does the IUD work? whereas women will ask "personal" questions like Does it hurt? In mixed groups, the man (or men) may tend to dominate the discussion. In this case, the facilitator-counselor uses a variety of techniques to keep the discussion focused on the kinds of issues or concerns that women typically express when they are in a single-sex group. It should be noted that not many men have shown up for group counseling, so we haven't yet had to deal with a group in which men are a majority. The comments from women who have undergone group counseling with their partners are very promising. Often women say, "Now he will not make me use the pill or the IUD."

Adolescents' Family Planning Questions and Needs

PROFAMILIA also has several clinics for young people (ranging in age from thirteen to nineteen). These were initiated in 1990 in response to the continually climbing rates of sexually transmitted diseases (STDs), including AIDS; unwanted pregnancy; and unsafe abortions among this age group. Young people were becoming sexually active without protection against STDs or AIDS and were getting pregnant because they did not use contraception.

In order to reach these youngsters, the content of the counseling in the youth centers is different from our approach to older clients. PROFAMILIA staff try to challenge and change some of the language and ideas that young people have about sexual behavior, men's and women's roles in sex and sexual decision making, and reproductive functions such as pregnancy and menstruation, as well as dispel the large amount of misinformation many young people have. On the one hand, young girls and their parents avoid talking about sex. Mothers tell their daughters only *cuidate* (take care of yourself). They also use negative language for reproductive functions, such as *está enferma* (she is sick, meaning that she has her period) or *me la perjudicaron a mi hija* (my daughter was hurt, meaning that she got pregnant). Boys, on the other hand, use words that suggest violent or aggressive sexual interaction with girls. *Coronar* (to crown) means to have sex without thinking about the consequences—without commitment. *Gozar* (to enjoy) means to get a girl at a party or social event and have sex with her. *Comer* (to eat) suggests that the boy forces himself on the girl, abuses or possesses her. All these words avoid the reality of sexuality. We seek to enable young people to talk about sex and its consequences more openly and accurately. In addition to contraceptive information and services, gynecological and general medical services, and pregnancy tests and other laboratory tests, these clinics offer counseling on issues such as sexuality, self-esteem, gender issues, sexual health, and decision making.

PROFAMILIA works with both individuals and couples. Unlike our older clients, young couples often demand joint counseling. We think that this is because girls have the self-esteem to request their partners' presence. Also, this new generation of young men are living in a society in which more women are educated, work outside of the household, and expect to be full citizens, equal to men.

Our counselors have found that the questions asked by young men and women are different from those of their elders. For example, it is common for young men to ask about the side effects of different contraceptive methods and how they are going to affect their partners. Young women usually ask about the failure rates of the methods or show strong concerns about the possibility of their mothers finding out that they are using a birth control method and ask, "Does it show?" But some of the questions are the same. We have found that both young and older men have similar concerns and prejudices about the use of condoms. It is common to hear boys say that they cannot use condoms with their partners because these are used only with prostitutes, or that condoms inhibit pleasure. As in other parts of the world, in

Colombia, we have found that both young men and young women are embarrassed about the use of condoms.

It should also be noted that working with young people has allowed, or even pushed, us to include sexuality issues in our work with adult clients. Building on these informal experiences, we have recently received a grant from the Ford Foundation to develop a model to work with young people in pairs (girl and boy) on sexual health. Our plan is to develop this program in our main clinic in Bogotá, test it in some of the other youth centers, and then adapt it for working with adults.

Rather than simply delivering family planning services within the existing social structure, PROFAMILIA has made a conscientious and concentrated effort to internalize respect for individual freedom, equality of women, and an understanding of male as well as female reproductive responsibilities to promote equality between the sexes.

*T*eaching Fertility
*A*wareness

How a Government Family Planning Program
Got Involved in Sexuality

Debbie Rogow

*A*lmost twenty years ago, I began teaching fertility awareness—instructing women how to observe their bodily changes during the month to determine when they were fertile. I volunteered to write about my experiences for this book because I remembered how valuable it was to women to learn about their bodies. But to tell the truth, I thought that it would be just one more paper to write.

In preparing this chapter, I met with my old fellow teachers, spoke with some old clients, and read through hundreds of follow-up forms and letters from clients. These clients had written—over and over again—that gaining this information about their bodies had been nothing less than a lifeline, a door to self-confidence, the foundation for a new understanding of their own sexuality. As I sat reading their comments, tears began streaming down my cheeks and I realized that this chapter was not just one more paper to write. Writing this chapter is a chance to reflect on and share perhaps the most meaningful work I have had the opportunity to undertake.

This is a story about how a public family planning program made a difference in the sexual lives of almost two thousand clients—a difference we never imagined when we began.

But Does It Work for Avoiding Pregnancy?

In 1980, we conducted a research study for the federal government to determine the use-failure and continuation rates among fertility awareness (FA) users. We found a use-failure rate of 9.9 percent and a one-year continuation rate of 67 percent. Taken at face value, 90.1 percent effectiveness indicates that knowing her fertile time makes a woman a more effective user of barrier methods or periodic abstinence. But this figure is even more impressive given that most of our study population belonged to groups at very high risk of unwanted pregnancy: close to half had had a previous abortion, and close to one-third stated that they only wanted to delay pregnancy for up to a few years. The report of this study can be found in *Advances in Planned Parenthood* 15, no. 1 (1980):27–33.

What Is Fertility Awareness?

Fertility awareness (FA) means becoming familiar with the changes in one's body during the ovulatory or menstrual cycle. Understanding these changes allows a girl or woman to identify when she is ovulating. Those signs that are most easily observed are changes in the cervical mucus (which women can observe when they urinate) and in the body temperature (which requires taking daily temperature readings). Some women also rely on other secondary indicators, such as changes in the location and feel of the cervix, abdominal pain at the time of ovulation, or the day of the cycle (calendar rhythm).[1]

Over the course of one cycle, almost any woman can learn to identify her fertile time. The period of time from menstruation to ovulation varies widely, but the time from ovulation to the next menstruation is virtually always the same (fourteen days), so a woman can predict her date of next menstruation. If she doesn't want to get pregnant, she can use a barrier method or avoid intercourse during her fertile time. If she does want to get pregnant, she can time intercourse appropriately.

Why and How We Began
to Teach Fertility Awareness

In the 1970s in the United States, right-wing political forces opposed to contraception and abortion were gaining tremendous influence. Along with successful assaults on abortion and less successful ones on contraception, this reactionary movement managed to secure substantial domestic and international funds for natural family planning (NFP). At the time, I was responsible for the education and training activities for the primary family planning program within the San Francisco Public Health Department in the state of California. My supervisor told me that word had come from the government that we had to cover all methods, including NFP; she asked me to call the local Catholic hospital and arrange for staff in-service training on the Billings or mucus method of family planning.

Aware of the political motivations behind this government directive and more than skeptical about the value of natural methods, I procrastinated. After several gentle reminders, my supervisor—who was also my friend and political ally, but a wiser woman than I—arranged the in-service training herself. Several weeks later, a married couple who worked with St. Mary's Hospital came to tell a couple dozen nurses and family planning counselors about the Billings or mucus method of NFP.

Two hours later, I sat stunned. I had an undergraduate degree in biology and had nearly completed my master's degree in human reproductive biology and population and family planning studies. No professor, no textbook, and no family planning provider had ever told me that the menstrual cycle was so much more than proliferation of the endometrium, ovulation, and shedding of the endometrium. No one had explained the symphony of changes my body went through every cycle and that, more important, several of them were easily observable. No one had told me that once I learned to watch for the changes in cervical mucus, *I didn't have to use a diaphragm or condom all month, after all.*

Our staff—a mix of English-, Tagalog-, and Chinese-speaking women and a few men aged twenty to fifty—quickly decided to take the three-session class on the Billings mucus method at the hospital. Aside from the lectures on sexual morality according to the Catholic Church (warning against the evils of masturbation, contraception, premarital sex, and abortion), most of us were very enthusiastic and began charting our cycles (excluding the men, the menopausal women, and the women taking the pill). We couldn't believe how easy it was to see the changes to which we had been oblivious our whole lives!

To prepare ourselves to offer similar classes, we found a consultant, Karen, who had experience teaching women, from a secular or nonreligious vantage point, how to identify ovulation. First we ran into the problem of terminology. The government had already accepted the Catholic Church's position that NFP meant the whole package—the education about one's body plus enforced abstinence during the fertile time. Under this view, the only people who would learn about their bodily changes were the ones who agreed never to use a barrier method. But our only goal was to teach women about their bodies so that they could make their own decisions about their sexuality and their contraceptive method (be it the condom, diaphragm, or periodic abstinence). Karen suggested the term "fertility awareness," and we agreed.

Karen also trained us to teach women about fertility signs other than mucus, such as changes in body temperature during the cycle. She even relied on changes in the location and feel of her cervix to tell when she was ovulating.

Together with Karen, we developed a curriculum, teaching aids, a user's manual, and supplies for teaching. The supplies we used included a giant sample chart that we made ourselves, some audiovisual slides ordered through NFP programs, a film using microphotography to show ovulation, blank charts and colored pencils, and a microscope and slides so users could put samples of their mucus on slides and see for themselves the dramatically different cellular structure of the different types of mucus. Then we began offering classes to women and their partners. After co-teaching with Karen for several months, a nurse and I began teaching the classes ourselves.

Each class consisted of three two-hour sessions, held every other week. In this way, most women went through a complete menstrual cycle during the instruction period. We also provided drop-in follow-up "clinics" and told all clients that they could

contact us at any time for further consultation. For research purposes, we also conducted routine telephone or mail follow-up
with all clients for at least one year.

We began a class series each month. Our first classes were
small, six or eight women. Soon the demand was so high that we
had to offer two new groups each month, with up to twenty-five
women in each group. Encouraged by our staff, about half the
women brought their male partners. In many cases, the couples
came shortly after an unwanted pregnancy and abortion; these
male partners were often particularly motivated to help find a
new contraceptive and make it work. Besides, the men found
information about women's bodies fascinating, and they enjoyed
participating in the group activities. By the second year, our
annual client load grew to about four hundred women (and two
hundred men)—more than double the number of female clients
selecting the IUD.

Most of our clients were referred by the family planning
nurses, who had begun routinely adding FA to the list of methods
available at the clinic. Some of the interested women were our regular clients who were "sick of the pill." Others were somewhat
interested in barrier methods and were amazed to hear that they
needed to use that method only three or four times a month. Still
others had come to the clinic for a pregnancy test or after an abortion; often, these women were interested in switching methods.
And some women came for help in trying to become pregnant. Of
course, people who completed the class also began sending us
new clients, but the support of a trained nursing staff in contact
with a hundred clients each week was the key to our success.

Although this was a government clinic, the clients ranged
from very poor to wealthy. Most participants, of course, were regular working people. Their ages ranged from eighteen to forty-
nine, though the average age was twenty-seven. And they came
from a variety of racial and language backgrounds. In fact, we
had to add classes in Chinese and Spanish to meet the needs of
our diverse population. The FA classes brought together poor,
uneducated women who were living on public assistance and
wealthy, professional women. Women whose lives normally would
not intersect on "equal ground" found themselves sharing the
same feelings and experiences, having the same questions about
their bodies.

Fertility Awareness in Developing Countries

Our experience taught us that women do not need to have much schooling to be able to identify their fertile times and understand what we teach about their bodies. A group of illiterate women I taught in Mexico understood the basic information at least as quickly as the university students who attended our public clinic in San Francisco.

With support from the United States Agency for International Development, Georgetown University's Institute for Reproductive Health provides training and technical assistance to developing country family planning programs interested in FA and NFP.

What We Taught

The course included information on female (and occasionally male) reproductive anatomy and physiology, with an emphasis on the ovulatory (or menstrual) cycle and the hormones that control the cycle. We spent the most time discussing those bodily changes that are observable: cervical mucus and basal body temperature. We explained how and why these signs change, how to observe the changes, how to keep a color-coded chart of the changes, and how to interpret the changes. We also engaged in various small group exercises in which participants shared their experiences related to contraception, explored their feelings about future and unplanned pregnancies, and shared their new experiences with FA. We also showed a film that used microphotography to show ovulation and fertilization.

What Our Clients Learned about Sex

You may be thinking that this curriculum doesn't seem to have much to do with sexuality. And that's what we thought. But we were wrong. Here are a number of typical examples.

At the start of each first session, we gave people the opportunity to talk about their past experiences with contraception. As participants went around in a circle, one person might mention, "I was on the pill for a couple of years and I decided to go off of it because I didn't think it was so good for my body. Now that I'm off the pill, I realize that my interest in sex is higher." The introductions would move around the circle, and a few minutes later another person would say, "I was so amazed by what Maria said before. I always felt like the pill depressed my libido but my doctor told me that it was probably just stress. Now I feel like I have my body back!"

During the discussion of anatomy, everyone would laugh about the fact that in high schools around the world, when we learned about the reproductive system, the clitoris was never mentioned. And almost nobody knew when during the cycle they were fertile.

Teaching about mucus required that we clarify the difference between the three common types of secretions women notice coming from their vaginas. First is the cervical mucus, a natural and healthy part of fertility. A second type is the vaginal secretion associated with sexual arousal. A third type consists of various discharges related to infection. We got very specific about how these differ. Becoming more knowledgeable and comfortable with their vaginal secretions made women feel less like their vaginas were "dirty." It also meant that many yeast infections could be identified by the woman at the early stage and treated with a douche and dietary changes.

We asked the participants to either abstain from intercourse during the learning month or to use nonlubricated condoms, which we distributed free of charge. In this way, they wouldn't be confused between semen, condom lubrication, and mucus while they were still learning to recognize their own mucus. It was important to give people—including the men present—the chance to talk about how they felt about this idea. By the beginning of the second session, two things happened. First, many of the participants shared that the decision about condoms and abstinence had provoked meaningful discussions with their partners about their sexual relationship. Occasionally, participants even shared that the abstinence period allowed them to experiment in their intimacy. And second, there were always more men in the second session than had come to the first. Women went home and told their husbands and partners, "Come to this great class! You're really going to like it and there are other guys there." This was a unique experience for these men.

At the beginning of the second and third sessions, as well as during subsequent follow-up consultations, we went over the women's charts with them in small groups. Part of charting involved recording their sexual activity. Participants enjoyed seeing all the symbols they had invented to mark this—some women put a heart, some women made an X, some women wrote "SEX!" But more important, they began discussing how they—together with their partners—made decisions about whether to have sex, what kind of sex to have, and so forth. One couple explained, "Well, we thought, okay, so we can't have sex, but we can still be, you know, affectionate with each other. So we spent some time just touching each other, sometimes in ways we really hadn't done before. And that got us talking about how, like, 'Gee, this is really nice. Why don't we ever do this? And doesn't this count as sex too?' We weren't so used to trying those things and talking about them."

What the Staff Learned about Sex and Gender

In addition to what the participants were learning about their own sexuality, we were learning a great deal about sex and gender. One particularly intriguing example was revealed to us during follow-up chart reviews. The majority of the women reported that they had the greatest interest in sex during the most fertile days. Since few of them were abstaining during the fertile time, it wasn't a matter of feeling sexually "deprived." The only explanation we could imagine was a hormonal one. The teachers had begun to notice this pattern in their own cycles too. And it did seem to make sense from an evolutionary perspective!

At that time, Australian researcher Lorraine Dennerstein had not yet published her groundbreaking work documenting this phenomenon (see her chapter "Female Sexuality, the Menstrual Cycle, and the Pill" in this volume), but we began to talk about it with our clients and to ask them to write down when they felt

Bringing the Information to Girls

After a few years of teaching FA to sexually active women and men, we began a program called FATE—Fertility Awareness Teen Education. We went to local high schools and taught girls about the fertility cycle and vaginal discharge—all the basics that the women had told us they wished they had known when they were young. Most of the girls had lives that were too erratic to involve regular charting, but they all valued learning about their bodies. Realizing that teenage girls had already internalized the idea that all vaginal discharge is dirty, we also began doing menstruation education for fifth and sixth graders. In this unit, we sought to demystify the whole cycle, explaining changes in mucus, oiliness of skin and hair, and so on, rather than simply portraying bleeding as the highlight of the cycle.

more and less sexual interest. This information was of more than academic interest. I remember one client who said, "I remember being very sexually attracted to a man at a party one time. Then, just a few days later, my husband was wanting to have sex and I wasn't feeling much of anything. I felt so confused and guilty. But looking back at the calendar, now I can see I was ovulating when I was at the party. I think I just get extra turned on at that time of the month!"

We also noticed that those women who didn't enjoy sex were "stretching" their fertile days as a way of negotiating a longer period of abstinence. For these women, FA became a conscious tool for increasing their sexual decision-making power. Becoming more sensitive to the experience of those women who were not enjoying intercourse was an important lesson for us: we stopped referring automatically to days when you "get to have sex" or "don't get to have sex."

Those women who were trying to become pregnant also noticed changes in their sexuality. Although they felt less spontaneous about having sex than previously, they talked about feeling more "in control" of their fertility. For those couples who had been trying for many months to conceive and were feeling so helpless, this sense of control was a valuable asset. (And many did become pregnant!)

As family planning workers, we began to incorporate some of these lessons into our general family planning services. We began to offer more women in the examination room the chance to see their cervixes in the mirror; IUD clients were particularly interested. We began to talk with women about expanding their say-so about when they had sex, so that they could prevent conception more effectively. And partly in recognition of the neglected role men play in sex and contraception, we began a men's clinic.

Treating Bodily Knowledge as a Precious Gift

Finally, we were constantly reminded that women cherish knowing about their bodies—and not only the clients who took several buses at night to come to our classes! Whenever one of the instructors was at a social event and someone inquired about her profession, a rapt crowd of women began gathering as soon as she began to answer. But certainly our clients gave us the clearest message of how much they valued this knowledge. By the late 1980s, money for public services was being cut, and our program was going to be eliminated. We wrote to a hundred female and male clients and asked them to send letters of support to government officials. We were surprised that eighty-one of them responded! Here are some excerpts from what they wrote:

Speaking from a male point of view, fertility awareness is a method that I can be involved in and which allows me to share some responsibility—and knowledge—in the process.

I know my body better. Women have a right to know their bodies more. The institutions which teach this method are contributing to the fabric of society.

I have gained knowledge about the cycles and function of my own body. This new and most important understanding between my body and me has helped me to prevent illness, maintain self-respect, enhance self-esteem, be more confident, and most of all take responsibility for staying well. It is with the deepest respect and sincerity that I say this information has helped me to be a more fully contributing member of society.

FA has had a very positive effect on my life. I have more body awareness, control over my life, and better birth control. I wish I had done this years ago.

I feel more in touch with my body and its functions. I know now what's going on with me at various times of the month.

Any family planning program and any sex education course should include fertility awareness information. What we learned has improved our understanding of the reproductive cycle and organs better than anything else we've ever done.

I consider myself well-educated, but the first time in my life that I became aware of the workings of my own body was when I took a fertility awareness class. Women deserve to know about such a safe, healthy, natural method!

Learning about my body gave me the most vital and useful information about my body I have ever gotten. Getting this information from a government clinic, and knowing that your highly qualified instructors were going out into the public schools to give classes, boosted my respect for the local government.

I consider myself an intelligent person, however, when I attended these classes I felt like I had been living in the Dark Ages, ignorant of my own body functions. Fertility awareness is for young and old alike, who want to work with their bodies instead of against them!

I say without hesitation that I learned 100 percent more about my reproductive "being" than I had known before.

I once got pregnant during my period, so I always thought I was really abnormal and always fertile. Now I understand that I have very short cycles and I do have some infertile days.

I didn't feel like I could ask my boyfriend to use condoms before, but since he understands my cycle, he's willing to use them during my fertile time.

Most of us learned that our genitals are ugly. Learning about my fertility cycle put me in awe of the female reproductive system. I feel so happy to have this knowledge.

All of a sudden you have to communicate with your partner—my boyfriend and I think that this was the most valuable part of the whole class.

After the first class, I started talking to Rebecca. At first we talked about past experiences with birth control. But I also got to under-stand how women have been robbed of knowing about their bodies and how this affects them sexually. We would do anything to sup-port the health center.

These were letters to the local government for budgetary sup-port. Imagine what these clients might have written if we had asked them to share how FA had enhanced their sexual lives!

———————————

I hope that family planning program staffs in other settings think about setting up programs to teach local women about their fer-tility. If FA is taught in groups, it is an inexpensive contraceptive method to provide. Such programs would certainly attract some new clients who are currently relying on "rhythm" and not even coming in to the clinic. Many people who are concerned about the side effects of modern methods would find that they have a broader range of acceptable methods. Class participants would have opportunities to explore their ambivalence about becoming pregnant. And many women would become staunch advocates of the family planning program. All these outcomes contribute to greater contraceptive use and effectiveness.

Others may learn, as we did, that FA is more than an approach to fertility regulation—it is a powerful tool for enabling people to become more comfortable with their own sexuality and their sex-ual relationships. Certainly, most people do not expect or imag-ine that they can improve their sexual lives. Such an opportunity comes as a rare gift—a gift that most public health programs never imagine giving.

Note

1. Different terminology has been applied to reliance on different signs: reliance on mucus signs is generally called the mucus method or Billings method; reliance on body temperature signs is often called the basal body temperature or BBT method; use of both methods is generally called the sympto-thermal method. The terms "natural family planning" and "fertility awareness" may refer to any of these approaches, although many church-based programs view natural family planning as prescribing specified sexual behavior as well.

Reproductive Health Interventions

*T*he Evolution
of a Sexuality
Education Program

From Research to Action

Margarita Diaz with Kirsten Moore

S ince 1987, the Family Planning
Clinic at the University of Campinas, Brazil, has operated a unique Sexuality Education Program (SEP) for women attending the clinic. Program founder and codirector Margarita (Maggie) Diaz reflected on the evolution of the program and her involvement with it.

Getting Started

Kirsten: Can you tell us how you identified the need for a sexuality program?

Maggie: I am a nurse-midwife and work in the family planning clinic attending patients. I had worked in the clinic for seventeen years as a family planning counselor and noticed that many women complained about problems in their sexual lives. Two of my colleagues, Patricia Goodson and Carlos Cavalcante, and I decided to document and analyze their sexual problems through a research study [Table 1]. We developed an interview questionnaire

Table 1 Sampling of Responses from a Study on Sexual Complaints of Women Using Contraceptives

Question	Response	
	Frequently/Sometimes	*Never*
Have desire/libido (n=378)	85%	15%
	Always/Almost Always/Sometimes	*Never*
Have orgasm (n=378)	88%	12%
	Good/Normal	*Poor*
Quality of Sexual Relationship (according to woman) (n=378)	90.2%	9.8%
	Good/Normal	*Poor*
Partner's opinion of sexual relationship (according to woman) (n=323)	92%	8%

and interviewed a random sample of 462 women attending the clinic who were using different contraceptive methods (NOR-PLANT® implant, injectable, pill, IUD, and diaphragm).

We found several things. Many women described their sexual lives as good. Those of us conducting the research first imagined that "good" meant the presence of orgasm and libido, but this was not the case. A lot of women who said that their sexual lives were good also said that they never felt orgasm, that they often felt no desire to have intercourse. They thought that their sexual lives were good because their relationships with their partners were good; their partners were affectionate, gave them lots of love, and treated them with respect. Even when they never or rarely felt the desire to have intercourse, their partners respected their desire to say yes or no and continued to give them a lot of love and compassion. These women always used the words "love" and "affection" to describe their relationships.

On the other hand, of those interviewed, 37 percent said that they had real problems—often, many problems. This was interesting, because some of these women felt desire and had orgasm but described their sexual lives as bad or average because they felt that their partners didn't respect them. These women described their relationships as lacking in love and compassion, as well as in

Table 2 Changes in Sex Life According to Contraceptive Method Used

Method	Improved	Worsened	No Change	No Information
Oral contraceptive (n=71)	s29.6%	14.1%	46.3%	7.0%
Injectables (n=134)	20.9	11.9	61.2	6.0
IUD (n=92)	30.4	13.0	55.3	3.3
Barrier methods (n=25)	24.0	4.0	68.0	4.0

sharing of responsibility within the house. In these relationships, the partner decided when to have intercourse.

Fifty percent of the women interviewed who had sexual complaints initially believed that their complaints were related to their contraceptive methods [Table 2]. Many times this was the only way women found to begin to talk about their problems in a family planning clinic—to say that they were related to a method. I think that it is easier for women to say, "Since I began using the pill, my libido is low," than to complain about their sexual experiences or their partners.

Kirsten: Do you have an idea of how many of their complaints of low libido were actually the perceptions of women themselves versus those of their partners?

Maggie: Women's perceptions are typically influenced by their partners. He believes—or wants to believe—that the method is causing the problem. Whenever our clients have sexual problems, the man always says that it is the woman's fault. In our experience, he never says that it is their problem as a couple or that it is his problem. He always says that it is the woman's problem, and I think women come to believe this themselves.

Objectives and Structure

Kirsten: What were the initial objectives of your program: to provide educational support for women experiencing some level of sexual dysfunction? to help women achieve more emotional satisfaction from their relationships?

Maggie: Initially, we designed our education program to give attention to the women who complained about sexual problems—that 37 percent who complained of lack of orgasm and desire or who identified some specific problem in their sexual lives. But we found that many women who said that they had problems didn't have any specific problems or were not sure if they had problems—they never had the opportunity to talk and ask questions about sex.

So we now have a more open recruiting process. We offer all women the opportunity to participate in the class. We learned that most women appreciate an opportunity to discuss sexuality.

The same staff member who will coordinate the group interviews the woman and gives her information about the content and kind of work performed in the course. A few women who are not comfortable participating in a group are offered individual counseling.

Kirsten: How did you establish the SEP within the clinic?

Maggie: After the research and elaboration of the objectives and activities of the SEP, we conducted a training course for all the nurses and social workers in the clinic to sensitize them to issues of sexuality and to identify people interested in acting as one of two coordinators of the sessions. We selected three nurses, one social worker and one educator-researcher and conducted a second training course, including addressing their own sexuality, to pretest the program.

One nurse and the sex educator-researcher left, at which point I trained Débora Bossemayer, who had previous training as a sex educator. She began by observing our group and soon took on the role of facilitator-coordinator and now trains other professional staff.

Kirsten: Can you describe the structure of the SEP sessions?

Maggie: Each session runs for two and a half hours in the morning. At the end of each session, the women are given some tasks to complete before the next meeting. The classes meet once a week for four weeks. We provide coffee, and the women organize to bring some food to share with one another.

Two people facilitate the sessions, and we begin with up to ten women in a group. However, our clinic is not located very conveniently, so the cost and time involved in transportation have affected attendance during the course.

We create a comfortable climate by using a variety of exercises to introduce people to one another. In the first exercise, I take a ball of string and say my name, what I do, the things that I like and don't like, and any other information that I want to share with the group. I then throw the ball to another woman, who says her name and gives some information about herself, and so on until everyone has introduced herself and is holding a piece of the string. It is very funny, because sometimes the ball falls to the floor and everyone laughs. Once everybody has been introduced, we untangle ourselves, throwing the ball back to the person who threw it to us, remembering her name and something else that was said. Everybody in the group helps out.

After introductions, we ask: "If we wanted to learn how to weave or sew, how should we begin? The women say: "We need to know about the machine, the pieces, the fabric." Then we ask: "If we need to learn about sexuality, what do you think we should know?" And usually they say, "the body." We then start with a model of a woman.

The main thing we work on is self-esteem, their concepts of beauty, messages about beauty we receive from the media, and so forth. After this, we discuss our body and how it functions, answering all questions and clarifying doubts. We always use a participatory approach and have materials like photos, a flip chart, and models to facilitate the learning.

Kirsten: It sounds like a "sexual literacy" course. What things do women generally know about their bodies? What are common misconceptions or gaps in their knowledge?

Maggie: I think that a basic level of sexual literacy exists among the women. I also think that just giving women information will not solve their problems. The most important goal of the group is to empower women so that they can solve their own problems.

Approximately 40 percent of the women in the initial research study and SEP complained about lack of orgasm. We use a lot of the techniques of Lonnie Barbach [1976] to help women have orgasm. One of the techniques is to discover and know your own body. At the end of the first meeting, we encourage the women to go home and to look at and touch every part of their bodies—to masturbate. The assignment is to touch the body, feel the sensation on the hand, arm, breast, all over the body to see what they feel in each part of the body and which part they like most.

The majority of these women have never touched the clitoris and don't know the purpose it serves. The perception exists among women that they can feel only in the vagina and can achieve orgasm only through intercourse. They focus their sexuality on the genital region and don't explore other parts of their bodies. Often, after the first meeting and a woman has achieved orgasm through touching her clitoris, she tells us that she has not previously allowed her partner to touch her because she thinks this is not appropriate.

Kirsten: What information and experiences do you give her to go beyond a basic level of sexual literacy?

Maggie: We try to extend the concept of sexuality to all kinds of desire, such as listening to music, remembering some pleasant things, watching TV, and feeling desire for a man. We explain that culture forbids the concept of desire for women. We give them permission to feel pleasant things, *not only related to sex with partners.* Women are not aware that all parts of their body, especially the stimulation of other senses through touching or music, are part of their sexuality. So we do exercises that don't have to do with the body but have to do with recognizing one's own desires outside of sex. For example, at the end of the second session, we give the women another exercise to do with their partners. The woman is to touch the body of her partner all over and her partner is to touch her—without having intercourse. We encourage her to tell her partner what feels best, what each likes most.

We also talk about how pain, stress, worry or illness can interfere with their sexual responses.

Kirsten: How do you get a woman to define her problem for herself?

Maggie: Women need to think about why they have sexual problems. They need to understand that their problems are often the result of a process, begun early in life, that forces women to repress their sexuality. In our society, there are very different expectations of men and women: A girl is expected to say "stop" if her boyfriend is touching some part of her body. If she allows the touching to continue (because it feels pleasurable to her), society—and possibly even her boyfriend—considers her a "bad woman." Consequently, many women repress or control their sexual responses because of what society or their families have told them. Once they realize they have done this, the importance of their sexual problems diminishes.

Because gender imbalances hold women responsible for everything in the home, women generally consider themselves responsible for any sexual problems. We encourage women to reflect on these assumptions, and we work on their self-esteem. This increases their confidence and enables them to talk to their partners about the problem.

Kirsten: I notice in the third meeting you have an exercise called "Learning to Trust." Who are they learning to trust?

Maggie: This is a simple exercise. One woman, who is blindfolded, is led around the room by another woman for several minutes. After this, we discuss the experience and why it is important to trust each other in this exercise and what this has to do with trust in their sexual partners.

We also encourage them to have the confidence to express to their partners what they want, what they feel, and what they don't want. Some women never considered talking about this with their partners. In this meeting, we ask about their sexual history and their lifetime experiences, and they share their first sexual encounters. This moment is very important because this is when women tell about experiences of violence—being raped by their fathers, sometimes by other members of the family, boyfriends or husbands. All this affects trust.

Kirsten: This sounds like a difficult process to manage. How do you facilitate the painful emotions that come up at this point?

Maggie: When they need more help, we refer them to another professional, for example, a psychiatrist or a sex therapist. Because we have two facilitators, if this moment brings out a lot of emotions and someone begins to cry, one of us will go out of the room with her and give her support. But after that, we usually come back to the group and continue working. We never had such a bad experience that we were unable to handle it.

Kirsten: Do the women like talking to one another? Have you ever had a case where two women knew each other outside of the group and felt that they just couldn't share?

Maggie: They seem to love sharing their sexual experiences with other women. Usually they meet each other for the first time when they start in the group. In the two cases where two women knew each other previously, they did not seem inhibited or have any difficulty participating fully, so I don't think this would be a problem if, for example, we worked in the community.

Problems

Kirsten: What kinds of problems have you encountered in implementing the SEP? From clients, staff, or within your own framework?

Maggie: Unfortunately, one problem is client load. We have a lot of women interested in joining the program. When we first started, we conducted more than six sessions a year (reaching sixty women). We would do one a month and then take a week off—about eight or ten a year. But now Débora and I travel a lot, and the other social workers and nurses are not always available to conduct the group. So we have a list of women waiting and we have a shortage of trained facilitators. This year we will be able to work with only four groups, fewer than forty women.

Also, women have problems attending the sessions on a regular basis. Bus transportation is so expensive and they need to take two different buses each way to get to the clinic in the university hospital. To complete one group, we schedule double the number of people we want (if we want eight, we schedule fifteen) because we know that half of them cannot come. Often, after they come once, they call and say they would like to keep coming but can't because their employers won't give permission to go to the hospital four times in a month.

My dream is to work in the community; we think this is appropriate for a group working on sexuality. Then we could work with the women not only in places such as mothers' clubs but also within schools. It is easier for us to go the community than for them to come to the hospital. As a university-based medical clinic, we have not yet been able to organize this.

Kirsten: Are you training other professionals in your clinic in the SEP to increase the pool of facilitators?

Maggie: As of now, we have four nurses (I am one), a social worker, and two psychologists—all women—who have been trained and regularly work as facilitators. There are also a nurse, two psychologists, and a physician who have had some training in sexuality and sometimes coordinate groups, but because they are involved in other activities, they are not always available. Facilitators receive theoretical training, after which they observe a session and later coordinate other sessions.

We are still looking for funding to develop a training curriculum that includes gender and sexuality for traditional family planning counselors. In our own clinic, training for family planning counselors includes only one module on sexuality.

We also receive requests from other family planning clinics to train their professionals in running a SEP.

Kirsten: How did you get the staff at your clinic or within the SEP to participate in the program? You mentioned that during training, educators had a chance to explore their own attitudes about this issue. Did you experience any tensions or resistance among staff?

Maggie: Active resistance doesn't exist. But one very noticeable thing happened. After doing the initial research, I personally recruited women for the SEP because they had voiced their complaints to me during a family planning consultation. When I stopped working in the clinic and only conducted the SEP, the number of women with sexual complaints suddenly decreased. Why? The nurses and physicians working in the clinic said that the women didn't complain anymore: "I don't think they have any problems." So we put a poster in the waiting room that said "If you have any doubts or if you would like to talk with us about your sexual life, please call Maggie or Débora," and the number of women registering increased again. My guess is that the nurses and physicians don't have any time and they don't create an opportunity during the consultation for women to complain about their sexual lives.

Kirsten: You mention that one of your reasons for getting into this was the link women made between using contraception and their sexual problems. Have you noticed that women at the end of the counseling and education change their contraceptive behavior? Do they become more satisfied that their problems weren't method related to begin with?

Maggie: I think if all clinic staff were trained in sexuality, the results would probably be better. Those of us working on sexuality in the clinic are a small group, and the rest of the staff are not prepared. We have trained the nurses who do the counseling and education work, but the women are in touch with a lot of people in the clinic, and it is not easy to control all the messages they receive. We are a university hospital, and it is very difficult to influence the residents who are rotating through other services. As a result, many times, if a woman using the pill comes to the clinic and complains about a decrease in her libido, the doctor only thinks to change the pill dosage. This reinforces the notion that only the pill affects sexuality and does nothing to address the other causes that may contribute to her lack of desire. Many times, women are still told that condoms negatively affect their sexual pleasure.

Evaluation

Kirsten: You conducted an evaluation of the program and found that many women felt that their problems were solved. How do they describe their problem as being solved?

Maggie: We found that 30 percent of the women said that their problems had improved completely. In this case, typically, the problem was only a lack of information or that they never felt orgasm because they never allowed their partners to touch them.

So those women who don't have any problems in their emotional relationships begin to feel and say that their problems are solved. Another 60 percent felt that they had solved their problems partially. They now feel orgasm but want to have a more equal relationship with their partners. They understand that they need to talk a little more; they need to get respect.

Kirsten: Along those lines, how far can you get by reaching just women in your education program?

Maggie: In fact, many of the women feel that it is important for their partners to also participate in a similar group for men. Recently, we began working with a male physician—a gynecologist and sex therapist—on gender. We trained him to conduct some of the sessions with women (we were curious to see what would happen). It was good in some aspects, but overall, we found that his presence inhibited the women from openly sharing in the group. So our plan is to have him work with men-only groups. These men do not necessarily have to be partners or husbands of the women who have sexual complaints. The intention is to offer this sex education course to all interested men with the hope that ultimately they will play a more active and informed role in the decision-making process about contraception and sexuality. Through our efforts to focus on gender and male involvement, we hope that our work with men will complement our work with women.

Also, when women don't solve their problems by the end of the group, we offer them the possibility of counseling with a specialist in the clinic. But usually the problem is with her partner, not the woman, and our specialist is a woman, so the men won't go to her. That is another reason that we began working with this male physician.

Kirsten: In your initial study and intervention, the number of women who thought that their sexual problems were linked to their contraceptive methods dropped from 50 percent to 5 percent. Do you find that women who participate in the SEP want to switch methods because they become more comfortable with a barrier method? Does using a condom become more of an option for women after the exercise of touching their bodies, for example?

Maggie: I think so. I think that those who participate have more interest in changing and the freedom to change methods, even when they realize that the method is not related to their sexual problems. Since they have been given permission to touch their bodies, they now have no problem using methods such as the diaphragm or condom. We have more women accepting these methods.

Débora remembers a woman who came to the group this year. She and her partner were using withdrawal because they didn't like to use a condom. This method was causing sexual problems for the woman, but still, they didn't want to use any other method. After the group, they decided to use a condom.

Kirsten: Do you think that offering a SEP improves women's access to contraception? For example, do women come to the clinic just because they know that this will be offered?

Maggie: Yes. Many women who had never come to the clinic for family planning services heard about the SEP group from a friend or another woman and were interested and called for more information. Other women who attended the SEP but were not using contraception came to the family planning clinic later.

Lessons Learned

Kirsten: In your experience, are the complaints Brazilian women have similar to complaints of women in other countries?

Maggie: Yes, I think so. In Latin America, I do training for family planning providers in Peru, Chile, Colombia, and so forth. Providers in other countries say that the complaints of women are the same, and they always ask us to provide training on how they can help women. In the last year, I have begun to include a module about sexuality and another about gender to help providers understand about the women who come to the family planning clinic and why it is important to talk about sexuality and contraception with them.[1]

In 1992, we participated in the Association for Voluntary Surgical Contraception's counseling workshop in Istanbul and met other nurse-midwives from Africa and Asia. At the beginning of this meeting, only those of us from Latin America talked about sexuality. We said, "It is important to include sexuality in the content of family planning training and as a matter of counseling," but this was not really picked up by the group. On the third day, however, after I presented a paper on our program experience, they came to us and said, "In our country, the problems are the same. Women feel used by their husbands, and they never feel orgasm or desire. But they need to feel this." They recognized that this is a very important issue. It was a communication breakthrough for us.

Kirsten: What were the surprises in all this—in the research, implementation, or evaluation—for you?

Maggie: I thought, as do many other professionals, that the only parameters, the only variables that mean satisfaction in sex are desire and orgasm. I learned a lot from the women. Now I realize that desire and orgasm do not necessarily mean satisfaction in a woman's life. They are two variables, but not necessarily the only variables.

This realization contributed to a change in the program's structure. When I did my preparation work, I was very worried about sexual dysfunctions and the techniques to correct them. But once I began working with the group, I realized that it was more important to start building women's self-esteem and change how they feel about themselves in order for them to find their own solutions. This is most important, because once I give them the elements of sexuality, they find their own solutions. Because I am a nurse and we study to be paternalistic and solve others' problems for them, I never believed that they would be able to solve their own problems.

Kirsten: Can you remember a woman who had what you thought was a clinical problem but who was able to solve it on her own when she had some help with her self-esteem?

Maggie: Yes, there are many cases. I remember a twenty-five-year-old woman who came to the group complaining about not having orgasms with her husband. During the group sessions, she told us that she was also having sexual relations with her father and that this had been going on since she was a girl. She explained that she had orgasms with her father, but not with her husband.

When she began in the group, her self-esteem was very low. She felt "dirty and guilty for this situation," and she felt that "all the other people were aware" of her situation. In the group sessions, we focused on improving her self-esteem and addressed her feelings of blame.

Some months after the sex education course, she came back to talk to us. Her physical appearance clearly showed that she had changed. She seemed to be a new woman. She told us that after her participation in the group, she was able to have a different relationship with her father and that he never again asked her to have sex with him. Now she can comfortably visit her father with her husband. In addition, her relationship with her husband has improved, communication in the relationship has improved, and she is now enjoying sex with her husband and reaching orgasm.

Kirsten: Looking back over your experiences, is there anything you would do differently next time?

Maggie: When we started the program, we were oriented toward clinical sexual education. Now the perspective of gender is stronger, because our own conscience, information, and learning during the last year told us that this is important. Now the goal is to empower women. We also look forward to working with our male colleagues in reaching out to the women's partners.

Kirsten: Any closing thoughts?

Maggie: Of all the things I have done in the clinic, this program gives me the greatest satisfaction. I am now a trainer in family planning and no longer work in the clinic attending patients. One of the connections I maintain with the clinic is the SEP because I find this work very important. As a trainer of providers, I am incorporating what I learned from the women in the SEP about sexuality and gender into my curriculum.

In the evaluation questionnaire, we ask the women what they learned as a result of this group and if they would like to say something to us. One woman told us that we "had planted a seed" and that she "is never going to let it become dry again." We think that what the women say in their evaluations represents the value of our program better than the numbers.

Notes

We would like to thank Debbie Rogow for her help in arranging this interview, smoothing over our language barriers, and sharing her comments and insights with us.

1. Those interested in receiving more information on this curriculum should contact Margarita Diaz in care of The Population Council, One Dag Hammarskjold Plaza, New York, NY 10017, USA.

Reference

Barbach, Lonnie. 1976. *For yourself: The fulfillment of female sexuality.* New York: Doubleday.

Integrating Laobe Women into AIDS Prevention Strategies

in Kolda, Senegal

Cheikh Ibrahima Niang

*A*frica has over half of the world's HIV-positive individuals, making it the continent most severely hit by the AIDS pandemic (Ona and Platt 1989; Mertens et al. 1994). In Africa, the virus is transmitted primarily through heterosexual contact (Kippax, Crawford, and Waldby 1994), and the power that men exercise in sexual relations has been documented as an HIV risk factor for women (Obbo 1993; Ankrah 1991). In spite of this, initial research on HIV and AIDS focused primarily on mapping the spread of the epidemic rather than identifying the behaviors or power imbalances that may place people at risk of HIV. In the late 1980s, a number of studies finally began to examine sexual behavior in order to determine and understand the social and cultural factors that promote the spread of the epidemic or hamper its prevention (Hrdy 1987; Scott and Mercer 1994).

In 1987, the World Health Organization developed a model instrument for quantitative research studies: knowledge, attitude, and behavior (KAB) surveys that consist of using standardized questionnaires, a research tool commonly used to determine attitudes and behaviors related to family planning. These surveys were initiated in several countries by the early 1990s, with the objective of making comparisons at the national and international levels. However, recent studies have shown the limitations of the KAB approach and questioned its validity and reliability (Schopper et al. 1993). Specifically, the studies tended to project sociocultural standards, taboos, values, and attitudes rather than reflect individual behavior and the realities of the context in which behavior occurs. Additionally, they did not sufficiently explore existing local networks and communication channels relating to sexuality, which provide a valuable source of information. Finally, these research efforts did not sufficiently explore opportunities for interventions that are urgently needed, given the nature of the AIDS pandemic.

In 1990, the International Center for Research on Women (ICRW) initiated the Women and AIDS Research Program to identify factors that influence women's risk of HIV infection and opportunities for AIDS prevention. The program identified two main gaps in existing AIDS prevention efforts with regard to women. First, although epidemiological research indicates that women of all ages and socioeconomic backgrounds are infected with HIV through sexual contact, prevention efforts focused primarily on commercial sex workers. Second, existing interventions paid little attention to the broad social, economic, and cultural context in which high-risk behavior occurs. The program identified the lack of reliable data on women's sexual lives and on the ways in which socioeconomic and cultural factors are determinants of their sexual experiences as deficiencies in HIV prevention efforts. To rectify this, the program supported researchers and practitioners to undertake seventeen research projects in Africa, Asia, the Pacific, Latin America, and the Caribbean (Rao Gupta and Weiss 1993).

In Senegal, the Women and AIDS Research Program supported a research team to work closely with traditional women's associations (the Laobe and Dimba groups) to identify HIV risk factors and to integrate these women into the development and implementation of HIV prevention strategies. This chapter focuses on the research process with the Laobe women, a traditional association of women who control the production and distribution of erotic goods and advice. The work with the Laobe women was particularly illustrative of the principles behind the ICRW project, because it involved in-depth descriptive research on sexuality and sexual behavior conducted by a local researcher, with the opportunity for direct intervention. The research process was unique because it utilized traditional associations and modes of communication to design an innovative intervention. Additionally, the research did not focus on commercial sex work in the traditional sense, yet it exposed some of the complexities behind the commercial and noncommercial exchange of sexual services and products.

Context of the Research

The Laobe are an ethnic group originating in the northern part of Senegal. They migrate from place to place and engage in itinerant activities. The Laobe women play a unique and influential role in the sexual and commercial arenas in the town of Kolda, through the production and distribution of erotic articles and advice. Although some authors regard the Laobe as a lower-level caste within the social organizations of the Wolof and the Peul (Diop 1981), Laobe women are sought after and highly esteemed as wives (they are thought to bring good luck to the men who marry them) or as occasional sexual partners (they are regarded as the most expert in providing sexual pleasure). Kolda, where the research was conducted, is situated in the southern part of Senegal. It has about 40,000 inhabitants who belong to the following principal ethnic groups: Peul, Mandingo, Balant, Wolof, Toucouleur, Manjack, Diola, Baïnounck, and Laobe (Diop 1981).

There is a gender-based local division of labor and activities, and women are generally considered to be responsible for domestic needs such as clothing, expenses of social ceremonies, children's needs, and food. Current economic conditions have made it necessary for women increasingly to resort to adaptive strategies to fulfill these responsibilities. These strategies include small-scale retail trade, itinerant trading, and the commercial and noncommercial exchange of sexual services. In fact, sexuality tends to be controlled by women as a commodity for exchange with men to enhance their economic position; the sexual realm is one arena in which women have some power to fulfill their economic and social needs.

The forms of marriage and marital partnerships are varied and somewhat fluid. The most widespread form of marriage in Senegal is polygamy. In the *département* of Kolda, about 60 percent of all married women live in polygamous households (Ministere de l'Economie, des Finances et du Plan 1992). Furthermore, according to the Senegalese Survey of Fertility (*Enquête Sénégalaise sur la Fécondité* [ESF]), after the first two years of marriage, there is one divorce for every ten marriages, and 20 percent of marriages end in divorce within six years (ESF 1985). Divorced women are often regarded as being relatively liberated from family control; they enjoy greater sexual freedom, which makes them more available for occasional sexual relations.

In Senegal, as in many other societies, it is often considered indecent to talk about sex or sexuality in explicit terms. There is a strong propensity to observe taboos concerning any reference to sex. Parallel with this social modesty, however, there is a complex symbolic language that serves to communicate matters of sex and sexuality. For example, in one tradition, a husband has only to place a razor blade near the toilet, where it will be noticed by his wife, to indicate that he wishes her to cut off warts around or in the vagina, a practice believed to facilitate penetration. Symbolic communication and other ways of enhancing sexual activity make use of the objects and information over which Laobe women exercise a quasi-monopoly, particularly in the Wolof and Peul societies. Additionally, although not explicitly stated, sexuality and sexual technique are generally viewed as a positive part of human life to be enhanced, celebrated, and valued.

Research Methodology

Recognizing women's risk of infection in this context, we were interested in finding culturally acceptable ways of gathering information and developing interventions related to HIV prevention and safer sex—in particular, eroticizing the condom. The cultural context made this strategy seem plausible. Given the influence that Laobe women have in the sexual arena as providers of sex and sexual products and advice, they were identified as a logical and important medium through which to introduce HIV prevention strategies into the community. The research project with the Laobe women had three objectives:

1. To understand the Laobe women's attitudes and practices concerning sexuality;
2. To analyze their interaction with society as a whole; and
3. To integrate condoms for men into the range of products the Laobe women distribute.

The project relied on traditional anthropological research methodology, and the research team consisted of a male anthropologist, who worked primarily with the male partners of Laobe women, and a female physician and female sociologist, who did the bulk of the work with the Laobe women. The female researchers spent a great deal of time building relationships and trust with the Laobe and felt at ease talking "woman to woman."

Initially, observations of Laobe women were made at marketplaces and along the itinerant trade routes they frequented. These observations were accompanied by informal interviews with eighteen Laobe women. Subsequently, in-depth individual interviews (using a semistructured interview guide) were conducted with five men who were occasional sexual partners of Laobe women, with five neighborhood leaders and their first wives, and with sixteen Laobe women selected on the basis of "snowball sampling." Specifically, we made contact with the leader of the Laobe women in the market at Kolda. She then introduced us to her friends, three other Laobe women, who in turn introduced us to their friends, until finally interviews with sixteen Laobe women were attained.

After the qualitative research, we prepared a questionnaire and administered it to 250 men and 250 women selected at random in the population to establish general trends in attitudes and behavior regarding sex and sexuality, as well as the extent of interaction between the community and the Laobe women.

Our Research Partners: The Laobe Women

At the start of our work, the research team defined a unique protocol of exchange with the Laobe women. The basic principle was that the researchers would learn from the Laobe women, to better understand their culture and role in society. The Laobe women were enthusiastic about being recognized as "those who teach" about sexuality and traditional erotic culture. Conversely, after the collection of data from the Laobe women, the researchers would share further information about the status of women and sexual behavior in other cultures and about sexually transmitted disease (STD) and AIDS prevention. This was particularly important for the well-being of the Laobe women, because they do not identify themselves as "commercial sex workers" or "prostitutes," even though they may provide sexual services. They are therefore not eligible for the STD services that are available and mandatory for prostitutes in Senegal.

According to our questionnaire, over half of our entire sample (both men and women) and almost three-quarters of the women buy erotic products from Laobe women. For example, the Laobe women produce and sell a variety of incenses *(cuuray)* to perfume their dwellings and drive away insects and also to arouse men's sexual desire or to create an environment favorable to amorous foreplay. According to one Laobe informant, the type of incense a woman places in a room where a man visits her may indicate whether she wants to see him again. Fragrant powders *(gongo)* also have an important erotic function. Every woman is supposed to have a particular style in combining fragrances. The Laobe women sell the basic ingredients and advise each woman, depending on her age, status, and circumstances, how to personalize her perfume. Laobe women say that a perfumed powder appropriately prepared by a woman should not leave any man sexually indifferent, if it is prepared with his arousal in mind. Additionally, Laobe women concoct plant-based drinks and other potions to augment the sexual attractiveness of women and attract the sexual interest of men. They also sell substances to be introduced into the vagina for erotic purposes, such as powders, small stones, and herbs.

Laobe women also decorate small loincloths used as underclothing. These come in different styles and serve different functions in amorous foreplay. They have various names that anticipate the sexual act and are decorated with drawings of sexual acts or male and female genitalia. These small decorated loincloths are seldom sold at markets but are delivered by the Laobe to the homes of the women who order them.

The most important specialty products of the Laobe are unquestionably their bead necklaces and belts. The necklaces serve as jewelry for women and children and are also used by the latter as talismans to protect against the so-called evil winds. Bead belts vary in shape, size, and significance, depending on the woman's age, her marital status, and the purpose for which the belt is worn. The belts are considered the most intimate articles of women's apparel; the symbolic language of sexual relations uses many references to them. The sound made by the beads hitting one another is considered very erotic, capable of stimulating the most intense sexual desires in men. The Laobe women arrange these beads in a way that produces the desired sound when they walk or dance. The beads are thought to bring good luck to those who obtain them. When a belt worn by a Laobe woman accidentally breaks in public, men and women rush to pick up the beads and guard them jealously.

Laobe women are much sought after for dressing women's hair (plaits) and leading family ceremonies, such as baptisms or weddings. During the course of wedding ceremonies, and particularly on the day after the wedding night, Laobe women conduct singing and dancing sessions, during which they compose poems. These poems praise the bride for her sensual and erotic qualities and constitute veritable hymns to sexual relations, including explicit language describing the sexual organs of men and women. Men, with the exception of musicians, do not participate in these ceremonies. Besides these ceremonies, Laobe women organize their own dance sessions, which are regarded as occasions for demonstrating their erotic talents; everything in the dances and songs evokes the sexual act.

Identified Risky Sexual Practices

In Senegal, there are several monographs that present specific categories of women identified socially as trading in sex (Gamble 1957). However, these studies focus only on one category of women, or "prostitutes," who are often viewed as marginal in society. Women's exchange of sexual services for money, material goods, or other services is, in fact, a much more complex phenomenon and is widespread across a range of social classes. This exchange can be an integral part of sexual networking and providing for the family.

Our qualitative and quantitative research results confirmed the existence of imbalances in socioeconomic and cultural power between men and women and highlighted how these imbalances translate into sexual behavior and exchange that place women at increased risk of HIV. The eroticization of relationships serves more than a sexual function in a context in which economic power is held essentially by men. When women are abandoned (most often for other women), they experience difficult psycho-affective consequences, and the resources the men contribute to their households are diminished. In order to prevent being abandoned and having their resources diminished, many women try to satisfy the erotic desires of men by engaging in sexual practices that place them at risk of HIV, such as cutting vaginal warts or introducing substances into the vagina.

Multiple Partners and Sexual Exchange

In order to avoid the high rate of nonresponse recorded by the KAB studies (Ministere du Plan et de la Cooperation du Senegal 1990), our questionnaire did not include direct or leading questions concerning personal sexual behavior. Rather, we asked our interviewees for their opinions about the behaviors of others, asking, for example, Do you think that many unmarried/married women/men at Kolda change their partners frequently? The majority of the sample responded in the affirmative.

According to the survey, the principal motivations for both unmarried and married women to have multiple sexual partners are related primarily to their economic needs and security. In particular, such behavior enables them to satisfy their needs for clothing and toiletries and to provide for their families. Seeking personal sexual pleasure accounted for less than a fifth of the responses.

The widespread pattern of unmarried women with multiple partners may represent a strategy of substituting for social mechanisms that are failing or are in transition. This strategy is used not only by divorced women. For example, with the current trend away from early marriage, an unemployed and unmarried woman who has reached the age when she ought to be able to rely on a husband may be embarrassed to ask her parents for money to pay for her clothing and toiletry needs. She therefore must "fend for herself" by using her sexuality to acquire financial means. Having several lovers and using a great deal of imagination to keep them from finding out about one another may be an element in the search for optimal combinations of resource possibilities, although sentimental motivations cannot be totally excluded.

Similarly, with regard to the principal motivations for the extra-marital relations of married women, the most frequent answers related to meeting toiletry, clothing, and food needs. Another motivation that did not appear in the quantitative analysis but was referred to several times during the qualitative interviews is the exchange of sexual services for money so that women can fulfill their social obligations during family ceremonies. These are expensive occasions, and, depending on their position within the network of family relationships, women have obligations to provide gifts and incur ceremonial expenses for the family in order to avoid loss of prestige.

Vaginal Cosmetics

The introduction of substances into the vagina for erotic purposes has been identified in certain countries as a practice that increases the risk of infection with the AIDS virus by irritating or upsetting the natural chemical balance of the vagina and increasing the risk of other infections (Runganga et al. 1992; Brown et al. 1993). In Kolda and various other localities in Senegal, we learned that the vagina is not considered a simple, natural part of the body; it is viewed as an erotic "work of art" that can be enhanced by the use of perfumes and the introduction of other substances (some women place incense between their legs in order to perfume the vagina). This practice is called *Safal* in the Wolof language, which means "heightening the quality of the taste." The substances introduced may be roots of certain plants that have been dried and specially prepared by Laobe women; powders and pebbles imported from Mali or from the Middle East; or cones, lozenges, and other pharmaceutical products that have a therapeutic purpose. The practice is believed to augment the male partner's pleasure by simultaneously constricting the vagina and increasing vaginal lubrication.

One of our Laobe women informants explained the practice as one in a range of sexual strategies that women use to get and keep sexual partners. "Men are the ones who run after the girls. When a girl is young and unmarried, she should attract the man by letting him fantasize about what sexual relations with her would be like. On the other hand, a married woman is expected to maintain her position by acting in such a way that the man always feels he is rediscovering sexual pleasure every time he has sexual relations with her, and she should show him that sex with her is the best, so that he will not be tempted by other women."

Of the 250 women in our sample, over three-quarters responded to the question regarding whether they introduced substances into their vaginas for erotic purposes. Of these, over a third stated that they had engaged in this practice at one time or another, and these respondents included practically all ethnic groups present in Kolda. However, a significant difference was found between married women (about 24 percent of all affirmative replies) and unmarried women (about 20 percent). Women between thirty-one and forty years of age were the largest group who engaged in this practice.

Introducing and Eroticizing the Condom

Our research team worked with the Laobe women to associate condoms with one of the products they sell—the loincloth—thereby eroticizing the condom. The Laobe women with whom we worked now call the condom "keep it hard," a name coined with reference to the name of the loincloth with which it is linked. The loincloth bears erotic drawings and is called "make it hard," implying that the man's erection should be hard and that condoms can help maintain erections.

Additionally, Laobe women use their own image to promote the condom. They are perceived as being endowed with great physical beauty and knowing a great deal about how to maintain this beauty and the good health that goes with it. They therefore emphasize that women must use the condom in order to stay beautiful and healthy. Laobe women promote condoms not only among other women who buy their products, particularly the customers who buy the loincloths, but also among men who want their products, advice, or sexual services.

The Laobe women play an important role as direct sources of information and as intermediaries for communication and information about sexuality and sexual behavior in the population as a whole. The work done at Kolda enabled us to identify erotic practices in the community that involve risk of HIV infection. These practices, deeply rooted in the local cultures, have become strategies used by women to influence the sexual decisions of their male partners, including limiting the number of partners they have. Additionally, we identified patterns of sexual behavior that seemed to arise in response to economic and social motivations, in a context characterized by a scarcity of resources and a growing number of domestic needs. In a context in which sexual products and technique play an important role in human relations, our work with the Laobe women created interesting possibilities for HIV prevention—namely, the eroticization and introduction of condoms and safer sex practices, such as nonpenetrative sex.

However, the intervention faces several challenges. One problem is the sustainability of any intervention involving Laobe women because of their extreme migratory mobility and our anticipated need to work with new groups of Laobe women. Additionally, although women may become interested in the idea of using condoms, they must negotiate condom use with their male sexual partners. Within marital relations, we found that women seem to have little power to make their partners use condoms. In extramarital relations, however, they seem more capable of doing so. (Although extramarital relations are never mentioned explicitly, the implicit references are unmistakable.) It is in these relationships in particular that Laobe women are promoting the use of condoms.

Although the intervention does not challenge, and in fact may reinforce, existing gender-based power imbalances in the social and economic arenas, it does offer the possibility of an immediate tool that will enable some women to protect themselves from HIV and other sexually transmitted infections. Additionally, the intervention introduces a conversation about condom use and safer sex into a complex arena of sexual communication and exchange.

In the next stage of the project, we will evaluate the process of introducing and eroticizing the condom through traditional associations and modes of sexual communication within a context of growing economic and social pressures on women. We will examine the immediate outcomes of the intervention on attitudes toward condoms, condom use, knowledge of HIV and other STDS, and health-seeking behavior. Additionally, we will analyze the sociocultural impact of the intervention on communication patterns, gender relations, and future HIV prevention strategies for women.

Note

All the data presented in this article are taken from a project carried out with the financial support of the U.S. Agency for International Development, which we received through the International Center for Research on Women, located in Washington, D.C. The ICRW also contributed indispensable technical support for the accomplishment of this project; in this connection, we extend our thanks especially to Geeta Rao Gupta, Ellen Weiss, and Daniel Whelan. Additionally, I would like to thank Sia Nowrojee, consultant to the Population Council, for reviewing and improving the quality of this paper.

References

Ankrah M. 1991. AIDS and the social side of health. *Social Science and Medicine* 32(9):967–80.

Brown, E. J., et al. 1993. Dry and tight sexual practices and potential AIDS risk in Zaire. *Social Science and Medicine* 37(8):989–94.

Diop, A. B. 1981. *La société Wolof.* Paris: Karthala.

Enquête Sénégalaise sur la Fécondité. 1985. *Nuptialité et fécondité au Sénégal.* Paris: Presses Universitaires de France.

Gamble, D. P. 1957. *The Wolof of Senegambia.* London: InterAfrican Institute.

Hrdy, D. 1987. Cultural practices contributing to the transmission of human immunodeficiency virus in Africa. *Reviews of Infectious Diseases* 9(6):1109–19.

Kippax, S., J. Crawford, and C. Waldby. 1994. Heterosexuality, masculinity and HIV. *AIDS* 8(suppl. 1):S315–23.

Mertens, T. E., et al. 1994. Global estimates and epidemiology of HIV infections and AIDS. *AIDS* 8(suppl. 1):S361–72.

Ministere de l'Economie, des Finances et du Plan, Senegal. 1992. *Recensement général de la population et de l'habitat de 1988*. Dakar: Author.

Ministere du Plan et de la Cooperation du Senegal. 1990. *La société Sénégalaise au SIDA*. Dakar: Author.

Obbo, C. 1993. HIV transmission: Men are the solution. *Population and Environment: A Journal of Interdisciplinary Studies* 14(3):211–43.

Ona Pela, A., and J. J. Platt. 1989. AIDS in Africa: Emerging trends. *Social Science and Medicine* 28(1):1–8.

Rao Gupta, G., and E. Weiss. 1993. *Women and AIDS: Developing a new health strategy*. Washington, D.C.: International Center for Research on Women.

Runganga, A., et al. 1992. The use of herbal and other agents to enhance sexual experience. *Social Science and Medicine* 35(8):1037–42.

Schopper, D., et al. 1993. Sexual behaviors relevant to HIV transmission in a rural African population. *Social Science and Medicine* 37(3): 401–12.

Scott, S. J., and M. A. Mercer. 1994. Understanding cultural obstacles to HIV/AIDS prevention in Africa. *AIDS Education and Prevention* 7(1): 81–89.

A Community Study of Gynecological Disease in Indian Villages

Some Experiences and Reflections

Rani Bang and Abhay Bang

*I*n third world countries, most women tend to encounter the health care system only when they are the target of family planning programs. Little attention has been given to the reproductive health of nonpregnant women. One reason for the relative neglect of gynecological care is a failure to appreciate the extent of unmet needs in rural areas (Bang, Bang, et al. 1989).

In Gadchiroli, a remote, backward district in the central part of India, where we run a nongovernmental organization called Society for Education, Action and Research in Community Health (SEARCH), we did a community-based study of gynecological problems of rural women, the first study of its kind in the developing world. In the study, we sought to determine: (1) the prevalence, types, and distribution of gynecological diseases in rural women; (2) the awareness and perceptions of the women about their gynecological and sexual disorders; and (3) the proportion of women who have access to gynecological care.

The study team (a female gynecologist with ten years' experience as a consultant, a physician, a pathologist, a laboratory technician, a nurse, and female social workers) visited the field camp and conducted the study. Female social workers, village leaders, and volunteers invited all females who were older than twelve years old or who had reached menarche to participate in the study, whether or not they had symptoms. A field camp was set up in the village, with facilities for private interviews and pelvic examinations, a pathology laboratory, and an operating theater. Information was obtained on personal history, socioeconomic status; perceptions and practices regarding gynecological symptoms; past experience of care; and obstetrical, gynecological, and sexual history. The women then had general physical examinations including speculum examinations and bimanual examinations of the pelvis; unmarried girls with intact hymens had rectal rather than vaginal examinations (Bang, Bang, et al. 1989). Women who were found to have disease were offered treatment.

The findings were startling. Ninety-two percent of the women suffered from gynecological diseases. Each woman had an average of 3.6 diseases, but only 7 percent of the women had ever sought medical care.

This study generated interest in women's gynecological diseases as a public health problem in various parts of the world. Many groups interested in women's health are now initiating similar types of studies in their own areas (see the chapter "Involving Women in a Reproductive Morbidity Study in Egypt" in this volume). But epidemiological and anthropological studies on reproductive health are relatively new, and research methods have not been perfected. Hence, along with hard data, observations and experiences about the process need to be documented and shared. In this chapter, we recount some of our personal experiences during the process of conducting this study, with the hope that they may be of use to others. Methodology will gradually evolve out of such soft data. We do not, however, intend to suggest that others should necessarily repeat what we did. There could be a hundred other ways of reaching the same goal.

There is one possible exception, however. During the evolution of the idea for this study, as well as while working on it, we realized that reproductive health involves both males and females. To be successful, any study of reproductive health should involve a team of male and female researchers. We have experienced the fruitfulness of combined perspectives in our own work, time and again.

Getting Started

The Story behind the Study

We, Rani and Abhay, were classmates during medical school. Subsequently, Rani did her M.D. in obstetrics and gynecology, and Abhay, though inclined to pursue public health, gained an M.D. in internal medicine. When we decided to marry, we didn't realize the public health potential implicit in our particular combination of professional backgrounds and interests. But, as a couple sharing the same profession, we often talked at the dinner table about various types of patients seen during the day. Rani enjoyed telling stories and anecdotes about cases from the clinic; Abhay enjoyed listening to them and thinking them over. One evening, Abhay observed that it seemed from Rani's description that the majority of women in society were suffering from one gynecological problem or another. How could it be such a frequent occurrence?

Clinic records did not reveal what proportion of women in the area had gynecological diseases. Could Rani substantiate our suspicions? Rani counted the number of women residing in a housing colony whom she had recently treated for gynecological problems. Surprisingly, it turned out that almost half of the women in the colony were suffering from gynecological diseases. That fact was astonishing.

Abhay said, "I don't know of any estimate of the burden of gynecological diseases in a community. Maybe no one has realized the magnitude and frequency of this problem. If what you have experienced is representative, then gynecological diseases may turn out to be a major public health problem. We should intensively and systematically study a community or a defined population to estimate the prevalence and incidence of gynecological diseases. It may be an eye-opener!"

Preparation for the Study

Later, when we were studying at Johns Hopkins for master's degrees in public health, we did a computerized literature search on population-based studies of gynecological diseases in developing countries and found that there were none! There were many studies on screening populations for cervical carcinoma or syphilis, but no estimates of the vast array of gynecological problems of women— such as white discharge, vaginitis, cervicitis, pelvic inflammatory disease, or menstrual problems. Our belief that a study on the prevalence of gynecological diseases needed to be done became stronger.

We were fortunate to meet Professor Carl Taylor at Johns Hopkins School of Public Health. He introduced us to established research methods in public health and also guided us in developing a study protocol for the community study of gynecological diseases. We learned from him the absolute prerequisites of clearly stated, measurable objectives; a study design; sampling; definition of various diagnostic entities; and data collection instruments, including the creation of dummy tables.

The reasons that no one had conducted such a study soon became obvious to us. Intending to help us develop the protocol, Professor Taylor introduced us to a senior American gynecologist who had headed obstetrics and gynecology departments in developing countries for years. He kept wondering why we wanted to estimate prevalence and incidence. He thought that instead we should take direct action by treating the gynecological diseases of women who came to clinics or hospitals. He also said, "How does it matter if many women have white discharge? Just as many people get the common cold or have nasal discharge; is it of any consequence? You are wasting your time measuring trivialities!"

As we attempted to raise funds over the next two years (1984–85), we frequently heard similar discouraging comments. "Measuring prevalence of gynecological disorders? Why? What for? Aren't there more serious diseases?" But Professor Ramalin- gaswamy, who was then director general of the Indian Council of Medical Research, and the Ford Foundation's New Delhi office decided to put trust in us and in our ideas. We got the necessary financial support.

Selection of Villages

In 1986, we started SEARCH and moved to Gadchiroli, a district that was relatively new to us. Our clinical work in the hospital helped us rapidly gain the confidence of the local population, and people from surrounding villages started contacting us about various problems. Gradually, the personalities of individual villages became known to us. We finally selected two villages—Wasa and Amirza—for the study of gynecological diseases.

They were average, representative villages as far as socioeconomic and demographic characteristics were concerned. They were relatively distant from town, but not too remote. They had united communities and backgrounds of collective action. For example, the entire Amirza village had once boycotted voting in an election because the government had not constructed the much needed approach road. A community study of gynecological diseases required a collective decision and the cooperation of the whole village, since all women, whether they had symptoms or not, were to be examined in order to estimate true population prevalence. Wasa and Amirza had educated village leaders who could understand the need for such a study and actively mobilize the village community.

In Wasa, a small mission hospital was used as the base to conduct the study. In Amirza, Lambe Guruju, a bachelor teacher, vacated his own house and made the necessary renovations to enable us to conduct the study. Each woman participating was required to visit five rooms: registration, interview by a female social worker, history and examination by a female gynecologist, pathology laboratory, and dispensary. The interview and examination were conducted in privacy. A woman cannot be at ease if she feels that there is a threat of being overheard or watched during such an interview and examination.

Interacting with the Community

Community Participation

Why should villagers participate in such a study? This was a million-dollar question and one that we thought was important to address directly with the community. Due to the aggressive family planning program, people are always afraid of veiled family planning activity. It is necessary to remove this apprehension before beginning any study of gynecological diseases.

With the help of village leaders, group meetings of villagers were held, separately for women and men, to explain the need for and the nature of the study. The village people, especially the leaders, were informed that this was a research study that would help their women and also have the policy impact of improving the health of womankind elsewhere. Such meetings helped in two ways. Villagers did not harbor suspicion about being used—this was a sort of informed consent of the community. And they felt proud that they were helping to bring out information on women's reproductive health to the whole world. It was not just our study or research project; it was their research project.

The inauguration of the study was organized by the villagers with tremendous enthusiasm and fanfare. The whole village observed a holiday, and community dinners were served to about a hundred guests in both villages. The idea and nature of the study were again explained. This also helped remove the suspicion and fear in women that our study could be a family planning camp under some different garb.

Involving Men

It was essential to involve men for several reasons. They are the decision makers in the family and, if not convinced, they might not allow their women to participate in the study. However, they worry about the health of their wives, sexual relations, and the health of their progeny, and most of the women communicate with their husbands about their reproductive health problems. In our study, when we asked, "Have you spoken to anybody about your gynecological complaint?" 80 percent replied yes. When asked with whom, 76 percent responded that they had communicated with their husbands.

In another vivid example, a woman came to us for white discharge. When asked how she first noticed it, she responded that she and her husband both took baths every night and were very particular about their sexual cleanliness. But they noticed a foul odor at the time of intercourse and were worried. Each thought that it was not his or her problem. To prove it, they smelled each other's genitals and discharge and reached the conclusion that something was wrong with the wife. Therefore, she came for the checkup.

But many men remain ignorant about reproductive health and women's suffering. If they are made aware, they can help and can persuade their women to seek health care. For example, when we organized a camp for village chiefs and showed them slides on reproductive health, they remarked, "Oh! We never knew that our women suffer from such problems! Now we know the causes and understand that these can be easily detected and treated."

Village Volunteers

The village volunteers, who were all young men from the community, were a great asset in conducting the study. Why did these young men, unpaid for this work, take an interest in the study of women's gynecological diseases? Months later, they told us, "We educated, unemployed youth while away our time and hence are usually considered vagabonds in our own village. One day, we were told that two America-returned doctors were coming to Amirza for some work. We awaited you with the idea of doing some innocent mischief. When you came, we couldn't believe that you were such America-returned doctors—wearing simple Indian-style dress of *khadi*. You spoke to us in local dialect. At that moment, we decided to help you in whatever you wanted to do!" What mattered most to them was not the topic of the study or the potential significance of the research but how we dressed and talked! Those young men, besides their contribution to the study, have taught us a lot. Three of them later became our full-time workers and took a leading part in a campaign against alcohol.

These volunteers did the population enumeration and made a list of all women in the village eligible for the study. They suggested the idea of giving each woman an appointment for her examination. They gave several reasons. Since women have household work and also work in the field, they can't abandon their routines and wait at the study site indefinitely for their turns. In addition, women in the area have a notion that they should come for abdominal and pelvic examinations with an empty stomach. Hence, unnecessary waiting should be avoided.

Later, we learned another reason that women must be told at least a few days before they will be examined. Some women hesitated about participating in the study on the day of the appointment because they were not "clean and ready." We observed that practically all rural women came with clean-shaved pubic areas; rural women consider it indecent to expose their hairy vulvas. Since women remove the hair by plucking it out with their hands—quite a painful and time-consuming job—they definitely need prior notice to clean themselves.

The volunteers gave each eligible woman an identity card with the date and approximate time to come to the study site written on it. The study was conducted three days a week for five months. The volunteers would go to each woman on the evening prior to her appointment and remind her of the next day's appointment for the study. If they found any resistance, they tried to persuade the women by getting help from other women or leaders, if necessary. There was a waiting list, and if one woman could not come for any reason, the next one on the waiting list would be called. This was a skillfully handled, organized operation.

Providing Treatment

All the women participating in the study who had any disease were given treatment, free of cost. This was both an ethical and a practical necessity. And although the study addressed only gynecological diseases, people's health needs know no such boundaries. Other types of diseases needed equal attention. Hence, Abhay treated the medical problems of the women in the study and also provided services to husbands and other family members. This had a positive impact in eliciting cooperation.

For example, in Amirza, the landlord's wife, an elderly woman, had been sick and inactive for fifteen years. She had tried all sorts of therapies without any relief. Abhay diagnosed her as suffering from myxedema (hypothyroidism) and treated her. The response to treatment was so dramatic that the woman's total appearance and life were changed. This gave us an instant reputation in the village as "good doctors." Such a reputation helped elicit wider participation in the study, though it was not the sole determinant.

Women who were found to have gynecological problems were asked to come back with their husbands and other close family members. The problem was explained to them with the help of sketches. Women and men were shown abnormal findings in the pathology tests, such as worms in stools, microfilaria in blood smears, and *Trichomonas vaginalis* and *Candida* in vaginal smears.

Because of these explanations, people were convinced about the need for, and usefulness of, laboratory tests.

Nonparticipation

Since the study was population based, requiring the participation of all or most of the eligible women (regardless of the presence of symptoms), our two greatest challenges were full participation in all aspects of the study and unbiased participation in the perception study. Several issues hindered participation. Because we wanted to do perception studies simultaneously with the medical exams, we did not explain to the women how the internal examination was done or educate them about the anatomy, physiology, or diseases of the reproductive organs prior to the study. Since only 7.8 percent of the women examined had received previous gynecological care, most were totally ignorant about the process of gynecological history taking and pelvic examination. After the first few days of the study, a rumor spread in the village: "Oh! It's very vulgar! *[Nanga nanga ahe.]* They ask obscene questions; that lady doctor wears a big gunny bag [glove] and inserts the whole arm inside the vagina!" Women who heard these rumors were afraid to participate in the study.[1]

When we heard this, we sent our social worker to explain the truth. We showed the women leaders, the *dais* (traditional birth attendants), and the friends accompanying the women being examined how the internal examination was done. We showed them gloves and explained why we needed to wear them. This, of course, helped a lot. Many women had cervical erosion or cervicitis, and when other women saw this, they were convinced of the need for and importance of an internal examination. We learned that women did not have much of a problem being observed by other trusted village women. In retrospect, we believe that we even could have fixed a mirror so that women could see their own examinations in progress.

If we had provided adequate education and explanation before starting the study, problems of misunderstanding would not have become a major threat. Researchers who are interested in measuring gynecological morbidity without doing perception studies should first use various methods (slides, posters, group discussions) to explain the whole process to women. If there is a risk of modifying perceptions with these explanations, the perception study should be done first, with the gynecological morbidity study done only after an educational phase.

Another problem arose in Wasa, the first study site. Whenever we found unmarried girls manifesting physical evidence of having had sex, our own ideas of morality would compel us to preach to the girl about the risks of such behavior. The result of our behavior was that everyone, especially the unmarried girls in the village, came to know that by examining them, the lady doctor could find out the secrets of their sexual lives. The unmarried girls started avoiding participation in the study.

In one family, there were two unmarried girls eligible for the study. The mother came for her examination, but the two daughters never turned up, despite repeated efforts of village leaders, volunteers, and social workers to convince them. In the end, the father of those girls told our social worker, "See! I know my daughters are not good. If they go for examination, the lady doctor is sure to know about their affairs, and my image in the doctor's eyes will be lowered. So it is better that I don't send my daughters for examination."

We had learned our lesson. In the next study village, Amirza, we had to train ourselves to keep our mouths shut and refrain from preaching, even though we saw evidence of premarital sex. The participation of unmarried girls was quite high in Amirza.

Gynecological disease is a sensitive area of inquiry. In spite of our best efforts, only about 60 percent of the eligible women in these two villages participated in the study. One way of handling the nonparticipation of the other 40 percent was to investigate whether nonparticipants were in any way different from the participants. As we described in a paper published in *Lancet*, a random sample survey showed that this was not the case (Bang, Bang, et al. 1989).

Talking to Women

Problems of Language

In taking the women's sexual and health histories, we learned about the importance of knowing the local usage of language for effective communication. Women often present their complaints in the form of symptoms that, in their culture, mean something different from their literal meaning. In our area, if a woman has a white discharge, she will say, "I have weakness." If the doctor does not take this as a clue and ask her the leading question, "Do you have white discharge?" the real complaint is missed.

We recollect now that when we were working as resident doctors in the medical college, Nagpur, which is 200 kilometers from Gadchiroli, at least 50 percent of the female patients in the busy medical or gynecological outpatient department were diagnosed as having "general debility," and were treated with vitamins. No disease could be detected in these women, whose main complaint was "weakness." Now we understand what they wanted to communicate. In retrospect, we see how futile were the vitamins dished out to thousands of such women in one single hospital, day in and day out, when they really sought care for the unspeakable symptom of white discharge. Since we doctors learn medicine in English and do not know the subtler meanings of the terms women use, such as "weakness," communication is faulty.[2]

Medical personnel and social workers need to know the local terms for specific medical problems. Gadchiroli has a rich local vocabulary, for example, *balant dosh* for puerperal psychosis, *padar* or *pandhara pani* for white discharge, *khaira dharane* for pain in one leg during pregnancy, or *mama-bhachich dukh* for the afterpains of delivery.

It is important to understand not only the spoken language and its complexities but also "sign language." Women often don't speak out their symptoms but make signs or gestures, by which the health care provider is supposed to guess the symptom or the disease. For example, in a case of a prolapsed uterus, a woman may not utter a single word but convey the problem with a particular sign, using her hands. There are some symptoms that the patient is not supposed to state at all. In the case of sterility, the sterile woman signals other women to talk while she keeps mum.

Some words also have double meanings. For example, while eliciting the medical histories, we asked, "How many children do you have?" In the local language in Gadchiroli, it is constructed as, "How many boys do you have?" (*Tumhala kiti mulan ahet?*). Because the word *mulan* means "boys" as well as "children," women often told us only the number of boys they had. Therefore, we had to ask them separately for the numbers of boys and girls and for the numbers of dead children, stillbirths, and abortions. Women generally avoided talking about pregnancy loss because, as one woman expressed it, "What is the use of telling that? It has gone to God!"

Underreporting of Disease

We also began to see the prevalence of underreporting or under-recording of symptoms. There are a number of reasons for this. Definite perceptions exist about what is "normal" and what is "abnormal" in terms of gynecological health. For example, women in our area believe that heavy menstrual flow is normal and desirable and would not report it as a complaint. Since they linked sterility with black-colored menses, instead of talking about sterility, women complain of "black menses." We medical professionals might ignore dark-colored menses, considering it normal.

We also learned that women often reveal one set of symptoms or history to the doctor and another to the social worker. For example, while examining one woman who came to us at the study site, we found that she had fresh injury marks on her body, which made it look as if someone had beaten her. When asked about the marks, she said without any hesitation that her husband had beaten her. We were annoyed and gave her a dose of feminist reason: "It is criminal to beat a woman like this, why do you tolerate it?" She very calmly said, "Oh! What is wrong in that? He came home tired from the field in the evening, and my food was not ready, so he beat me as he was very hungry. It was not his fault. It was natural for him."

As soon as we finished her examination and sent her for pathology tests, the social worker came to us excited and said, "Did she tell you her story?" When we answered yes, the social worker said, "But do you know why he beats her?" We said, "Yes, because she does not cook the food on time! But this is no way to treat a wife. We will call the husband and talk to him." The social worker laughed and told us the story that the woman had told her: that she had conceived in spite of her husband's vasectomy, through an illegitimate relationship. The pregnancy was quietly terminated, but the husband came to know about it. From then on, he suspected her fidelity and regularly beat her. However, the woman continued her illegitimate relationship with her lover, who had accompanied her that day to the study site and was still sitting in the corridor. Thus, it was important to compare both histories in this measurement of reproductive morbidity.

There was always underreporting of stillbirths. *Dais* refused to admit having ever conducted a delivery resulting in a stillborn baby. We initially suspected that *dais* concealed this information to keep up their reputations as successful *dais*. But later on we realized that *dais* had no concept of uterine power in the mechanism of labor. They believed that the babies came out as a result of their own bodily movements. They asked us, "If the baby dies inside the womb, how can it come out? It is impossible! It must be alive to come out, and die later on."

In general, women in traditional Indian society are conditioned from childhood to tolerate pain and discomfort without making any fuss. Therefore, they don't report symptoms even if they have them. They believe that it is women's destiny to suffer from these problems. Many women said, "Under any circumstances, we can't afford to take to bed as sick, because then who will do the household work?" So they continue to suffer and work, which makes family members believe that they do not have any problems. And some women fear that if they reveal that they have a gynecological problem or disease, their husbands may desert them. Besides, when traditional Indian men or women go to medical practitioners, they do not necessarily voice their symptoms or complaints. When the doctor asks about their complaints, they say, "*You* tell us what problem we have!" People believe that it is the job of the medical professional to recognize the complaints or disease of the patient. The attitude is, if the patient has to tell his or her complaints, what is the doctor there for?

Finally, in spite of all the precautions taken to record symptoms, there can still be women who have "silent disease." In this study, we found that 45 percent of the women with gynecological diseases were asymptomatic.

Taking Sexual Histories

We saw that women, and men, too, are often ignorant about the technical language for orgasm, foreplay, and other aspects of their sexuality. We have to explain to them what we mean before we inquire about such issues. Our experience has been that once they do open up, people talk freely about their sexual lives and problems.

We learned that women experienced anxiety and stress because of disturbed marital relationships. For example, one young woman from Wasa, aged twenty-two years, complained of severe weakness and loss of weight. She looked quite ill and tense. On medical examination, no abnormality was found. We called her back for a special appointment and talked to her in private. She told her story with tears in her eyes. She had been married seven years ago. She and her husband loved each other. Their house had only one room with no privacy, and the young woman's mother-in-law slept in the same room, with her head near the legs of the couple, so they could not have sex without waking her. The mother-in-law asserted her power by controlling the availability of sex to the young couple. The husband would climax within two minutes, and the young woman was never satisfied. (God knows about his satisfaction!) But because of shyness and guilt, the young couple would not protest to the old woman—despite their severe anxiety. The young woman told us, "My mother-in-law openly says that she never got any sexual satisfaction from her husband and this son of hers would not give any to her daughter-in-law."

Even old women gave histories of regular sexual relationships. The old women would sheepishly justify, "Chikhalala pani suta-narach," which meant "Mud will always hold some water in it." This was their way of saying that even when old, the body will always have sexual desire, and both men and women will always have some secretions.

———

After the study was completed, the findings of the study (except those about premarital sex) were shared with the villagers through group meetings of women, men, village leaders, and dais, as well as through a health awakening, or jatra. The cost of the study, including laboratory tests and treatments, was told to the people too. They were pleased about being taken into our confidence.

Notes

1. We found it perplexing that women considered our inquiry into their gynecological and psychosexual problems vulgar, since their own gossip was far more open and direct about sexual matters. When we pointed out this contradiction, many women said, "Our vulgar talk has an erotic function, it gives us pleasure, excitement. But why should a doctor talk about these things?" So the problem was one of the expected role of the doctor.

2. This failure of communication may be one reason that public health professionals have not realized the magnitude of the gynecological problems that exist. It may be possible that women all over the world are being sent home from clinics with vitamins and tonics when they have come seeking care for gynecological problems. This may also partly explain our finding that even though 92 percent of the women in our study had gynecological problems, only 7.8 percent had ever undergone pelvic examinations and received treatment.

Reference

Bang, R. A., A. T. Bang, et al. 1989. High prevalence of gynaecological diseases in rural Indian women. *Lancet* 1(8629):85–88.

Involving Women in a Reproductive Morbidity Study in Egypt

Hind Khattab, Huda Zurayk, Nabil Younis, and Olfia Kamal

The Giza Morbidity Study, a study on reproductive morbidity, was conducted in 1989–90 in two rural villages in the Giza governorate of Egypt. The main objectives of the study were to determine the prevalence of gynecological and related morbidity conditions[1] in the community through a medical evaluation, which included a physical examination and laboratory testing; as well as to test an interview-questionnaire in comparison with the results of a medical evaluation, as a potential instrument for community diagnosis and screening related to gynecological and related morbidity conditions.

An important goal in the Giza Morbidity Study was to achieve high participation rates in the gynecological exam. A major component of the research design required each woman to respond to a questionnaire-interview and be ready to undertake a medical examination and laboratory testing. Therefore, we needed to establish a climate of rapport and mutual trust within the study community from the start. We wanted the women involved to feel that they had a meaningful stake in what was going on (Raeburn 1992). Therefore, field-workers sensitive to social traditions and community concerns, and familiar with obstetric and gynecological conditions, had to present the medical and interview tools of the research in a culturally appropriate manner. In a later stage, following the study, these field-workers would also help disseminate correct and appropriate medical information to overcome the observed lack of awareness among women concerning their health needs and priorities (Khattab 1992). They also acted during the study as intermediaries between women and medical professionals, who were often seen as distant and patronizing.

We adopted an action-oriented approach. Our premise was that the women who constituted the study community were active participants in the project, not subjects to be manipulated for research purposes, and that it was important for the community or population to gain not only from the results of the research but also from the process itself (Harris 1992). To meet this objective, the research team arranged to provide treatment for all diagnosed diseases among participating women and to refer cases that needed more specialized medical investigations to the collaborating university hospital.[2]

Preparing the Field Team

This chapter focuses on the field techniques used to involve the women in the study sample in the various stages of the research procedure. The principal task was to make sure that the field team was well prepared to enter the study community and able to apply a disciplined, appropriate, and efficient procedure for the implementation of the research objective and tools. They were the study project's visible face—the catalysts between the research study team, the medical and health professionals, and the village community.

The first step was preparing the field research team for community involvement. They had to be grounded in the techniques of community participation, since their field task would consist of gaining the trust of a village community, interviewing over five hundred women in the study sample, and asking each to have a medical examination, with follow-up of all phases of required treatment. They were also expected to smooth over problem areas, notably when dealing with fearful women, reluctant families, or hostile husbands. Field-workers would have daily and intimate contact with the two villages for over a year.

Six field-workers, one field supervisor, and one field manager formed the field team. They were all young Egyptian women with social science degrees and experience of varied duration in community research and community development work. However, none of them had previously been involved with the medical aspects of women's reproductive health.

Beyond the mandatory exposure to the objectives of the study and the details of the study instrument to be administered, the members of the field team were given an intensive course on medical aspects of women's reproductive health. This covered a review of symptoms, pelvic examination, laboratory test procedures, and common treatments. It was given over a period of several days by the two obstetrician-gynecologists on the research team who shared a belief—not commonly found in the regional medical profession —that nonmedically trained persons would be able to absorb and understand the facts of medicine and medical practice sufficiently to complete the assigned research task, which included asking about medical symptoms, delivering prescribed medication to women, and supporting them during treatment at home or in a hospital.

Outreach communication methods for use with the community, the women, and their families were reviewed and rehearsed with the anthropologist on the research team. It was necessary to hold several sessions because the success of the field-workers' contact in the community, particularly with the women and their families, was crucial to the smooth progression of the various stages of the research project. Moreover, contact with the women involved discussing topics that were intimate and sensitive, relating to the details of their reproductive lives and health and the privacy of marriage. From previous studies, it was realized that women acknowledge with reluctance their own health needs, giving priority to the health needs of the family, and that special care would have to be taken to keep them involved.

Participatory training in observation, participant observation, and intensive interviewing techniques was held for almost four weeks. The anthropologist on the research team guided the field-workers on how to solicit women's participation for all stages of the study without imposing any part of it that participants might feel uneasy about. It was considered more important to establish a healthy and respectful communication with the women than to emphasize participation.

This approach had a positive influence on participation. Despite the relatively large size of the study sample and the complicated data collection process required, nonresponse was kept to a minimum, with many women who had initially refused to take part in some or all of the research tasks coming back to give their full support. By the end of the field study, an impressive 91 percent participation rate had been achieved.

Entering the Community

The initial entry into the community required the consideration of four aspects: obtaining the cooperation of the physicians and staff at the two village health centers and their participation in the study, getting official permits for study implementation and for the physicians' participation, gaining the confidence and support of formal and informal village leaders, and familiarizing the village women with the field team.

The research team had decided early on that the medical examinations would be undertaken at each of the two village health centers by the respective female physicians there, each of whom had been in charge of the clinic for many years. They were both already well known to the village women. It was believed that familiarity with them would make the gynecological component of the medical examination less threatening, and the choice of women doctors eliminated the potential problem of gender interference.

Informal visits to the two health centers assured the team that the health center physicians and staff would be willing and committed participants in the study. The research team was able to introduce themselves and clearly present the study goals. They were also able to observe the clinic facilities and check equipment and supplies, which made it clear that upgrading the physical facilities would be necessary.

Obtaining permits in Egypt is not an easy task, and it was clear that the research project would have to rely on the networking skills of team members who were well known in official circles and who had some experience in dealing with the Egyptian bureaucratic apparatus on other projects. A number of visits to both the Ministry of Health and the Central Agency for Public Mobilization and Statistics were made by the research team as a whole. This was a deliberate strategy that paid off, in that team members' academic qualifications and professional standing created a favorable impression and highlighted the credibility and seriousness of the project and appeared to help move the files smoothly through the steps required.

During the five-month waiting period for official permits, the field team—under the leadership of the anthropologist on the research team—took the opportunity to present the purpose of the study and to introduce themselves to the community, in particular to the formal and informal community leaders and to the village women and their families. Formal leaders included members of the village council, the Omda or village headman, and the Imam of the mosque. They were visited individually, and when introducing the study to them, the field team emphasized its contributions to improving the awareness of health problems of women not only in the community but also in Egypt as a whole and possibly in other countries of the region. It was explained, however, that the study's first responsibility was to the village women themselves, for whom free medical examinations were provided and free treatment offered. Lower-grade health center personnel, both medical and paramedical, who were believed to be instrumental to the study in their informal leadership roles were also approached.

Getting to Know the Women

Getting to know and beginning to earn the confidence of the women in the study sample were the field team's earliest and most pressing concerns. It seemed to be a good idea for contact to take place as soon as possible in the process of setting up the field research schedule. This opportunity presented itself in the task of mapping the villages to select the household samples. The field team members were charged with undertaking the mapping, accompanied by the health center registrar in each of the two villages. As members of the team walked through the streets, they were introduced personally by the registrar to the village men and women living there, which lent legitimacy to their presence. In its earlier training sessions, the team had been encouraged to stop and talk to the women, ask after their health and general well-being in a friendly, nonaggressive manner, and seek to establish cordial relations with them. The process of walking the same street twice or more over several days to greet the women over and again slowed the mapping task but proved exceedingly useful in gaining acceptance in the villages.

A second opportunity to familiarize the field team and the women with each other came with the pretest of the study procedures for daily field activities. This involved interviewing selected women on the gynecological component of the questionnaires and accompanying them to the health clinic for medical examinations and laboratory tests. During the two-week pretest period, six women were interviewed and accompanied to the health center on two selected days a week for the medical examination. Less than three weeks later, women were presented with the results of the laboratory tests and the medical examination and given the prescribed medications. The speed with which this phase was conducted was a great asset in convincing the villagers that the study group was serious and intended to help.

This opportunity to learn more about the women themselves, to sound them out on their reactions to the study and their responses to the invitation to undertake medical examinations, proved invaluable in refining the field plan. For example, it was learned that "Thursday is cooking day because butchers slaughter on that day . . . and women will not be free to talk." The field team also learned that "women are usually free after eleven in the morning, because children are at school, men are at work, housework is almost done. Work activities in the field or in peddling are also less intensive." The team also learned that women could talk while washing but never while baking, for fear of the evil eye.

More important, a number of remarks indicated why women were reluctant to undertake a medical examination. Health professionals were perceived as insensitive. Comments such as the following were common: "I am afraid . . . because the physician inserts a cold, hard metal object into a woman which hurts a lot." "I feel embarrassed and very uncomfortable lying down with my legs up during the examination." "The last time I had a gynecological examination, I bled and my belly hurt for a few days." After probing, it became evident that some of the women's fears and discomforts were the result of previous personal experience with health services, both public and private, although a few were based on hearsay by relatives, neighbors, and friends.

The field team was aware that the pretest of field activities was a significant testing ground for the smooth progression of the project. It was used by the community to assess the serious intent and commitment of the study. If the women who participated in this phase were satisfied, they would become advocates for the study in its next phase. This was indeed the case for some participants. One satisfied woman told her daughter (who was reluctant to participate in the study): "Look what they have done for me . . . they brought me medication from the pharmacy which costs a lot of money. You have no excuse not to go, I'll stay with your children, I'll carry out your daily chores, just go and think about your own health." This positive attitude, however, was not always the case. A few women remained frightened, protesting loudly and complaining during the medical examination, scaring off other potential participants who were waiting in the clinic for their turns.

The field-workers had to respond vigorously and decisively to reduce the fear and discomfort surrounding this experience. First, the physicians were made aware of the problem and were asked to be more gentle during the physical examination and to give each woman enough time to feel relaxed and safe. Moreover, the field team suggested to participants that a social researcher could attend the various medical investigations with them, if they so chose. Visiting the doctor accompanied by a relative or a friend is a common practice in the culture, and the suggestion was taken up by most of the women.

The issue of showing appreciation to the women selected to participate in the pretest and in the full study was resolved by discussing the matter with the women themselves. This was also useful in underlining the project team's commitment to involve the village women in a way that would be acceptable and useful to them. A consensus was reached that the best way to show appreciation would be through a gift that included two boxes of laundry soap powder, two bars of scented soap, and two packets of biscuits for the children. This present was deemed appropriate by all, since soap promoted hygiene and sanitation and biscuits had nutritional value.

The Data Collection Procedure

During a first visit to a woman in the sample, the field-worker would explain all stages of the study and seek her agreement to participate. If the woman refused, the field-worker would not insist but would inform the woman that the team would be working in the village for several months, and that the same interviewer would stop by again to see if the woman had changed her mind. With time, women exchanged experiences and the refusal rate dropped; the final refusal rate was a low 9 percent. Many of the women who at first refused to take part accepted on the second approach or even sought out the interviewer themselves. In fact, many women who were not part of the sample came to the health center requesting the medical examination. Unfortunately, they could not be included in the study because of our limited resources. They were told, however, that a medical service was available to them at the center during clinic hours.

Once a woman agreed to join the study, the field-worker tried to complete on the spot, whenever possible, the first general component of the questionnaire on the socioeconomic conditions of the family, and the second component on obstetric morbidity during the last pregnancy, for women whose last pregnancy had occurred in the past two years. If the woman was not able to spare the time to reply to both components together, the field-worker would make an appointment for a more convenient time. The field-worker also made an appointment with the woman to fill in the component on gynecological symptoms, which had to be on a day that the woman could also accompany the field-worker to the health unit for the gynecological examination. Such an arrangement was necessary because the gynecology-morbidity component collected information on current symptoms, which was compared with the results of the gynecological examination performed on the same day. Following the interview on gynecological morbidity, the field-worker took the woman to her appointment at the health unit. In most cases, it was possible to walk to the unit from the woman's house. If the house was on the outskirts of the village, the team car was used. The field-worker used the journey to the health center—whether on foot or by car—to ease the woman's mind about the medical examination she was about to undergo. At the health center, if everything had proceeded smoothly that day, the woman would not have to wait long. Following the medical examination (which included a general and a gynecological component) and laboratory tests (blood, urine, Pap smear, swab), the woman was taken back to her house by the field-worker herself in most cases. Before leaving the health center, she was given her gift of thanks neatly packed in a nylon bag.

This phase was particularly stressful for the members of the field team, who had to bring a designated number of women to the health center at specified times during an allotted three days per week. On those days, each field-worker had to carefully plan her schedule in terms of administering the interview to each woman, taking her to the health center and back whenever possible, and repeating the process until the day's quota was completed. Often the field-worker would arrive at a woman's house at a specified appointment time only to find the woman involved in some chore and unable to accompany her.

In some cases, the field-workers had to visit a woman three or four times or more before she was free to go for the medical investigation. Most of the younger women had to secure the permission of their mother-in-law before they could go. On several occasions, the mother-in-law would say, "She cannot go because she is cleaning the house." Or, "She will be free in two hours, after she finishes washing and the laundry." In one instance, a potential participant who had fixed a date for the medical examination apologized, saying, "I cannot go just yet. My mother-in-law died just a few days ago. How can I think of myself when her blood is still hot?"

In these cases, the field-worker would not press the woman but would make another appointment with her. The field-worker would then have to adjust her schedule for the day to replace the canceled appointment so as not to disrupt the physician's schedule. Field-workers developed a mechanism for these adjustments, but the process remained stressful.

Dealing with Problems

The data collection phase went relatively well, particularly after the first three weeks, when word of the activity spread among the village women. However, the field situation was not always without obstacles. One difficult moment occurred when rumors threatened to impede the progress of the project. For example, it was reported that there was an unidentified epidemic in the village and that the field team was there for this purpose. Another rumor was that the field team was taking blood samples to sell abroad. Others reported that the team was promoting family planning "like the rest of those who come here" or that the team intended to operate on women to sterilize them.

The field team's constant presence in the village helped refute most of these rumors. However, it took time, effort, and tact. One immediate action was to repeat the announcement that participants had the option to refuse to give a blood sample. Once this was made clear, the large majority of women consented to have their blood tested. Also, the strategy of including infertile as well as menopausal women in the sample helped convince the villagers that the project was genuinely not interested in controlling the number of pregnancies or children families intended to have. The fact that the health center physicians themselves examined the participating women refuted the rumors concerning the use of villagers to train students. Moreover, the researchers requested that the Ministry of Health postpone other research or health-related projects in the area, to control unforeseen factors that might jeopardize the study. Officials were most cooperative in that respect, and no permits for training or research were granted during the full course of the work.

Undoubtedly, the cooperation of the paramedical personnel working at the health centers and who were part of the field team provided the field-workers with a great deal of support in the initial period, not only in lending legitimacy to their presence but also in refuting rumors about the project.

The Field-Workers' Continuing Contribution

Completing the collection of information from the women did not mean the end of the field-workers' relationship with them. Throughout the duration of field activities, the field-workers made it a point to frequently ask after the women whenever they were in the vicinity of their houses. On one occasion, a field-worker heard of the death of the brother of a potential respondent. She immediately went with her colleagues to pay their condolences. A few days later when the field-worker met the woman in the street, she was asked, "When are you coming to take me to the health center? You know, I told my husband the other day that I cannot refuse to go with you when you cared enough to sympathize with me in my grief." Thus, continuity in relationships with the women was not only emphasized by the study supervisors but also demanded by the women themselves. This meant an ever-increasing workload for the field-workers, which they handled efficiently and cheerfully.

Moreover, the field-workers had to be constantly attentive to a range of life cycle events such as deaths, marriages, and births and aware of economic conditions, social and family structures, and cultural norms related to reproductive health, all of which were often behind women's refusal to seek medical help. At the beginning, for example, it was difficult to persuade older women or women married to older men to participate in the project. One woman said, "I am old, such medical problems are for the sexually active, not for me." Another woman said, "How can I go to the health center for gynecological investigation when everybody knows that my husband is incapacitated. This will suggest behavior that is incriminating." A third woman said, "My husband is away in Libya. Why should I go for a gynecological examination now?"[3]

The field-workers were also responsible for delivering treatment or medication prescribed by the physician and for planning hospital referrals and follow-up during recuperation for the few cases in which this was recommended. It was felt that working with the community created a moral responsibility to treat the women who were revealed to have reproductive health conditions that needed further investigation, even in a hospital setting and to the extent of surgery, within the limits of project resources.

When laboratory tests and medical examinations were completed, the results were presented to one of the research team physicians acting as a medical field supervisor, who would diagnose the case and prescribe the medication. The field-workers would then buy the medication, writing the name of the woman and the mode of use on every box. They would then go to the woman's home, give her the medication, and describe the mode of use. Field-workers were also instructed to check on the correct use of the medications. When sexually transmitted diseases were diagnosed, medications were also sent for the husband.

If further medical investigations were deemed advisable, the senior physician on the research team would recommend referral to the collaborating university hospital. The field-worker would then prepare the woman's medical file and send it to the hospital to fix an appointment. Meanwhile, she would be preparing and persuading the woman and her family to take this new and often disquieting step in treatment.[4]

These activities were not part of the research task, nor did they contribute to the pool of hard data collected. They were, nevertheless, an important means by which the action-oriented nature of the study was demonstrated.

Notes

1. Gynecological morbidity as covered by the study refers to conditions of ill health that are not related to a particular pregnancy episode. They include reproductive tract infections, cervical ectopy, and cervical cell changes and prolapse, as well as other related morbidity conditions such as urinary tract infection, anemia, hypertension and obesity. (Younis et al. 1993).
2. Moreover, the team committed itself to disseminating research findings, when these became available, by organizing workshops and producing a variety of publications aimed at the medical community, at health program managers, and at policymakers. Indeed, as soon as the preliminary study results were in hand, the team began to share the findings with the larger community of professionals concerned with women's health, from both medical and social science disciplines. An intervention program, based on the study results and on further in-depth qualitative research, was subsequently designed to improve women's knowledge of their own health needs, to create awareness of reproductive health conditions, and to empower women to seek reproductive health care services.
3. These statements clearly indicate the impact of culture on women's health perceptions and behavior and demonstrate the need to be sensitive to such issues in the design of field research. Women acknowledged reproductive health problems only if they were permissibly sexually active. Those who were not sexually active were expected to live with their problems without complaining or seeking medical help.

Morbidity was not seen to be independent of sexual activity or related to past practices.
4. These situations are well exemplified in the case studies published in Khattab (1992). They reflect the full extent of the social constraints imposed on women in seeking health care for themselves.

References

Harris, E. 1992. Accessing community development research methodologies. *Canadian Journal of Public Health* 83(suppl 1):562–66.

Khattab, H. 1992. *The silent endurance: Social conditions of women's reproductive health in rural Egypt.* Amman: UNICEF; Cairo: Population Council.

Raeburn, J. 1992. Health research promotion with heart: Keeping a people perspective. *Canadian Journal of Public Health* 83 (suppl 1):520–24.

Younis, N., H. Khattab, H. Zurayk, M. El-Mouelhy, M. Fadle Amin, and A. M. Farag. 1993. A community study of gynecological and related morbidities in rural Egypt. *Studies in Family Planning* 24(3):175–86.

Biomedical Research

Female Sexuality, the Menstrual Cycle, and the Pill

Lorraine Dennerstein

Knowing how the female sexual response changes in relationship to the menstrual cycle is profoundly important. This knowledge may help women understand their own sexual behavior and feelings. It may help reduce the unrealistic expectations for women to maintain sexual interest throughout the menstrual cycle. It raises important questions about how synthetic hormones—by altering the natural cycle—affect sexual response.

Although most research identifies a peak in female sexual response at the time of ovulation, the existing research is hardly uniform regarding the influence of the menstrual cycle on female sexuality. For the most part, this is because of major methodological difficulties inherent in this type of research.

One central methodological question is how female sexual outcomes should be measured. Many studies have used frequency of intercourse. Hedricks et al. (1987) and Morris et al. (1987) both found, for example, that intercourse was most frequent at the time of ovulation. However, frequency of intercourse is not an adequate measure. In many societies, men have the greatest voice in choosing when to have sex, and women may be discouraged from initiating or refusing sexual activity. Thus, frequency of intercourse may tell more about *male* sexual drive and social needs and expectations than it does about female sexual interest. Furthermore, having intercourse may reflect a range of other unrelated interests women may have, such as trying to conceive, enhancing intimacy, achieving material gain, and so on. Finally, this type of study assumes that all sexual activity is necessarily penetrative.

Some studies have tried to distinguish self-reported female sexual desire (Adams, Gold, and Burt 1978; Stanlislaw and Rice 1988).[1] Stopes (1931) studied women whose husbands were away at war. She found two peaks of sexual desire reported by these women: one just before menstruation, the other two weeks later. Matteo and Rissman (1984) analyzed daily records of both sexual thoughts and sexual activities from seven lesbian couples (where gender power differences in sexual decision making were presumably greatly reduced). Significant peaks in orgasms and self-initiated and total sexual encounters were found around the presumed midportion of the menstrual cycle.

Other studies have focused on female sexual outcomes by measuring physiological responses (such as vaginal blood flow) in a laboratory setting (Morrell et al. 1984; Schreiner-Engel et al. 1981). In this artificial setting, the stimulus is provided by fantasies, audiotapes, and erotic videotapes. The few studies carried out with this methodology (Meuwissen and Over 1992; Schreiner-Engel et al. 1981) found no consistent pattern of variation in vaginal arousal during the menstrual cycle. Moreover, such studies may tell us little about the real-life changes experienced by women or about the responses of women who would not volunteer for the bodily intrusions required by such research.

The second central methodological issue in this kind of research is the need to secure adequate endocrine measurements to assess the menstrual cycle phase and influence. Because women's cycles vary in length, duration of menses, and time of ovulation, adequate endocrine measures are required to avoid erroneously assigning peaks and troughs in sexual desire to the wrong phase of the cycle (Doty 1979; Udry and Morris 1977).

Adams et al. (1978) used the basal body temperature method as a crude indicator of endocrine levels and, in particular, of the ovulatory phase of the cycle. They reported that female-initiated sexual behavior (including masturbation and the use of erotic fantasy and literature) peaked around ovulation. Unfortunately, users of the basal body temperature method are not always able to identify the precise day of ovulation; accurate identification was only 34 percent in a study conducted by Lenton, Weston, and Cooke (1977).

Sanders et al. (1983) and Udry and Morris (1977) did early exploratory research involving the use of endocrine tests to identify cycle phase. They found peak levels for sexual interest in the follicular phase (after menstruation), followed by a fall at the time of ovulation. However, these studies relied on fairly crude measurements: Sanders did not use daily tests, and Udry and Morris gathered daily endocrine data on only a small subset of their sample.

Dennerstein et al. (1994) conducted a study that utilized more adequate measures for both the independent and the dependent variables (identifying the cycle phase and women's sexual outcomes). In this study, 168 women collected daily, twenty-four-hour urinary samples over an entire menstrual cycle; total estrogen and pregnanediol levels were measured. These women also recorded their sexual interest and mood on a daily basis throughout the cycle. Results showed a statistically significant rise in sexual interest during menses, sustained higher levels of interest during the follicular phase, a small ovulatory peak, and a sharp decrease following ovulation. This pattern was present independent of whether women suffered from premenstrual symptoms.

In summary, Dennerstein's findings—along with those of many of the studies discussed above—indicate that female sexual interest peaks at the most fertile time of the cycle. Although this arrangement appears to foster perpetuation of the species, it places individual women at great risk of *unwanted* pregnancy, because women themselves most desire sex when they are potentially fertile. Thus, there are some special challenges for those women relying on periodic abstinence (during the ovulatory phase) for family planning.

Although there appears to be a strong pattern of change in sexual interest with menstrual cycle phase, correlation with actual hormonal levels of estrogens or pregnanediol was weak (Dennerstein et al. 1994). This suggests a link to other substances that vary consistently with the menstrual cycle and that may play a major role in the neuroendocrinology of female sexuality. There are few studies that have measured such substances (for example, androgens or oxytocin) on a daily basis throughout the menstrual cycle. This is an important area for future research.

Sexuality and Oral Contraceptives

As mentioned in the previous section, the knowledge that naturally produced female hormones affect sex interest in a consistent way during the menstrual cycle raises important questions
about what kind of effect synthetic hormones (particularly oral
contraceptives) may have on female sex interest. Oral contraceptives are thought to suppress follicle-stimulating hormone and
luteinizing hormone (hormones that promote the growth and
the expulsion of the egg, respectively); this results in lower levels
of estrogens and progesterone produced by the body. The pill
also suppresses the midcycle ovarian increase in androgens, a
group of hormones that may counteract the midcycle increase in
female sexual interest (Bancroft et al. 1991a, 1991b).

Certainly there is strong anecdotal evidence that some women
perceive that oral contraceptives adversely affect their sex interest
and response; others perceive a positive benefit, and still others
perceive no change. The current state of knowledge from research
seems to confirm this experience: findings indicate a great deal of
variation in how much oral contraceptives affect sexual response
among individual women and in the nature of that change.

Among the prospective studies, Cullberg (1972) found that
women using oral contraceptives reported significant negative
effects on mood but not on sexual behavior, as compared with
women on placebo. Leeton, McMaster, and Worsley (1978) found
a significant decrease in sexual response during oral contraceptive
use. The Leeton group did a cross-over study—women spent time
on the pill and on a placebo—but the sample size was very small.[2]

Graham and Sherwin (1993) also found that women with premenstrual symptoms suffered decreased sexual interest after
starting the pill (in this case, triphasics). This effect was independent of any effect on mood. The World Health Organization is
currently supporting a prospective study in the Philippines that
hopes to examine the effect of oral contraceptives on sex interest
among women.

In 1980, Dennerstein et al. conducted a clinical trial to attempt
to evaluate whether oral contraceptives affect sexuality. In this
year-long, double-blind, cross-over study, we found that women

taking ethinyl estradiol experienced a beneficial effect on sexual desire, enjoyment, and vaginal lubrication as compared with placebo. Women taking norgestrel reported an adverse effect. Because this study was carried out among women who had undergone hysterectomy and bilateral oophorectomy (to control for hormonal variation) and were in stable heterosexual relationships (to reduce social factors), it constrains our ability to draw conclusions about women with normal ovarian function who are mediating a wider range of psychosocial influences, such as those associated with new relationships or unstable relationships.

The findings with regard to the effect of oral contraceptives on the cyclical nature of sexual interest are more consistent than those regarding the effect on overall sexual interest. Adams et al. (1978) found that non–pill users reported a midcycle peak in the frequency of female-initiated sexual behaviors; pill users did not report this peak. Similarly, Alexander et al. (1990) found that pill users did not show the cyclical pattern for sexual desire evident among nonusers.

The current state of knowledge about oral contraceptives suggests that they suppress the cyclical nature of female sexuality but that there is a great deal of variance among individual women in any effects (positive or negative). Longitudinal studies of large and representative groups of women in their reproductive years are needed to determine the side effects of oral contraceptives, including on sexual response. Such studies should include baseline recording over at least one menstrual cycle prior to beginning any medication; use of double-blind methods and placebo is also important.

Notes

1. Leiblum and Rosen (1988) provide a working definition of sexual desire as "a subjective feeling state that may be triggered by both internal and external cues, and that may or may not result in overt sexual behavior."

2. A number of cross-sectional surveys on sex interest among pill takers have also been carried out, with mixed results. However, such studies have limited validity, because they cannot sort out differences that were present before the study. The population of women who choose

to begin oral contraceptive use and who then continue such use may be very different from women who do not choose this method or who discontinue its use because of side effects (which may include an effect on interest in sex).

References

Adams, D. B., A. R. Gold, and A. D. Burt. 1978. Rise in female initiated sexual activity at ovulation and its suppression by oral contraceptives. *New England Journal of Medicine* 299(21):1145–50.

Alexander, G. M., B. B. Sherwin, J. Bancroft, and D. W. Davidson. 1990. Testosterone and sexual behavior in oral contraceptive users and nonusers: A prospective study. *Hormones and Behavior* 24(3):388–402.

Bancroft, J., B. B. Sherwin, G. M. Alexander, D. W. Davidson, and A. Walker. 1991a. Oral contraceptives, androgens, and the sexuality of young women: I. A comparison of sexual experiences, sexual attitudes, and gender role in oral contraceptive users and non-users. *Archives of Sexual Behavior* 20(2):105–20.

Bancroft, J., B. B. Sherwin, G. M. Alexander, D. W. Davidson, and A. Walker. 1991b. Oral contraceptives, androgens and the sexuality of young women: II. The role of androgens—double blind comparison with a placebo. *Archives of Sexual Behavior* 20(2):121–36.

Cullberg, J. 1972. Mood changes and menstrual symptoms with different gestagen/estrogen combinations. *Acta Psychiatrica Scandinavica* 1972 (Suppl):236.

Dennerstein, L., G. D. Burrows, G. J. Hyman, and K. Sharpe. 1980. Hormones and sexuality: effects of estrogen and progestogen. *Obstetrics and Gynecology* 56(3):316–22.

Dennerstein, L., G. Gotts, J. J. Brown, C. A. Morse, T. M. Farley, and A. Pinol. 1994. The relationship between the menstrual cycle and female sexual interest in women with PMS complaints and volunteers. *Psychoneuroendocrinology* 19(3):293–304.

Doty, R. L. 1979. A procedure for combining menstrual cycle data. *Journal of Clinical Endocrinology and Metabolism* 48(6):912–18.

Graham, C. A. and B. B. Sherwin. 1993. The relationship between mood and sexuality in women using an oral contraceptive as a treatment for premenstrual symptoms. *Psychoneuroendocrinolgy* 18(4):273–81.

Hedricks, C., L. J. Piccinino, J. R. Udry, and T. H. K. Chimbira. 1987. Peak coital rate coincides with onset of luteinizing hormone surge. *Fertility and Sterility* 48(2):234–38.

Leeton, J., R. McMaster, and A. Worsley. 1978. The effects on sexual response and mood after sterilization of women taking long-term oral contraception: results of a double blind cross-over study. *Australian and New Zealand Journal of Obstetrics and Gynecology* 18(3):194–97.

Leiblum, S. R., and R. C. Rosen. 1988. Introduction: Changing perspectives on sexual desire. In *Sexual desire disorders,* edited by S. R. Leiblum and R. C. Rosen. New York: Guilford Press.

Lenton, E. A., G. A. Weston, and I. D. Cooke. 1977. Problems in using basal body temperature recordings in an infertility clinic. *British Medical Journal* 1(6064):803–5.

Matteo, S., and E. F. Rissman. 1984. Increased sexual activity during the midcycle portion of the human menstrual cycle. *Hormones and Behavior* 18(3):249–55.

Meuwissen, I., and R. Over. 1992. Sexual arousal across phases of the human menstrual cycle. *Archives of Sexual Behavior* 21(2):101–19.

Morrell, M. J., J. M. Dixen, C. S. Carter, and J. M. Davidson. 1984. The influence of age and cycling status on sexual arousability in women. *American Journal of Obstetrics and Gynecology* 148(1):66–71.

Morris, N. M., J. R. Udry, F. Khan-Dawood, and M. Y. Dawood. 1987. Marital sex frequency and midcycle female testerone. *Archives of Sexual Behavior* 16(1):27–37.

Sanders, D., P. Warner, T. Backstrom, and J. Bancroft. 1983. Mood, sexuality, hormones and the menstural cycle. 1. Changes in mood and physical state: Description of subjects and method. *Psychosomatic Medicine* 45(6):487–501.

Schreiner-Engel, P., R. C. Schiavi, H. Smith, and D. White. 1981. Sexual arousability and the menstrual cycle. *Psychosomatic Medicine* 43(3): 199–214.

Stanislaw, H., and F. J. Rice. 1988. Correlations between sexual desire and menstrual cycle characteristics. *Archives of Sexual Behavior* 17(6): 499–508.

Stopes, Marie. 1931. *Married love.* London: Putnams.

Udry, J. R., and N. M. Morris. 1977. The distribution of events in the human menstrual cycle. *Journal of Reproduction and Fertility* 51(2): 419–25.

*H*ormones and Female Sexuality

Developing a Method for Research

Murray Anderson-Hunt, with Lorraine Dennerstein, Lyn Hatton, Jennifer Hunt, Joanne Mahony, Delys Sargeant, and Nancy Stephenson

W omen's reproductive health and sexuality remain controversial areas of research because their analysis and development involve critical assessment of contemporary cultural thinking and biomedical research methodologies. Designing a research methodology that conforms with valid, scientific principles and also shows respect for women's intimate experiences is certainly a challenge.

The Key Centre for Women's Health in Society is an academic center of excellence that undertakes both undergraduate and postgraduate teaching and research in women's health. The center's objectives include promoting the use of a research model whose content is defined by women and that is informed by feminist, social, biomedical, and community perspectives, with the end result of empowering women to better care for their own health.

This chapter shares our experience of trying to incorporate these ideals and objectives into a research project focused on a protein-hormone called oxytocin and its effects on women's sexual feelings and behaviors. We hope that our description of the process of conceptualizing and carrying out research about human sexuality will contribute to an understanding of the physiological basis of our sexual experiences in the wider context of the social forces which affect our lives.

I chose the headings, "People," "Process," and "Product: An Interesting Model" as the framework for this chapter because they helped me focus on important issues about women's sexuality without decontextualizing intimate aspects of human experiences.

My involvement in this research project began while I was still a general hospital doctor, before I had commenced my psychiatry training. The incident that sparked my interest concerned a woman's experience of intense sexual desire and arousal after using the protein-hormone oxytocin, which presumably interacted with a progestin pill she was taking for contraception (Anderson-Hunt and Dennerstein 1994).

Oxytocin is a protein-hormone and is synthesized in certain nerves, beginning in the hypothalamus and ending in the posterior pituitary gland. Oxytocin is also produced in gonadal tissues in both women and men, and it is similar in structure to vasopressin (also known as antidiuretic hormone, or ADH). As a neuropeptide, oxytocin acts on the smooth muscle cells of the uterus and of the breast ducts to cause contraction of these tissues, resulting in well-documented effects in the expulsive, second stage of labor and in the lactokinesis—or the "letdown"—of milk with nipple stimulation during breast-feeding. Commercial pharmaceutical preparations of synthetic oxytocin are most commonly used in women to induce labor and to assist with the letdown of breast milk. Oxytocin is known to rise during sexual arousal and peak during orgasm in both women and men (Carmichael et al. 1994) and probably causes the rhythmical contractions of the uterine muscles during orgasm.

After hearing this woman's experience, I studied an array of research articles about hormonal and other chemical substances involved in reproduction and female sexual arousal, particularly oxytocin. Most of these studies involved various mammals, from simple rodents to higher primates, and seemed to confirm an interaction between oxytocin and sex steroid hormones (for example, progestins) in these animals (Carter 1992; Insel 1992; Pedersen et al. 1992). Recent reviews describing the functions of oxytocin, particularly in mammals, have suggested that this peptide has multiple roles in a wide range of social, maternal, and reproductive behaviors, including grooming; nesting; mother-infant bonding and other affiliative behaviors, such as adult bond formation; gamete transport; and sexual satiety.

The initial case report suggested that the interaction between sex steroids and oxytocin augments the physiological and possibly psychological aspects of female sexual arousal and climax. In addition, anecdotal stories from lactating women who had experienced feelings similar to sexual arousal while breast-feeding were further evidence that oxytocin may indeed affect women's sexual arousal. This could be the result of a process in which steroids "prime" certain tissues, initiating the formation of oxytocin receptors on cells, which in turn are "triggered" by the circulating oxytocin and augment physiological and possibly psychological aspects of female sexual arousal and climax. Given all this evidence and information, I became interested in learning whether this woman's experience might be a window into understanding oxytocin's effects in women. Simply put, might oxytocin act as an aphrodisiac?

Choosing an appropriate research methodology to establish whether oxytocin creates or contributes to women's sexual responsiveness has been a difficult exercise. I realized that because oxytocin probably has a significant physiological role in the human sexual arousal process, my research project would have wide clinical, ethical, and psychosocial implications, particularly if one considers the gender and power issues in intimate relationships as well as in the larger society. If the naturally occurring oxytocin, when administered as a "drug" to women, can alter their sexual mood, then issues such as whether this hormone or other drugs with similar effects should be available (or even researched) enter a complex political arena, because they imply the possible control and exploitation of women's sexuality by chemical means. It was important to me that my research model reflect an understanding of its possible social significance.

People

*No understanding of women will ever be possible until women themselves
begin to tell what they know.*
　　　—Paraphrase of John Stuart Mill, *The Subjection of Women*

I am a psychiatrist in training at the Key Centre. It surprises both
men and women that, as a male doctor, I choose to study and
work in a unit that was established primarily for the research and
teaching of women's health. Their surprise becomes more apparent when they realize that my research interests are the experience and psychoneuroendocrinology of women's sexual desire
and arousal and how these aspects of female sexuality interact
and change during the life cycle.

I have always believed that the starting point and focus for this
research should be women's own thoughts and feelings about sexuality. Even before I took the case report and the abstracts of selected
articles to my colleague, Lorraine Dennerstein, I had begun to talk
with friends and colleagues about the potential uses and misuses of
this preparation or any other chemical that might act as a female
aphrodisiac. From the beginning, it was clear that this was a controversial area for research and a political "hot potato." It became
more unlikely that particular aspects of the project would proceed
unless the value of the hypothesis and its implications were explicitly debated and a way was found to incorporate the ethical and
social dimensions into the research process sensibly and sensitively.

Eventually, with Professor Dennerstein's prompting, I enlisted
a number of individuals as a reference group for this research.
The role of this group was to establish a reasonably broad, cross-
sectional view of the general community's opinions about issues
surrounding research into the biochemical control of women's
sexual functioning and arousal.

Jennifer Hunt, the mother of two children, confirmed these
experiences as common among women. As the convener of the
management collective of the local Women's Health Service, she
was the first person to discuss the major issues involved in the relationship between hormones and control of women's sexuality. Lyn
Hatton, coordinator of Women's Health Service and a mother,
helped me consider these issues in further depth, as did Nancy

Stephenson. Nancy is a community psychiatric nurse and a lecturer in mental health nursing at Deakin University. Her enthusiasm for this research and her ability to clarify methodological issues have been invaluable, particularly in formulating nonsexist methods and nomenclature that conveys respect for women.

I had often talked with members of the local chapter of a community support and education group and particularly with Joanne Mahony, who is a mother of two children and has a special interest in breast-feeding and the interactions between mother and infant. Her main contribution was to emphasize the psychosocial factors that may lead to decreased sexual arousal after childbirth. She also made suggestions about how to consider and study women throughout the postpartum period.

As a physiologist and founder of the Social Biology Resource Centre, Delys Sargeant is an expert in the field of sexuality. She encouraged us to reconsider the very words used to define different aspects of women's sexual responses, particularly the concepts of arousal, desire, and fantasy. Her experience as a social health educator—in particular, promoting understanding of sexual health among health practitioners—leads her to challenge the continuing, male-centered interpretations of sexual arousal in women.

Process

When a subject is highly controversial, and any question about sex is that, one cannot hope to tell the truth. One can only show how one came to hold whatever opinion one does hold.
        —Virginia Woolf, *A Room of One's Own*

The quote from Virginia Woolf's book indicates that this *process* of clarifying issues, developing perspectives, and doing studies in sexuality research is just as relevant as the *content* of the ideas themselves.

Concerns That Emerged from the Background Research

Although we believed that the interaction between sex steroid hormones and sexual response was well supported by experimental evidence in animal studies, this could not be considered justifiable ground for predicting such a response in women or for officially approving the use of such hormones in clinical circumstances. If, after further research, the hypothesis proves to be valid, this might lead to the licensing of these preparations (perhaps in some sort of combination) for the specific purposes of enhancing women's normal sexual experiences or restoring sexual interest and enjoyment in women whose sexual response is diminished by hormonal contraception or some sexual dysfunction. However, no controlled trials with women currently exist from which to draw firm conclusions about these potential uses of oxytocin.

My informal discussions with colleagues and friends reinforced concerns about the potential misuses of hormones or other chemicals that might act as an aphrodisiac. Staff members at the Key Centre also raised the question whether clinicians would consider the hormonal interaction a therapy for an illness or dysfunction or a recreational preparation, improving wellbeing by augmenting the quality of sexual experience. They were surprised that other potentially prosexual substances had not been topics for philosophical or ethical debate despite their apparent relationship to other reproductive interventions involving hormonal or drug treatments and to alternative therapies for improving sexual functioning.

Initial Design of the Research Project

A number of parallel strands of thought emerged as possible directions for the development and research of the original idea.

Initially, our research plan involved three components, similar to other traditional research projects. The first component would be a literature review to examine the range of usual sexual responses during the menstrual cycle, during lactation, and in the puerperium, and the effects of hormones during these times. Current knowledge of changes in sexual arousal caused by these hormones and chemicals would be examined, and the possible role for oxytocin in this pathway designated. This would give us a baseline against which to measure our findings.

The second component would be an open study to determine whether the observation noted in the original case report could be replicated. The conditions surrounding the experiences of the first woman would have been duplicated as closely as possible in an open-trial situation. Other women who had stopped breast-feeding but were on the mini-pill (which contains progestins only) would be given oxytocin. If the results from this open study were sufficiently encouraging, we would have initiated the third component—a double-blind study to test the hypothesis in two cohorts of women.

Locked-Away Knowledge versus Open Sharing

The possible commercial applications of our research findings suggested that it might be appropriate to approach a pharmaceutical company, outline a project proposal, and request funding for research. However, precisely because the concept had marketing potential, we decided to formulate a provisional patent application to protect the idea from being used by a company, even if it rejected our research proposal, and to give us the control to choose the companies or groups of researchers that we felt would deal most appropriately with the information, in keeping with the ethical concerns we had considered.

We were determined to reveal the specific details of the hypothesis and the method itself to pharmaceutical companies only if they were prepared to enter into a confidentiality agreement.[1] Despite our significant effort to achieve this, there was great reluctance among senior staffs of drug companies to sign such an agreement, even after face-to-face contact and their verbal assent.

In the meantime, we had applied for and obtained a provisional patent application that effectively gave us and the University of Melbourne the "intellectual property" protection of this method for augmenting female sexual responsiveness. However, obtaining the patent, which represented ownership and control of information about women's sexuality, presented a paradox for the kind of research process we were trying to develop.

The Key Centre's research staff promotes the goal of women determining their own health needs, defining their own concepts of illness or well-being, and setting priorities for research—not necessarily from a biomedical perspective. Although our design reflected the distinction between biological *determinism* and biological *determinants* in the investigation of female sexuality,[2] the proposed model seemed to conflict or be inconsistent with current directions in women's health research. We were caught between the need for "locked-away" knowledge (referring to the secrecy and confidentiality of the intellectual patent designed to protect the hypothesis) and the alternative perspective of "open sharing" of knowledge, particularly with women involved in the study.

These tensions became even more apparent when we began the process of setting up the studies. This involved recruiting women as subjects who met the criteria outlined above; developing an appropriate self-reporting questionnaire; and obtaining the proper informed consent after adequate explanation of the nature, possible effects, and side effects of the hormones. It also involved the granting of an ethics committee's approval. The purpose of such a committee, which may be based at a university or at a hospital, is to ensure that appropriate background evidence exists for such a study, that the research methods are sound, and that the issues of respect, consent, and confidentiality are addressed.

Because of the intellectual patent and the then-current stage of project development, we were not able to offer the ethics committee adequately detailed information about the research proposal or the full background to the research. In my opinion, it may also have seemed to the committee that our research design went something like this: the purpose of our study is to examine the manipulation of women's sexual drive and moods, using contraceptive and other synthetic, hormonal drugs to produce evidence for the potential commercial exploitation of an unrecognized interaction, after clinical trials conducted by a male doctor involving young, healthy, lactating mothers as experimental subjects.

Discussions with senior endocrinology research scientists (such as Professor Henry Burger from the Prince Henry's Institute for Medical Research) confirmed our emerging understanding that there might not be any long-term value in protecting an "invention" of this type. Also, the arrangement did not readily allow the general dissemination and publication of our work and hypotheses in peer-review journals, nor encourage other researchers' opinions about its possible development or suggestions for alternative research directions and methods. It was becoming increasingly apparent that the intellectual patent on the hypothesis was too protective and prevented the provision of complete and appropriate information to the ethics committee, community discussion or reference groups, scholarship or research foundations, and, importantly, potential subjects of any research to enable them to give truly informed consent. We decided to allow the provisional patent application to lapse and to change our agreement with the University of Melbourne to allow for a gradual open-disclosure policy.

Current Research Directions

Despite all these difficulties, we decided to take proactive steps to clarify and explore the issues relevant to this debate because a number of other prosexual drugs are currently being tested by various pharmaceutical companies.[3] It is only a matter of time before these products enter the commercial market, and if there is an apparent absence of a contextual framework, any response women may have might be seen as only reactive and irrelevant to further research.

Thus, we proceeded with the literature review and submitted the original case report (Anderson-Hunt and Dennerstein 1994) and the updated literature review (Anderson-Hunt and Denner-stein forthcoming) to journals for publication. At present, we are concentrating on validating a method of assessing experiences using subjective, self-rating scales, and it is our aim to eventually develop an appropriate method for our research.

We approached a number of women with whom we had already talked to establish a reference group for the ongoing project. After an initial meeting with some members of this group, notes were prepared, outlining and clarifying the major points of concern. The contributors were asked to comment on these notes, and a synthesis of their responses is presented in the next section. We consider this to be a significant achievement, as it has become increasingly apparent from our discussions and from the current literature that a debate about the ethical dimensions of this type of research is almost nonexistent, save for isolated passages in general "reproductive technology issues" books.

Product: An Interesting Model

Marta: I went into hospital to have our baby, but Thomas has transferred Helen's baby into my womb.

Mary: Why would he do that?

Marta: To see if he could do it.

—Sandra Shotlander, *Angels of Power*

The impact of this quotation lies in Thomas's arrogant presumption that just because some form of reproductive technology is possible, it is appropriate to use it. The idea of a female aphrodisiac has acted as a unique catalyst to explore this assumption. This discussion has given rise to a framework that, we believe, can be used in other discussions of women's sexuality. Our intention in using this framework is to clarify certain issues, not necessarily to resolve the difficulties raised.

When talking about our research and hypothesis both in informal discussions with colleagues and friends and in more formal debates with the reference group and Key Centre staff, we found that people tended to address five main topics: sexual/erotic, history/folklore, affiliative/bonding, cultural/social, and exploitative/

**Interactive model of perspectives about aphrodisiac
and prosexual substances**

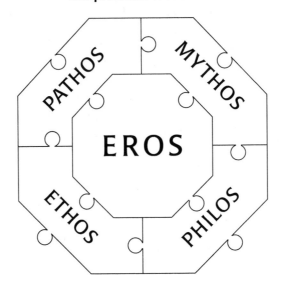

negative influences. These have been synthesized into a simple and aesthetic framework, represented in the figure above, in which we used the Greek words *eros, mythos, philos, ethos,* and *pathos,* respectively, to refer to the aspects named above.

Some men and most women slowly moved clockwise around the schema, considering each theme in place and almost always in the same order as in the figure, though it may have taken them a few minutes or sometimes days. (Not surprisingly, however, some women who had earlier considered power, control, and exploitation in social health and human relationships went immediately from *eros* (sexual/erotic) to *pathos* (exploitative/negative) and returned to examine other aspects of prosexual substances later.)

This progression was so distinctive that our model literally created itself. It just required us to categorize and arrange the dimensions. The interactive nature of the perspectives is illustrated by the jigsaw puzzle effect in the figure. We placed *eros* at the center because it acts as the focus for most conceptualizations of sexuality. There has been and probably always will be debate about its importance and role in discussions about sex, sexuality, and gender, but it is usually considered first, even if the intention is to negate or downplay its significance in a particular arena of human sexual experience.

Incidentally, in our view, it is unlikely that this paradigm would have been developed or that the broader contextualization of these ideas would have occurred if we had been considering an aphrodisiac for men, although in retrospect, we believe that this model applies to any prosexual drug or hormone combination for either sex.

Eros

The central perspective of the model involves the sexual and erotic aspects considered in our discussions, which we termed *eros*. When the oxytocin–sex steroid interaction was mentioned as a potential aphrodisiac, the first response of both women and men was to ask about its effects on sexual arousal and its efficacy. For most, the second question was, "Where can I get some?"

At this point, concepts of power and control over sexuality usually entered the conversation. Almost all the men, despite being gently encouraged to consider other aspects of the concept of aphrodisiacs, remained fixed on the *eros* perspective. We believe that this attitude reveals the appeal of being able to influence women's sexual arousal on demand, suggesting control over their sexuality.

Mythos

The long history of aphrodisiology involves mystique, folklore, rumor, and a lot of wishful thinking; most of the so-called aphrodisiac substances that supposedly lead to immediate bliss have questionable efficacy, and some have significant side effects (Money, Leal, and Gonzalez-Hedyrick 1992; Rosen and Ashton 1993). We used *mythos* to refer to the historical, legendary, and current views of aphrodisiacs.

The concept of aphrodisiacs has had many meanings over the years, and the question What is an aphrodisiac? is interesting. Although it has usually been considered a substance, it can also be an experience or an expectation based on previous experience, music, foods, or even scents. There is a long list of aphrodisiacs that might improve potency or increase sexual desire for either sex, but for some men, aphrodisiacs for women imply a way of controlling women's sexual moods and arousal to service their own desires.

Philos

When weighing the value of such research, we considered oxytocin's potentially positive role in affiliative aspects (*philos*). The psychosocial basis of the bonding and attachment processes in humans has been considered and theorized in more depth than the biological pathways underpinning such behaviors. But we do know that oxytocin is purported to be one of the major hormonal neuromodulators involved in the physiological pathways of a number of aspects of bonding behavior and reproduction. Other neuropeptides (such as vasopressin and endogenous opioids) and phenylethylamine also seem to be emerging as major players in this research into neurohormonal mechanisms and pathways for such emotions as lust, love, grief, and jealousy.

We concluded that the biological basis of attachment, for example, understanding the chemistry between and within people in "love" and "loss" situations, is a worthwhile area of inquiry. However, a purely biochemical view of "love" is clearly inadequate without consideration of the complex interactions that make up human bonding and sexual experiences. Therefore, the broader cultural and anthropological dimensions of relationships merit discussion when considering the research and use of drugs that may affect sexual relationships.

Ethos

We used the term *ethos* to categorize the possible contextual and technical ramifications that research into prosexual drugs might have in a culture. As mentioned, most women but only some men were able to consider aphrodisiacs in a wider context. This is of particular concern to Key Centre staff, but the dilemma for us remains how to analyze intimate human experience in its appropriate context without losing an objective scientific perspective.

The potential of using either a naturally occurring hormone such as oxytocin or alternatives to synthetic oxytocin may have considerable appeal. Contemporary research has used other hormonal methods, such as androgens or higher doses of estrogen and progestins, to augment female sexual responsiveness. Other prosexual drugs have been described in scientific reviews. However, a concern with the impact of such substances has not been reflected in these other scientific studies.

The original research design involved some women who were breast-feeding. This introduces a number of separate issues regarding their involvement in drug or hormone trials, including the concern that lowered sexual arousal during lactation or the postpartum period may be related to psychosocial difficulties or could be considered a "usual" physiological state rather than a dysfunction requiring therapy.

An additional concern is the need for informed consent and information availability—important considerations in any trial situation. And yet, this creates a further research dilemma because providing information about the possible effects of oxytocin on a woman's body chemistry and moods prior to the trial might bias her answers.

Pathos

When certain women considered the concept of a drug that affected sexual desire, their understanding about sexuality, gender, and female-male relationships prompted them to immediately consider the downside to this whole idea. We collected these concerns under the heading *pathos* because the term itself implies sadness and tragedy.

In many cultures, women lack an autonomous or independent voice regarding their own sexuality, sexual interactions, and sexual expression. Few women—heterosexual or homosexual—have expressed a "need" for an aphrodisiac. This lack of autonomy is particularly problematic, as there may be pressure from partners or from society in general to take such a substance. A woman may internalize these pressures to conform to an image of greater well-being and sexual functioning and decide to take such a drug.

Availability of such preparations may create more problems than solutions for women. Not only are there expectations for a woman to have a successful career, manage a home, be a good mother, be thin, and always be "sexy," but now there might be pressures to be sexually aroused on demand and to perform at a constant sexually active peak by using chemical assistance. We are particularly concerned about the potential exploitation of women in unhappy relationships, although anyone might be forced to give in to strong demands.

Moreover, a decreased sexual desire may be the result of a complex set of psychosocial factors: previous sexual difficulties or abuse, postpartum problems such as stress, tiredness, overwork, concerns about body image, anxiety about the infant, and so forth. An aphrodisiac will not help a woman resolve these issues.

Yet it is important to remember that women can act as agents in this decision. A woman may choose to use this combination of progestins and oxytocin during menopause—a time at which one-third of women report a decrease in sexual functioning (although this, too, may put further pressure on menopausal women to have some form of estrogen replacemement therapy). Or a woman may choose to use it because she has tried other methods to improve a hypoactive sexual desire related to some other causes without success.

The question of who makes this decision—a woman, her partner, her peers, her medical practitioner, or someone else—is an important one. Who controls the information about prosexual drugs also remains a sensitive concern. These issues of power and control mean that the role of any substance in human-human sexual interactions should be questioned carefully.

Discussion

Redesigning and reformulating our project is an ongoing process. The review of the research literature continues alongside the process of clarifying the contextual issues, paradigms, and language used in sexology research. Surprisingly, there was an unexpected benefit to keeping the details of our work in-house all this time. We learned that the value of the hypothesis and its implications needed to be explicitly debated and a way found to incorporate the ethical and social dimensions into the research process. Although we were not able to resolve all these issues, we were able to clarify some important points of consideration for research of this type:

- For the first woman, the effect on arousal and desire was close to overwhelming, but this may not be the case in other women. However, if this is the "usual" response, then it may be exploited in intimate relationships or in a societal context in which women's sexuality is controlled or regulated.

- The unknown risks of ongoing use of any hormone must be considered; we still know little about potential side effects.

- Careful consideration needs to be given to whether these kinds of preparations will be used for recreation or therapeutic purposes. Each raises specific issues when it comes to regulating access and use.

- Regulation of such products should be on the political agenda, and an *informed* debate on the value of introducing such substances to a wider market should take place. This debate should happen sooner rather than later, as some test products are close to the marketing stage.

- This debate has to consider the responsibilities and ethical constraints of those who control and regulate the supply of such preparations as well as those individuals or institutions that research their effects.

By having to continually explore the impact of a potential aphrodisiac on women and the possible ramifications of introducing such a substance into any society, culture, or subculture, we engaged in a significant exploration of issues. This might never have happened if we had published the idea, gained early research funding, or had immediate ethics committee approval.

What We Learned

Our role at the Key Centre, as both a research and a training unit, enables us to inform other medical and social health researchers as well as to influence the general community's opinions about how women view developments that affect their sexual well-being. We believe that the definitions, terminology, and assessment measures of women's sexual experiences and behaviors need continual revision and reevaluation in light of what women tell us about themselves. For this reason in particular, we believe that our model—formulated through discussion with women and men—is useful. In addition, it fills a significant gap in the current literature of models that contextualize research on prosexual drugs.

We hope that by clarifying issues in this debate and by exploring some possible directions for the resolution of these difficulties, our work to develop a contextual framework for considering aphrodisiacs and prosexual substances in research and their use in any society will be of use in the study of other aspects of sexology.

Notes

1. A confidentiality agreement is a binding contract between two parties under which one party releases information to the second party on the understanding that the latter will not use or act on the information without acknowledging the first party as the owner of the information.
2. Biological determinism is a philosophical stance that suggests that the body has to function in a particular manner because it is structured in that way, whereas biological determinants are elements derived from a physiological understanding of a biological process and are thus free of any directive about how they have to function.
3. The most recent advances have been detailed further and reviewed in the article by Rosen and Ashton (1993), and it is evident to us that *pharmacosexology* (the study of the role of drugs in sexual behavior and their influence on sexual function and dysfunction) is a developing scientific field. These authors also emphasize the lack of trials and studies of prosexual substances involving women and consider methods of developing other prosexual drugs. The only dilemmas they note, however, are *clinical* ones, further illustrating the relative philosophical and sociological vacuum around the concept of researching aphrodisiacs.

References

Anderson-Hunt, M., and L. Dennerstein. 1994. Drug point: Increased female sexual response after oxytocin. *British Medical Journal* 309:920.
Anderson-Hunt, M., and L. Dennerstein. *Oxytocin and female sexuality.* Forthcoming.

Carmichael, M. S., V. L. Warburton, J. Dixen, and J. M. Davidson. 1994 Relationships among cardiovascular, muscular, and oxytocin responses during human sexual activity. *Archives of Sexual Behavior* 23:59–79.

Carter, C. S. 1992. Oxytocin and sexual behavior. *Neuroscience and Biobehavioral Reviews* 16:131–44.

Insel, T. 1992. Oxytocin—a neuropeptide for affiliation: Evidence from behavioral, receptor autoradiographic, and comparative studies. *Psychoneuroendocrinology* 17(1):3–35.

Mill, J. S. 1869. *The subjection of women.* New York: D. Appleton and Company.

Money, J., J. Leal, and J. Gonzalez-Hedyrick. 1988. Aphrodisiology: History, folklore and efficacy. In *Handbook of sexology.* Vol. 6, *The pharmacology and endocrinology of sexual function,* edited by J. Sitsen. Amsterdam: Elsevier Science Publishers.

Pedersen, C., J. Caldwell, G. Jirikowski, and T. Insel, eds. 1992. Oxytocin in maternal, sexual, and social behaviors. *Annals of New York Academy of Sciences* 652:1–492.

Rosen, R., and A. Ashton. 1993. Prosexual drugs: Empirical status for the "new aphrodisiacs." *Archives of Sexual Behavior* 22(6):521–43.

Shotlander, S. 1991. Angels of power: A modern myth in two acts. In *Angels of power and other reproductive creations,* edited by S. Hawthorne and R. Klein. Melbourne: Spinifex Press.

Woolf, V. 1929. *A room of one's own.* New York: Harcourt Brace.

*T*he Effects of Hormones on Male Sexuality

Findings from Clinical Trials on Male Contraception

Ann Robbins

*T*he evidence for the effects of hormones, particularly the sex steroids, on human male sexuality is intriguing. Many reports, both anecdotal and scientific, have documented the effects of androgen, the major class of sex steroid produced by males, on many aspects of sexual desire and performance. Thus, testosterone, one of the primary androgens, has been the focus of much of the experimentation on the biological basis of male sexuality. This chapter provides a brief overview of what we know about the influence of hormones, particularly testosterone, on male sexual drive and behavior, drawing from data collected in clinical trials on hormonal methods of contraception for men. Results from the other sources are reviewed as well. Because it is sometimes technically and ethically difficult to systematically analyze and interpret the biological influences on male sexual behavior, a discussion of various methodological issues is also included.

Evidence for Effects of Hormones on Male Sexual Behavior from Animal Data

The results from studies on androgen's effects on behavior in male animals are summarized here because these studies provide the reference and framework on which subsequent human data are based (see Meisel and Sachs 1994 for a recent review). In addition, the types of experiments conducted on animals provide important insights into androgen's direct effects on the brain, the organ that ultimately controls all behavior; such studies are not possible on human subjects.

Most of the animal data come from studies of rats and mice, but data have also been collected in dogs, cats, and monkeys. In all these species, castration reduces and usually eventually eliminates male sexual behavior. However, the length of time it takes for an observed reduction in sexual behavior depends on several factors. There is great variation among species, with the decline occurring within a week or so in rodents but sometimes not for months or even years in dogs, cats, and monkeys. The age of the animal at the time of castration and his amount of sexual experience prior to castration are also important factors. For example, a mouse with no sexual experience at the time of castration may never show sexual behavior, whereas a sexually experienced mouse may continue to exhibit mating behavior for several weeks following castration.

Restoring androgen to the castrated animal restores sexual function, but again, the time required for sexual function to return is influenced by several factors. For example, the length of time between castration and initiation of hormone replacement is critical; restoration is more effective the sooner androgen is replaced. Also, higher doses of testosterone are more effective than lower doses, although the amount of behavior generally does not increase above precastration levels, no matter how high a dose is administered. Interestingly, estradiol, usually considered the "female" hormone because it is produced predominantly by the ovaries, can be as effective as testosterone in restoring male sexual behavior.

Finally, data indicate that discrete, identifiable brain areas are responsible for producing sexual behavior in rodents and primates. These brain areas also contain specific proteins, called androgen receptors, that respond to testosterone. Thus the brain areas that contain androgen receptors are also important in controlling sexual behavior.

Methodological Issues in Human Research

Once the jump from animal to human studies is made, there are several important methodological issues to consider when studying male sexual behavior. Some of these are summarized below and have been reviewed by Bancroft (1990).

Components of Sexuality That Can Be Measured

Three components of sexuality can be measured in clinical studies on hormones: sexual behavior, physiological or biological responses, and psychological components. Behavior is usually measured by the amount or frequency of sexual activity, generally defined as intercourse or masturbation, with or without orgasm. Physiological measures include the strength and duration of penile erection and the level of hormones in the blood. Psychological variables that have been recorded are sexual desire, arousal, and motivation. Usually the frequency of occurrence of these feelings is documented, and the subjects are asked to rate the intensity of the feelings on a numerical scale. As this is highly subjective information, standardized scales have been developed, such as the Frenken sexual experience scales. These scales assess values about sexual morality, such as attitudes toward premarital sex; measure psychosexual stimulation, which reflects the extent to which a person seeks out or avoids audiovisual or imaginary sexual stimuli; and measure sexual motivation, which reflects sexual interactions with one's partner.

Methods for Assessing Sexual Behavior

Assessment can be done by a variety of methods, depending on which component of sexual functioning one wants to measure.

For example, frequency of sexual behavior (intercourse, masturbation) is often collected prospectively by daily self-report on a sexual diary card or retrospectively by interview or questionnaires. Physiological responses are typically collected in a laboratory setting and require special laboratory equipment or biological assays. For example, the rigidity of the penis and its circumference during erection (penile tumescence) can be measured by a commercially available device called "Rigiscan" (Burris, Banks, and Sherins 1989). Psychological variables can be measured by both types of methods: self-reporting in daily diaries or questionnaires that indicate the frequency and strength of the variables. Sexual arousal can also be quantitatively measured by such things as pupil dilation, changes in heart rate and blood pressure, or even brain wave patterns.

Each method of assessment has its strengths and weaknesses. In general, self-reports are subject to error, especially the "halo effect" of making data appear better than they actually are (for example, reporting more intercourse than actually occurred). In the emotionally charged area of sexual performance, this type of enhancement is especially probable. Also, retrospective methods are plagued by forgetting or selective remembering. Although laboratory data can be more objective, because these responses are collected in an artificial setting and measure a limited aspect of sexuality, it may be hard to extrapolate such data to real-life situations.

Proper Controls for the Interpretation of Clinical Data

One of the biggest problems in studying sexuality in humans through the scientific approach is eliminating both experimenter and subject bias. This is often difficult from both a practical and an ethical point of view. The best type of design is "double-blind," which uses a placebo. In this case, neither the experimenter nor the subject knows if the subject receives the hormone or the placebo. If this is not possible, the controlled study should at least include a pretreatment period (during which data are collected before the subject receives a hormone) or a comparison group of subjects who do not receive the hormone but are closely matched to the hormone-treated group in terms of characteristics such as age, race, socioeconomic status, and educational level. Also, the study must provide a mechanism to account and control for external variables that could affect sexual behavior, such as sickness, travel, or nonavailability of the partner.

Types of Clinical Studies on the Effect of Androgen on Male Sexual Behavior

The sources of human data that provide information on hormones and male sexuality include the following (see Hoberman and Yesalis 1995; Bardin, Swerdloff, and Santen 1991 for recent reviews): (1) correlative studies of aspects of male sexuality and testosterone levels; (2) clinical studies on men who, for a variety of reasons, lack testosterone and are given replacement androgens; and (3) clinical studies on men who have testosterone levels in or near the normal range but for a variety of reasons (medical conditions, enhancing athletic performance, contraception) have used exogenous androgen. All three approaches have strengths and weakness. Representative results from the first two types of studies are summarized below (also see reviews by Bhasin 1992; Carter 1992; Sherwin 1988).

Perhaps not surprisingly, a number of correlative studies have indicated a positive association between testosterone levels and sexual behavior. One study among adolescent boys indicates that the level of testosterone is predictive of sexual motivation and behavior (Udry et al. 1985). In addition, as men age, the absolute level of testosterone decreases, and a correlated decrease in sexual activity has been observed (Davidson et al. 1983; Tsitouras, Martin, and Harman 1982). Testosterone given to eugonadal men (men with normal testes) complaining of low sexual interest produced a significant increase in one measure, sexual thoughts (O'Carroll and Bancroft 1984).

The link between testosterone and sexual interest is also apparent to the men themselves. For example, in a placebo-controlled, double-blind study of testosterone supplementation in aging males (age range fifty-seven to seventy-five), twelve of the thirteen subjects were able to correctly guess when they were receiving testosterone rather than placebo injections (Tenover 1992). Their predictions were based on such things as increased libido and an increased feeling of well-being or aggressiveness in business transactions.

Hypogonadal men have extremely low levels of endogenous testosterone due to surgical castration or disease that has destroyed the function of the testes. Androgen replacement therapy administered to these men generally stimulates sexual interest and behavior compared with pretreatment levels (Burris et al. 1992; Kwan et al. 1983). However, increasing the androgen dose above a certain level does not increase sexual activity. In addition, normal sexual functioning has been observed in men without functioning testes, depending on the type of stimulus.[1]

Male Hormones and Male Contraceptive Methods

Male hormonal contraceptives target hormones in the brain-pituitary-gonadal axis (see figure next page). A specific part of the brain, the hypothalamus, produces gonadotropin hormone–releasing hormone (GnRH; also called luteinizing hormone–releasing hormone or LHRH), which causes the release of luteinizing hormone (LH) and follicle-stimulating hormone (FSH) from the pituitary gland. These hormones, in turn, are responsible for stimulating the production of testosterone and spermatogenesis from the testes. The proper balance of these hormones is absolutely essential for normal functioning of the male reproductive system. Hormonal methods of male contraception work by disturbing this delicate feedback system, resulting in suppression of spermatogenesis and testosterone production. This produces the contraceptive effect by reducing sperm levels but also results in a decrease in libido by reducing serum testosterone levels.

To date, clinical trials on male contraception have primarily studied the effects of exogenously delivered androgens in the form of injections, implants, and pills (Sundaram, Kumar, and Bardin 1993; Wang, Swerdloff, and Waites 1994). The increase of androgens in the bloodstream causes the GnRH cells in the brain

Schematic diagram of the brain-pituitary-gonadal reproductive axis

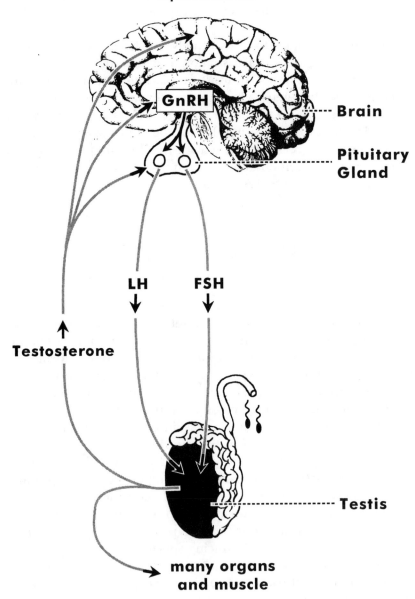

and/or the LH and FSH cells in the pituitary to decrease production of their hormones in response to the excess androgen, thus decreasing sperm production. Synthetic gestagens that have antiandrogenic properties have also been tested, with and without a concomitant androgen treatment (World Health Organization 1980, 1982; Knuth, Yeung, and Nieschlag 1989; Wu and Aitken 1989).[2] Clinical trials on products that target higher levels of the reproductive axis, such as GnRH antagonists or agonists or GnRH vaccines, have also been reported (Alexander 1994; Bhasin and Swerdloff 1986; Vickery 1986). It appears that these methods require the use of a concomitant androgen for normal sexual behavior (Bouchard and Garcia 1987; Bremner, Bagatell, and Steiner 1991; Pavlou et al. 1991).

Data from Clinical Trials for Male Contraception

What have we learned about male sexual behavior as a result of these studies? The most extensive report to date on the effects of hormonal contraceptives on male sexuality and the acceptability of hormonal contraception for men comes from a study by the World Health Organization (WHO) published in 1982. Since this study, a large number of studies in the contraceptive literature have reported results from individual clinics in which a small number of subjects used one of the regimens tested in the original WHO study. However, these studies do not adequately assess sexuality or acceptability. Moreover, they typically provide only the number of men who complained of changes in libido during the trial, and this number is small. Table 1 lists other studies of androgen or androgen plus gestagen regimens and the effects on libido when they were mentioned.

The 1982 WHO study was a multicenter, multicultural phase I clinical trial that examined several combinations of synthetic androgens and gestagens as well as a gestagen (cyproterone acetate) alone.[3] The experimental design included placebo control groups, pre- and post-treatment observation periods for each subject, and different doses for most treatment regimens. This strong design

Table 1 Clinical Trials for Hormonal Male Contraception: Androgen or Androgen Plus Gestagen

Reference	Hormone	Dose	Duration (mo.)	No. subjects	Libido Effects (no.)
Anderson et al. 1992	TE	200 mg I.M.	1–2	31	Increased sexual arousability No change in sex behavior
Handelsman et al. 1992	Testosterone pellets	6 × 200 mg=1,200 mg	6	9	Normal sexual function
Matsumoto 1990	TE	25–300 mg I.M.	6	51	Normal sexual function
Wallace et al. 1993	TE	200 mg I.M.	12	28	Not measured
WHO 1993	TE+DMPA 19-nor+DMPA	200 mg + 250 mg I.M. 200 mg + 250 mg I.M.	6 6	49 47	Decreased sex drive (2) Decreased sex drive (7)
WHO 1990	TE	200 mg I.M.	18	273	Increased aggression and libido (3)
Wu and Aitken 1989	TE+DMPA	250 mg + 200 mg I.M.	3	10	Decreased sexual function (1)

TE = testosterone enanthate; 19-nor = 19 nor testosterone-hexyloxy-phenyl-propionate; DMPA = depot-medroxyprogesterone acetate; IM = intramuscularly.

helped strengthen the analysis and interpretation of results, despite the small number of subjects in most treatment groups.

The trial was conducted at six sites (Bangkok, Santiago, Seoul, Toronto, Hong Kong, and London, although only placebo was tested at the London site), and the results from 119 subjects were reported (see Table 2 for a summary). Subjects were aged twenty-five to forty-five, with a baseline sperm count greater than 20 million per milliliter, considered to be the lower limit of the normal range. The trial schedule included a twelve-week baseline or pretreatment phase, followed by sixteen to twenty-four weeks (depending on the site) of treatment, and a twenty-four-week recovery or post-treatment phase. Data on sexual function and acceptability were collected by interview (questionnaire in Toronto) during all stages of the trial.

Two main end points were assessed: measures of sexual behavior (thirty variables) and measures of the subjects' acceptance of (seven variables) and beliefs about (thirteen variables) the contraceptive method they used. Of the thirty sexual behavior measures, sixteen of the variables were combined into the composite variable of "overall sexual energy," which was considered one of the best indicators of the entire spectrum of sexuality measures.[4]

The overall results (regardless of the treatment regimen used) indicated that only three of the thirty variables of sexual function changed significantly during the study: frequency of morning erection (decrease, < .001); change in sexual desire (decrease, < .02); and number of negative behavior events (increase, < 0.1).[5] None of the acceptability variables changed significantly. In contrast, all but one of the variables that measured the subjects' beliefs about the method changed significantly over the course of the trial. In most instances, the change was in the positive direction. The type of hormone regimen and amount of hormone accounted for 20 percent of the variation in "sexual energy" observed from baseline to treatment.

Overall, acceptability of hormonal methods of contraception remained high throughout the three stages of the study, with virtually no significant changes in acceptability variables across time. However, the one regimen that used cyproterone acetate alone, a synthetic gestagen that has a strong antiandrogen effect, was *least* acceptable. All the significant treatment effects from cyproterone acetate were negative. These results indicate that contraceptives based solely on hormones with strong antiandrogen effects adversely affect sexuality.

Table 2 WHO Study of Acceptability of Male Hormonal Contraceptives

Location	Androgen	Gestagen	Number of Subjects
Bangkok	TE (monthly injection)	MPA (daily oral)	25
Santiago	TE (monthly injection)	DMPA (monthly injection)	23
Seoul	Testosterone cypionate (monthly injection)	DMPA (monthly injection)	10
Toronto	Methyltestosterone (daily oral)	MPA (daily oral)	8
Hong Kong	None	Cyproterone acetate* (daily oral)	27
London	Placebo	Placebo	26

*See note 2 regarding comments on cyproterone acetate.

TE = testosterone enanthate; MPA = medroxyprogesterone acetate; DMPA = depot-medroxyprogesterone acetate.

Source: Modified from WHO 1982.

Subjects were asked to rate five statements supplied to them as predictors of their intention to use a new contraceptive in the future. During the initial two phases of the study (pretreatment and treatment), the subjects selected being "liked by women" as the best predictor of future use. During the post-treatment phase, the subjects stated that a belief that the method would "cause sickness or weakness" was the most important predictor, followed by being "liked by women." Interestingly, the predictor "increases a man's sexual desire" was not chosen by the subjects as predictive of future use. The authors suggest, however, that if this had been phrased as "decreases a man's sexual desire," it might have had more of an impact.

The overall conclusions from this, the most extensive study to date on the sexuality and acceptability measures during use of hormonal contraceptive methods for males, are the following:

1. Most regimens did not significantly affect overall sexuality. However, the one most likely to produce a negative change was an antiandrogenic gestagen delivered without concomitant androgen. This suggests that a decrease in endogenous testosterone, which could occur with this method (although testosterone level was not reported in this study), has negative effects on male sexuality.

2. Long-term hormonal contraceptive use is acceptable to men from several different cultures, and this acceptability remained high throughout all phases of the trial. The level of acceptability was inversely related to the number of effects on sexuality; thus, the lowest level acceptability occurred in the gestagen-only users, who reported the greatest number of negative effects on sexuality.

WHO subsequently conducted two large, multicenter, international trials on the use of testosterone enanthate (TE), a synthetic androgen, as a male contraceptive. The results of the first study have been published (WHO 1990), and the results of the second are currently being analyzed and written. Both studies followed a similar protocol. In the first study, TE (200 mg) was injected intramuscularly at weekly intervals until the men became azoospermic (defined as no sperm in the ejaculate in three consecutive specimens at two-week intervals). The second study also included subjects who became severely oligospermic (defined as a sperm count of less than 3 million per milliliter). Once the required effect on sperm was achieved, all contraceptive methods used by the man and his partner were discontinued, and the couple entered a twelve-month efficacy phase. At the end of this year, the men entered a recovery phase, which lasted until the sperm count returned to pretreatment levels.

In the results from the 1990 WHO study, effects of the treatment on sexuality were not reported. However, three of the 271 men enrolled in the study discontinued use of TE due to "increased aggressiveness and libido" (see Table 1). It is hoped that the overall results from the second WHO study will provide a more comprehensive analysis of the effects of TE on measures of male sexuality. Meanwhile, some of the participating clinical sites in the WHO study have initiated a "substudy" to specifically examine this issue. For example, Anderson, Bancroft, and Wu (1992) used a single-blind, placebo-controlled study design to assess the effect of TE on many aspects of sexuality in thirty-one men using the standardized Sexuality Experience Scales questionnaires. They reported that psychosexual stimulation, which reflects noninteractional sexual awareness and arousability, was significantly increased by TE. There was also a significant increase in "interest in sex" in one group receiving testosterone, although closer inspection revealed that this increase was largely due to the response of one subject. The enhancement in sexual feelings was not followed by increased sexual activity; there were no significant changes in frequency of intercourse, masturbation, or penile erections. Also, no significant mood changes, such as readiness to fight or irritability, were reported. Thus, the TE treatment increased testosterone levels above the normal range, but this supraphysiological dose, although stimulating some aspects of sexual desire, did not affect overt sexual behavior or aggressive feelings.

The Effect of Synthetic GnRH Used for Male Contraception on Sexual Behavior

Because the male contraceptive methods based on androgen alone are successful in producing azoospermia in only approximately 70 percent of men (Handelsman, Conway, and Boylan 1992), other methods are being developed. Synthetic GnRH methods that have been tested in clinical trials include GnRH antagonists and agonists (Bhasin and Swerdloff 1986; Bremner, Bagatell, and Steiner 1991; Vickery 1986). Antagonists block the effect of the endogenous GnRH, therefore shutting down the brain-pituitary-gonadal reproductive axis. GnRH agonists initially stimulate FSH and LH secretion from the pituitary, but within a short time, the overproduction produces negative feedback on the GnRH system, ultimately having the same effect as the antagonist in turning off the reproductive axis (see figure on page 284). Since both of these methods inhibit testosterone production as well as spermatogenesis, they must be used with concomitant androgen. The replacement androgen is given to counteract any negative effects on libido from the endogenous testosterone suppression, but in some cases, it can restimulate spermatogenesis (Bouchard and Garcia 1987). Thus, the androgen supplementation must be carefully titrated to provide enough to maintain libido but not enough to stimulate sperm production.

The effect on sexuality of a GnRH antagonist called Nal-Glu was measured in ten men (Pavlou et al. 1991). Libido effects were evaluated every two weeks by questionnaire and clinical interview and included assessment of subjective changes in libido, quality of sexual activity, and frequency and quality of erections and ejaculations. In the first two weeks of treatment, when Nal-Glu was delivered alone, there were complaints of libido changes (not specified in paper). However, during the eighteen weeks of treatment when Nal-Glu was given with a low dose of TE to eight subjects, no statistically significant changes in libido were observed. This lack of effect on libido was observed even though testosterone levels remained below the normal range for at least half of each week as a result of the regimen design.

A comparable trial with a strong experimental design tested the effect of using Nal-Glu alone, TE alone, and Nal-Glu plus TE over different periods of the study. Among the nine men, approximately half reported decreased libido and/or difficulty achieving erection during treatment with Nal-Glu alone (Bagatell et al. 1989). These problems were alleviated when TE treatment was combined with Nal-Glu; no subject reported altered sexual function or decreased libido during Nal-Glu plus TE treatment. Other studies have reported similar results (see Tom et al. 1992; Behre et al. 1992).

Implications of Male Hormonal Contraceptive Research for Sexuality

Although many aspects of clinical trials on male contraception are the same as those in trials on female methods, some unique aspects arise. For example, whereas the ability of a particular male method to decrease sperm production or lower endogenous hormone levels is assessed in the subject himself, contraceptive efficacy can be assessed only in a female partner.

An important difference between the history of male contraceptive trials and that of female contraceptive trials is the early emphasis on acceptability among males. This emphasis is due to the belief of the investigators (almost all males themselves) and the statements of potential male users that a method that decreases sex drive would not be acceptable. In female contraceptive trials, the acceptability of a method is normally not measured until later stages of clinical trials (for example, phase III or even postmarketing trials), but in the case of male hormonal contraceptive methods, assessments of how the method affects sexuality and how the men feel about the possible changes have been advocated and undertaken at very early stages of method development. Unfortunately, even today, relatively little work is being done on the effects of hormonal contraceptives and female sexuality (see the chapter by Dennerstein in this volume), possibly reflecting an implicit bias that sexuality in women is not important. Another possible explanation for the early emphasis on acceptability among men is that "sexual failure" is more obvious in men.

A final issue is that men who enroll in clinical trials and eventual users of a male contraceptive method may be a unique subset of contraceptive users. It is generally believed, although not yet known, that most men who are interested in this type of method are in long-term, monogamous relationships and are highly motivated. Thus, data gathered from clinical trials of male hormonal contraceptives offer interesting information on the effects of hormones on male sexuality, but the probable unique characteristics of the men who volunteer to participate must temper the urge to generalize the results to all men. Future studies and focus groups in which sexuality and mood are carefully monitored and critically analyzed are needed to determine if these results from clinical trials are representative of the effects of androgens on men in the general population.

Despite the differences between male and female hormonal contraceptive trials, there is one important similarity: the use of virtually any method, whether targeted for males or females, will have implications for the sexual partnership, and potential side effects may be viewed differently by the partners. For example, in the case of male hormonal methods, increases in libido or aggressiveness may be considered positive attributes by the male user but not by the female partner. It will be important in future clinical trials to include an assessment of the partners' impression of changes in these areas.

Although not absolutely dependent on androgen, human libido and sexual behavior are clearly modulated by this hormone. The data from clinical trials on male hormonal contraceptive methods indicate that methods that suppress endogenous testosterone negatively influence sexual desire and function and require androgen supplementation. However, the level of androgen required may be at the low end of the physiological range. Also reassuring is the fact that when synthetic androgens are used alone, there are no reports of hypersexuality, even when hormone levels are increased above the normal range. This suggests that in humans, as has been demonstrated in animals, there may be a "ceiling effect" of hormones; after a threshold level is reached, administering more hormone does not produce more behavior.

Notes

1. For example, hypogonadal men had the same frequency of erections in response to erotic films as normal men but were not as successful as normal men in obtaining erections when told to fantasize (Kwan et al. 1983).
2. Gestagens, also called progestagens or progestins, are a category of hormone steroids that are produced by the female ovaries and are important for gestation and the maintenance of pregnancy. However, due to the similarity of their chemical structure to androgen's, synthetic gestagens (for example, those that are made by drug companies) can also have androgenic or even antiandrogenic properties. Although classified as a gestagen in the WHO study, cyproterone acetate has very strong antiandrogenic properties, so that it blocks the action of the male's own natural testosterone. Because of these effects, cyproterone acetate and other gestagens with antiandrogenic properties have been used in the past for the treatment of hypersexuality and male sexual behavior.
3. In a phase I trial, which is the earliest stage of testing in humans, the biological effects and possible adverse effects of the hormone are tested and monitored, but not the efficacy. Thus, the subjects were instructed to continue to have their partners use an effective contraceptive during the trial.
4. The sixteen positive and negative variables that were combined to constitute the measure of "overall sexual energy" were the following:

> intensity of sexual desire
> intensity of sexual pleasure

importance of sexual pleasure
enjoyment of sexual thoughts and feelings
general satisfaction with partner
sexual satisfaction with partner
frequency of orgasms with partner
daily frequency of sexual thoughts/feelings
change in sexual desire
change in frequency of orgasms with partner
change in quality of sexual experience
number of erectile problems
number of premature ejaculation problems
number of negative behavior events
number of positive behaviors and circumstances
number of negative interpersonal and external events

5. The definition of "negative behavior events" is not given in the paper. The only information available is that it was derived from analysis of a nineteen-item checklist (also not given) of recently experienced events. Information in parenthesis indicates direction of change during treatment and the level of statistical significance, as derived from two-tailed paired t-tests.

References

Alexander, N. J. 1994. Contraceptive vaccines. In *Contraceptive research and development 1984 to 1994*, edited by P. F. A. Van Look and G. Perez-Palacios. Delhi: Oxford University Press.

Anderson, R. A., J. Bancroft, and F. C. W. Wu. 1992. The effects of exogenous testosterone on sexuality and mood of normal men. *Journal of Clinical Endocrinology and Metabolism* 75(6):1503–07.

Bagatell, C. J., R. I. McLachlan, D. M. de Kretser, H. G. Burger, W. W. Vale, J. E. Rivier, and W. J. Bremner. 1989. A comparison of the suppressive effects of testosterone and a potent new gonadotropin-releasing hormone antagonist on gonadotropin and inhibin levels in normal men. *Journal of Clinical Endocrinology and Metabolism* 69(1): 43–48.

Bancroft, J. 1990. Sexual behaviors. In *Measuring human problems: A practical guide*, edited by D. F. Peck and C. M. Shapiro. New York: John Wiley & Sons.

Bardin, C. W., R. S. Swerdloff, and R. J. Santen. 1991. Androgens—risks and benefits. *Journal of Clinical Endocrinology and Metabolism* 73(1):4–7.

Behre, H. M., D. Nashan, W. Hubert, and E. Nieschlag. 1992. Depot gonadotropin-releasing hormone agonist blunts the androgen-induced suppression of spermatogenesis in a clinical trial of male contraception. *Journal of Clinical Endocrinology and Metabolism* 74(1):84–90.

Bhasin, S. 1992. Androgen treatment of hypogonadal men. *Journal of Clinical Endocrinology and Metabolism* 74(6):1221–25.

Bhasin, S., and R. S. Swerdloff. 1986. Mechanisms of gonadotropin-releasing hormone agonist action in the human male. *Endocrine Reviews* 7(1):106-14.

Bouchard, P., and E. Garcia. 1987. Influence of testosterone substitution on sperm suppression by LHRH agonists. *Hormone Research* 28(2–4): 175–80.

Bremner, W. J., C. J. Bagatell, and R. A. Steiner. 1991. Gonadotropin-releasing hormone antagonist plus testosterone: A potential male contraceptive. *Journal of Clinical Endocrinology and Metabolism* 73(3): 465–69.

Burris, A. S., S. M. Banks, C. S. Carter, J. M. Davidson, and R. J. Sherins. 1992. A long-term prospective study of the physiologic and behavioral effects of hormone replacement in untreated hypogonadal men. *Journal of Andrology* 13(4):297–304.

Burris, A. S., S. M. Banks, and R. J. Sherins. 1989. Quantitative assessment of nocturnal penile tumescence and rigidity in normal men using a home monitor. *Journal of Andrology* 10(6):492–97.

Carter, C. S. 1992. Hormonal influences on human sexual behavior. In *Behavioral endocrinology,* edited by J. B. Becker. Cambridge, Mass.: MIT Press.

Davidson, J. M., J. J. Chen, L. Crapo, G. D. Gray, W. J. Greenleaf, and J. A. Catania. 1983. Hormonal changes and sexual function in aging men. *Journal of Clinical Endocrinology and Metabolism* 57(1):71–77.

Handelsman, D. J., A. J. Conway, and L. M. Boylan. 1992. Suppression of human spermatogenesis by testosterone implants. *Journal of Clinical Endocrinology and Metabolism* 75(5):1326–32.

Handelsman, D. J., T. M. M. Farley, A. Peregoudov, G. M. H. Waites, and World Health Organization Task Force on Methods of Regulation of Male Sterility. 1995. Factors in nonuniform induction of azoospermia by testosterone enanthate in normal men. *Fertility and Sterility* 63(1): 125–33.

Hoberman, J. M., and C. E. Yesalis. 1995. The history of synthetic testosterone. *Scientific American* 272(2):76–81.

Knuth, U. A., C. H. Yeung, and E. Nieschlag. 1989. Combination of 19-nortestosterone-hexyloxyphenylpropionate (Anadur) and depot-medroxyprogesterone-acetate (Clinovir) for male contraception: Influence on conventional semen parameters and sperm motion in 12 volunteers. *Fertility and Sterility* 51(6):1011–18.

Kwan, M., W. J. Greenleaf, J. Mann, L. Crapo, and J. M. Davidson. 1983. The nature of androgen action on male sexuality: A combined laboratory–self-report study on hypogonadal men. *Journal of Clinical Endocrinology and Metabolism* 57(3):557–62.

Matsumoto, A. M. 1990. Effects of chronic testosterone administration in normal men: Safety and efficacy of high dosage testosterone and parallel dose-dependent suppression of luteinizing hormone, follicle-stimulating hormone, and sperm production. *Journal of Clinical Endocrinology and Metabolism* 70(1):282–87.

Meisel, R. L., and B. D. Sachs. 1994. The physiology of male sexual behavior. In *The physiology of reproduction*. Vol. 2. New York: Raven Press.

O'Carroll, R., and J. Bancroft. 1984. Testosterone therapy for low sexual interest and erectile dysfunction in men: A controlled study. *British Journal of Psychiatry* 145:146–51.

Pavlou, S. N., K. Brewer, M. G. Farley, J. Lindner, M. C. Bastias, B. J. Rogers, L. L. Swift, J. E. Rivier, W. W. Vale, P. M. Conn, and C. M. Herbert. 1991. Combined administration of a gonadotropin-releasing hormone antagonist and testosterone in men induces reversible azoospermia without loss of libido. *Journal of Clinical Endocrinology and Metabolism* 73(6):1360–69.

Sherwin, B. B. 1988. A comparative analysis of the role of androgen in human male and female sexual behavior: Behavioral specificity, critical thresholds, and sensitivity. *Psychobiology* 16(4):416–25.

Sundaram, K., N. Kumar, and C. W. Bardin. 1993. 7 alpha-methyl-nortestosterone (MENT): The optimal androgen for male contraception. *Annals of Medicine* 25(2):199–205.

Tenover, J. S. 1992. Effects of testosterone supplementation in the aging male. *Journal of Clinical Endocrinology and Metabolism* 75(4):1092–98.

Tom, L., S. Bhasin, W. Salameh, B. Steiner, M. Peterson, R. Z. Sokol, J. Rivier, W. Vale, and R. S. Swerdloff. 1992. Induction of azoospermia in normal men with combined Nal-Glu gonadotropin-releasing hormone antagonist and testosterone enanthate. *Journal of Clinical Endocrinology and Metabolism* 75(2):476–83.

Tsitouras, P. D., C. E. Martin, and S. M. Harman. 1982. Relationship of serum testosterone to sexual activity in healthy elderly men. *Journal of Gerontology* 37(3):288–93.

Udry, J. R., J. O. G. Billy, N. M. Morris, T. R. Groff, and M. H. Raj. 1985. Serum androgenic hormones motivate sexual behavior in adolescent boys. *Fertility and Sterility* 43(1):90–94.

Vickery, B. H. 1986. Comparison of the potential for therapeutic utilities with gonadotropin-releasing hormone agonists and antagonists. *Endocrine Review* 7(1):115–24.

Wallace, E. M., S. M. Gow, and F. C. W. Wu. 1993. Comparison between testosterone enanthate–induced azoospermia and oligozoospermia in a male contraceptive study I: Plasma luteinizing hormone, follicle stimulating hormone, testosterone, estradiol, and inhibin concentrations. *Journal of Clinical Endocrinology and Metabolism* 77(1):290–93.

Wang, C., R. S. Swerdloff, and G. M. H. Waites. 1994. Male contraception: 1993 and beyond. In *Contraceptive research and development 1984 to 1994*, edited by P. F. A. Van Look and G. Perez-Palacios. Delhi: Oxford University Press.

World Health Organization (WHO) Task Force on Methods for the Regulation of Male Fertility. 1990. Contraceptive efficacy of testosterone-induced azoospermia in normal men. *Lancet* 336(8721):955–59.

———. 1993. Comparison of two androgens plus depot-medroxyprogesterone acetate for suppression to azoospermia in Indonesian men. *Fertility and Sterility* 60(6):1062–68.

World Health Organization (WHO) Task Force on Psychosocial Research in Family Planning. 1980. Acceptability of drugs for male fertility regulation: A prospectus and some preliminary data. *Contraception* 21(2):121–34.

———. 1982. Hormonal contraception for men: Acceptability and effects on sexuality. *Studies in Family Planning* 13(11):328–42.

Wu, F. C. W., and R. J. Aitken. 1989. Suppression of sperm function by depot medroxyprogesterone acetate and testosterone enanthate in steroid male contraception. *Fertility and Sterility* 51(4):691–98.

PART THREE

---

*Challenging
Entrenched Attitudes
and Behavior
Related to Sexuality*

The Varieties
of Sexual Experience

of the Street Children of Mwanza, Tanzania

Rakesh Rajani and Mustafa Kudrati

*How we think of children and youth will determine our ability to commu-
nicate with them, for it will determine whether we talk to them, or with
them; whether we are lecturing or whether we are engaged in dialogue.
Communication with children and youth has its special features and
characteristics; the essential challenge for us is to find ways of expanding
the dialogue, and the direction of greater inclusiveness and more meaningful—rather than token—participation.*

—Jonathan Mann, Second International Conference on
Street Youth, Rio de Janeiro, 1992

Recent attention to the dangers of AIDS and other sexually transmitted infections (STIs) has renewed the interest in young people's sexual practices and "risk behaviors." That many adolescents
have sex, despite official norms, is well known. The World Health
Organization (WHO) estimates that, in many countries, over two-
thirds of adolescents aged fifteen to nineteen years have had sexual intercourse, that adolescents and young people account for a
disproportionate share of STIs, that about half of all HIV infections have occurred in young people under twenty-five years old,
and that one-fifth of people with AIDS are in their twenties (Fee

and Youssef 1993 1; WHO 1992, 1). Available evidence suggests that this picture is generally true for Tanzania and the East African region as a whole (Demographic and Health Surveys 1986–89; Mbunda 1988; TAMWA 1993).

Street children throughout the world are particularly at risk for infection with HIV and other STIs for several reasons: the need to perform "survival sex" or prostitution, greater freedom to experiment with sex, lack of adult protection and socialization, and the inherent dangers of street life. A few studies are beginning to show worrying rates of HIV seropositivity among street children. For example, 7 percent of street boys aged six to fourteen years in Khartoum, 9 percent of street children in state penitentiaries in São Paulo, and 5.3 percent of runaway or street youth in New York have tested HIV-positive (Luna and Rotheram-Borus 1992; UNICEF 1990).

Numerous initiatives have been taken to respond to the crisis, and HIV and AIDS programs are now a common part of interventions for street children. A critical part of such programs' success is how adults relate to children when dealing with sexuality. Historically, sex and AIDS have carried enormously unhealthy moral baggage that has created fear, eroded children's confidence, and driven sexual activity underground. Even the best attempts of some pro-child social workers and children's advocates (including *kuleana* staff) have been ignorant of how street children's sexuality is manifested, which complex factors influence it, and how this varies in different contexts. Social workers often do not understood street children's lives, thoughts, feelings, and priorities and are locked into patterns that sabotage the potential for genuine partnership.

For example, AIDS educators frequently exhort street children to "wait until marriage" or, failing that, to "stick to one faithful partner." More "liberal" educators promote condom use but in the same breath strongly deride male children who engage in anal sex (see, for example, Aggleton, Homans, and Warwick 1988). Since multiple partnering and anal sex are both common sexual practices among street children, such educational exercises stigmatize, make illicit, and short-circuit healthy discussion of certain behaviors. Children are made to feel that their sexual expression is shameful. Instead of being challenged, dogmatic religious or macho viewpoints are reinforced as normative. In this

---

kuleana

kuleana's programs are organized through two interrelated centers. The center for children's rights implements integrated programs in health, innovative education, advocacy, counseling, business support, and community awareness for approximately 140 street children (aged five to sixteen) at any one time. About 100 of these children are also provided with access to a temporary night shelter, vegetarian meals, showers, and a place to wash clothes. The center for sexual health is involved in creative sex education, advocacy for young people, counseling, support for persons with AIDS, condom marketing, running a community resource center, HIV testing, and the production of low-cost, participatory health learning materials. Both centers are involved in research, networking, training, and building up local capacity. *kuleana's* programs are implemented in close cooperation with a range of institutions, including other NGOs, local government departments, and schools.

---

process, street children are denied the skilled, intelligent, and passionate support they require in dealing with sexuality.

kuleana *and the Street Children of Mwanza*

kuleana is a Swahili word meaning "to support" or "to nurture one another." We are a small nongovernmental organization (NGO) based in Mwanza, Tanzania's second largest city, with an estimated population of 600,000. We approach our work with a strong human rights perspective, particularly in relation to children and young people. A significant component of *kuleana's* work is preventing HIV and STIs among street children; this is a joint activity of the Center for Children's Rights and the Center for Sexual Health (see box).

The street children of Mwanza come from wide-ranging backgrounds within the northern lake zone of Tanzania. According to a UNICEF-supported situation analysis conducted by *kuleana*

(Rajani and Kudrati 1993), most street children in Mwanza are forced onto the streets due to a complex combination of factors. The most significant factor, however, is physical and emotional violence in the home (89 percent of the respondents cited violence as a reason for leaving home). Other factors include the emergence of more fluid family networks in newly urbanized families, the weaker position of women within the household, and the weakening of support structures and economic viability (including the death of caretakers) caused by the AIDS epidemic.

Of the 140 street children in the *kuleana* program, only fifteen are girls. This reflects the general ratio of boys to girls on the streets throughout East Africa. Boys generally have more freedom to leave home, experience street life as relatively less risky, and have a larger set of survival options available to them compared with girls. In contrast, girls are often forced into doing harsh and abusive domestic labor in the homes of their families, relatives, or others. Typically these girls are denied the right to education, leisure, and play. Initial evidence suggests that physical and sexual abuse is widespread, but girls in these situations are usually isolated and have little recourse to complain about abusive treatment. Their situation may be the most critical human rights issue in Tanzania today.

kuleana believes that building relationships of mutual trust and respect with street children lies at the heart of conducting effective research and promoting healthy sexual behavior. Strong and informal relationships between staff and children are encouraged. The ten *kuleana* staff members who work closely with street children have participated in training related to working with children in a nonpatronizing and supportive way, learning listening and facilitation skills, encouraging open discussion of sex, and using group-building dynamics.

Knowing that someone cares for them and listens to them over a sustained period of time helps build children's self-esteem. By consistently standing with the children, *kuleana* staff have helped reverse the marginalization that traps street children into abusive behavior. By providing meals (in exchange for responsibility) and a temporary night shelter, we have given children access to a place that is safe from violence and the gnawing pain of not knowing where their next meal is coming from. In learning to tell street children that their feelings of sexual desire are wonderful and normal and that their concerns about sexual violence are real and serious, we have managed to validate children's feelings and undo debilitating notions of shame.

Learning about Children's Sexual Experiences

Unfortunately, relatively little information is available about the specific nature of street children's sexuality and related health implications. When street children have sex, with whom, in what ways, with what frequency, and for what motives remain largely unknown. We also have little understanding of how street children conceptualize their own sexuality. *kuleana* decided to learn about street children's sexual practices in order to assess risk and design appropriate HIV and STI interventions and to better understand what motivates street children to have sex. Most importantly, *kuleana*'s research is situated within an environment of practical services, committed relationship building, and long-term advocacy. The research agenda and its specific trajectories are usually driven by what street children themselves define as priorities, interests, or concerns. We at *kuleana* believe that this sort of relationship is critical to effective research and is probably necessary if the intention is to serve the interests of the street children themselves.

Information about street children's sexual expression is acquired by *kuleana* over time, in four ways. First, most children are members of peer groups of about nine to twelve members. The staff person or counselor attached to the group uses a detailed baseline outline as a guide to find out about children's past and present lives in general. This is done in a gradual, informal manner and can take more than a year to complete. Frequent contact, a relaxed, nonjudgmental attitude, and trust are essential to this process. The information is collected as part of the normal group interaction, during weekly group "picnics," and in individual counseling sessions when a child is experiencing particular difficulty. Information is recorded in a personal file, to which other staff may add comments and observations.

Second, street children's experiences and views about sex are shared in open discussions on a regular basis. This takes place in a variety of structured and informal contexts, including regular classes in *kuleana*'s nonformal education program, some theater performances, special sessions on relationship skills or conflict resolution, and impromptu discussions facilitated by evening staff.

Third, two groups (of five boys and eight girls) have served as the primary consultants on information about street children's sexual practices. Close and trusting contact with the group of boys (aged twelve to fifteen) was first established in the course of carrying out a general situation analysis of street children in late 1992. Members of this group often view themselves as the "original" *kuleana* members and feel a special sense of belonging. This group participates in regular, in-depth discussions about sexual practices, views, and attitudes with core *kuleana* staff.

Informal work on sexual practices with girls began in early 1993 and focused on STI prevention, education, and treatment. A more organized girls' group (aged ten to sixteen) was formed in early 1994 in response to escalating acts of violence, including rape, against girls sleeping on the street. This group meets weekly with a core team of three female *kuleana* staff members. Although these sessions are highly focused and structured, they allow for considerable flexibility. Topics are often initiated by the girls and have included self-esteem, decision making, the meaning of friendship, STIs, pregnancy, contraception, condom negotiation, menstruation, and the feeling of being in love. The methodology used is participatory, and the use of singing, puppets, masks, role playing, and drawing is encouraged.

Finally, the *kuleana* clinical officer, a full-time staff person, compiles careful health records about each street child receiving medical attention, including occurrence of STIs and other physical signs of sexual activity. Notes are also made on street children's experiences with local health services.

Varieties of Sexual Expression and Risk Behavior

The necessity of selling sexual favors in order to survive is seen as a major risk factor in HIV infection among street children (Boyden and Holden 1991; Luna and Rotheram-Borus 1992; UNICEF

1990). Numerous studies report a recent increase in adults seeking younger sex partners who are perceived to be free of HIV. Adults exploiting children in this way pose a particular danger, because they probably have higher than average rates of HIV seropositivity. The physiological trauma (sores, bleeding) that is more likely to occur when bigger adults have vaginal or anal intercourse with smaller children also substantially increases the chances of HIV infection. In these fundamentally unequal relationships, children have little power to negotiate the terms of sexual encounters, such as the use of condoms or avoidance of rough sex practices.

However, too much focus on adult perpetrators and stereotypical prostitution can be limiting and misleading.[1] An overemphasis, for example, on the threat posed by external exploiters may give a false sense of security about sex with "friends." Our experiences and research findings at *kuleana* point to the need to pay more attention to children's sexual expressions with one another. Some of our key findings are presented below.

Prostitution

Most significantly, stereotypical prostitution probably accounts for less than 5 percent of all potentially risky sexual encounters among street children in Mwanza. During the course of the study, very few boys reported having engaged in this type of prostitution. Although it was reported more frequently among girls, it still constituted a relatively small percentage (less than 15 percent) of their total sexual activity. Slightly more frequently, both boys and girls reported reluctantly agreeing to have sex with male acquaintances with whom they were staying at night in exchange for warmth, safety from police, and meals. In these cases, the sexual partners were usually known to the children and were part of their network of relationships.

Rape

Rape was reported by both boys and girls.[2] In most cases, the assailant was older, known to the children, and attacked while they were sleeping. Rape of boys involved anal penetration, and rape of girls involved both anal and vaginal penetration. In the past twelve months, several cases of STIs in both boys and girls were traced to such incidents of rape. Sleeping together in groups is preferred, as it offers the safety of numbers. However, even in these situations, some children reported a reluctance to resist unwanted sexual advances for fear of being beaten later by their assailants when alone.

To the street children, the fundamental motive for ambush rape appeared to be the expression of physical power and its use as a weapon of terror. Many children exclaimed, "What could I do? He is the boss!" and "He rapes us because he wants us to know who is in charge." The threat of rape was also used to subdue children into obedience: "If I don't do what he tells me to do, he will treat me badly at night." Significantly, children always placed rape (conceptually) with other expressions of violence (beatings, fights, being locked up) and not in the same cluster of expressions used to refer to sex or play.

Kunyenga: *Initiation among Street Boys*

The street slang for nonmutual anal penetration is *kunyenga*. However, *kunyenga* is also practiced among street boys in initiation rites that are conceptually complex and different from the rape described above. Typically, a new child is lured over to "the rocks" (on the hills around Mwanza) by a group of boys who promise food and access to the "group secret." New children, who probably feel isolated and vulnerable, usually go along because of curiosity, wanting to belong, and the inability to say no. Once on the rocks, each member of the group anally rapes, or *nyengwas*, the new boy. The group explains this as a necessary and proper rite of belonging and threatens violence in case of resistance. It is explained as a way of telling new children that "our life is different from normal life" or, more specifically, that "we play by different rules."

Virtually all street boys have been *nyengwa*ed in this way. The children described the experience as confusing and somewhat scary but did not appear to be immediately traumatized by it. We were often told, "They fucked me," and we would see a bewildered face that seemed to say, I don't quite understand why, or what does this mean? Although *kunyenga* is an important rite of passage in identity formation, the children seemed to be uncertain about the function of this particular initiation rite. When asked why this practice was important, they responded, "We just do it" or "That's just how it is."

Belonging is established through the very assertion of authority. Exhibition of another's power over one's body appears to be the inevitable price of becoming a member of the group. How this practice influences future group dynamics, sexual relationships with friends, or the experience of intimacy remains unknown. We also do not know the effects of this form of *kunyenga* on children's emotionality, self-esteem, or sense of self, especially in the long term. Even though it clearly expressed the use of power, children conceptualized this initiation experience differently from other experiences of sexual violence, such as ambush rape at night, which were more strongly associated with being wronged or shamed. According to the children, *kunyenga* was different because it was "open" and "something that had to happen."

Kunyenga *at Night*

Another form of *kunyenga* takes place at night among (usually) same-size boys between seven and thirteen years old. Typically, a boy wakes up to find one of his sleepmates attempting to have or having anal sex with him (leading to ejaculation). About 7 to 10 percent of the boys were identified by their peers as being particularly prone to this "habit." In discussions, these boys consistently shrugged about their reasons for this practice: "Hey, I wake up, and just feel like doing it" or "I couldn't help it with the [physical] pressure." Other than going for the quieter (that is, more docile) children and avoiding someone bigger who may "beat you up," the choice of partners seemed quite arbitrary.

Our colleagues at *kuleana* have observed that street boys in Mwanza practice relatively little self-masturbation, and this form of *kunyenga* appears to be primarily about relieving sexual tension: "It's really a practical thing about what to do with a hard-on." The children who are used "as receptacles" (their own words) appear to be more irritated at being woken up and "*pizzed* upon" (in cases of ejaculation) than violated or traumatized: "Why does this asshole bother me when I'm trying to sleep? Why can't he go bug someone else?"

The line between this kind of *kunyenga* as relief of sexual tension and "comfort sex"—the sexual expression of affection and consideration among boys—is often blurred (see Bond, Mazin, and Jiminez 1992). *kuleana* staff and other children reported seeing children holding each other tightly, rubbing their genitals against each other, fondling, and engaging in anal sex. In these exchanges, both partners might participate equally, except during anal sex, when one was "active" and his partner might even "pretend to sleep."

These expressions often appeared to provide pleasure and to involve mutual consent. When asked, street boys typically described the experiences as "playing," that is, not something that should be taken seriously. They were very reluctant to admit gratification or an active role in *kunyenga* as comfort sex, because anyone willingly and actively pursuing homosexual relations is seen as *mhanisi* (the cultural equivalent of "faggot"), or "man turned woman." To be so labeled can have severe consequences: one can be rejected from the peer group or, worse still, be subject to increased vilification and physical abuse. Authorities such as the police have also been reported to treat those suspected of homosexuality with particular harshness. At a personal level, being *mhanisi* is experienced as the worst kind of humiliation.

The prevailing homophobia raises important questions about how children view their own homosexual relations. Clearly, one way in which children cope with this is to see homosexuality as "play between friends" (a legitimate activity among boys) rather than "sex" (illegitimate). The probable serious psychosocial effects of this dissonance, especially the long-term effects, remain unknown.

Boys' Sex with Girls and Women

Street boys in Mwanza also engage in vaginal sex, usually with street girls or marginalized young women who work as commercial sex workers. For most boys, this sex normally begins at around age fourteen or fifteen. In a survey of thirty-two boys aged fourteen to seventeen years, we found that twenty-five out of thirty-two (78 percent) had had sex with females; for most of those who had not done so, "it was only a matter of time" before they would. In most cases, both partners knew each other and came from similarly marginalized backgrounds. Condom use was sporadic; very few appeared to use them regularly, and not a single child reported using condoms consistently.

Sex with girls or women is seen as "real sex." It marks the transition into "manhood" and is an important way of distinguishing oneself from the "boys." Female partners vary; some boys described having "favorites," but "steady" relationships rarely last more than three months. Additionally, sex with women represents power in several ways. Because it usually requires money or relatively expensive favors (going to a movie, buying a meal), access to women implies enviable financial extravagance. "I take my woman to the video, and then I treat her to ice cream [a status product] and then we have sex" is a statement of pride and accomplishment.

In focus-group discussions, it was also quickly apparent that sex with women represented the power of having a body at one's disposal to relieve sexual tension. "Whenever I have [an erection] I have a woman to *pizz* into." This is widely perceived as more mature than masturbation or the "shameful" act of anal intercourse. "Buying" a prostitute meant having the power to have her do whatever the boy wanted her to do, at least temporarily. Finally, vaginal sex was seen to symbolize physiological strength, potency, and virility, characteristics critical to being a "real man." "I have my girl" often seemed to be the legitimizing punctuation to many a street boy's deliberately smooth macho walk.

This does not mean that street boys lack feelings of care and affection. On various occasions, boys appeared to be nervous and excited and enthralled by romantic feeling. We observed several relationships in which boys were "in love" and treated girls with apparent tenderness. But there was never any question that boys had to be in charge and "their" girls had to be subservient. When challenged, boys invariably responded that both boys and girls had a "right place" or well-defined roles and that they were simply playing their proper part. Patterns of male domination within their families or surrounding society were often invoked. Besides, it was remarked, "being soft makes you look like you're not a man, like you are a woman." Image was essential; a boy going through adolescence had to show his friends that he knew how to act his role.

How street boys conceptualize sex is critical to the design of effective programs. Our experience shows that street boys engage in a wide range of sexual activities with remarkable variation in motives. Significantly, our discussions with street children revealed that they employ different conventions in conceptualizing this range of activities. Whereas we had (initially) seen all the activities described as different clusters of sexual activity, street boys see them as separate and distinct activities, only one of which is actually defined as "sexual."

The Sexual Lives of Street Girls

In her review of the literature on sexuality, Dixon-Mueller (1993, 271) notes that "the sexual pathways that adolescent girls and boys follow are typically very different, with important implications for service providers." The contexts in which they have sex, the factors that regulate it, and effective ways of promoting sexual health are vastly different for street girls as compared with street boys.

Significantly, our study showed that sex plays a much larger and more central role in the lives of street girls, especially after puberty, as compared with boys. The frequency of sexual acts was higher, it occupied much more of their time, and it was clearly identified by girls as a high priority in counseling situations at *kuleana*. The incidence and recurrence of STIs were also proportionately much higher in girls compared with similarly physically mature boys. During the course of the study, over 80 percent of the girls had STIs at least once (several had two or more recurrences), as compared with 30 percent of boys who were estimated to have experienced STIs during the same period.[3]

Street girls in Mwanza have sex primarily with street boys and other men situated on the margins of society (for example, unemployed men and those working in low-paying, low-status jobs such as restaurant cleaners and porters). In two cases, girls had occasional sexual relations with men who were part of a group of homeless people with leprosy. During the study, only one girl (aged sixteen) worked in stereotypical prostitution at a bar. Girls reported engaging primarily in vaginal sex and, less frequently, in anal sex. Condom use was very erratic, regardless of the partner.

As is generally the case in many societies, in Tanzania, particular primacy is placed on females as sexual beings. Much of the rhetoric about what it means to be a woman, wife, or girlfriend revolves around satisfying one's male partner sexually and in other related roles (such as childbearing). *kuleana*'s experience in Mwanza shows that this is particularly true for marginalized females such as street girls. Importantly, in contrast to other women and street boys, street girls have a much narrower range of options for earning a living. Therefore, whereas other girls and women may be able to assert a different role for themselves, street girls have comparably fewer resources, clout, or protection. "If I was a school girl I could say don't bother me, I want my education. If I had a business I could say I was a businesswoman. If I had lived in a home then they wouldn't think of me [sexually] because they would know I have parents."

Pushed into these roles, street girls often have to accept conditions that are harmful to their health and self-esteem. As Dixon-Mueller (1993, 269) writes, "Girls and women often have little control over what happens to them sexually, that is, over men's sexual access to their bodies and the conditions under which sexual encounters take place." Street girls reported being frequently abused by their male partners. Relationships have very little mutuality; beatings, threats, rough sex, and other kinds of violence are quite common. Girls also have relatively little leverage in negotiating condom use and other safer sex practices.

However, the situation is more complex than it appears at first sight. Street girls appear to have internalized their role as sexual beings and to see sex as a way to meet their needs. Just as boys understand "being a man" as behaving in a dominant fashion, girls understand "being a woman" as pleasing men sexually. This is no accident. In both childhood and street experiences, girls have learned that self-esteem, acceptance, and love are usually available only through sex.[4]

At the same time, characterizing the street girls as passive victims is inaccurate. Far from being "crushed," they rarely seem depressed and are often extremely spunky and sharp. Even in some clearly unequal relationships, street girls can be tremendously savvy and are often able to extract considerable benefits for themselves. For example, street girls' relationships with men often involve complex practical exchanges. In some cases, street girls receive important benefits in the form of food, clothes, and entertainment. In other cases, boys or men who offer physical protection from a harsh world are particularly valued. "First he bought me these nice shoes. Then I like him because he won't let anybody else hurt me. Last night he chased away the guys who had been harassing me."

Despite their rather overwhelming experiences of sex as power, intimidation, and practical exchange, many girls continue to experience sexual feeling in terms of love, physical attraction, and yearning for friendship. In conversations, we hear remarks like, "He looks soooo nice!" "I want to be with him now!" or "You know, I really like him, I like the way he takes care of me, I think I want to be married with him." Relationships are also viewed as one way to re-create families that the street girls have lost or never had. The male partner is usually referred to as "husband" and less frequently as "father." "Family activities" of eating and sleeping together, shopping, planning dates, and taking care of each other when ill are seen as ways of expressing "family affection." (See Worth's chapter in this volume for a further discussion of this theme.)

As can be expected, the combination of damaging sexist roles and the internalized desire to seek fulfillment through them can be profoundly confusing for street girls. Because the continuum between love and abuse is so blurred, and because they have very low self-esteem, street girls often accept violence and humiliation in the pursuit of love and connection. Alternatively, girls may pursue sex in a cynical and calculated attempt to gain resources while continuing to think that the sexual experience needs to be "something special." This confusion often leaves them paralyzed, their ability to seek and create healthy options seriously undermined. One particularly disturbing effect seems to be a complete numbing out—separating one's mind from one's body and being incapable of refusing sexual advances and the abuse of one's body. Many street girls in Mwanza find it difficult to even conceptualize a desire to care for themselves.

The Difficulties of Working with Children on Issues of Their Sexuality

We have tried to show that street children's sexual expressions are varied and complex and that we need to understand them carefully and deeply if we are serious about our work. We at *kuleana* have been struggling with these issues over the past two years. Our ongoing work with the street children of Mwanza has provided us with unique opportunities to carry out innovative interventions. But, despite numerous successes, we are still trying to develop healthy sexual lifestyles among street children. We are the first to admit the enormity of this task.

So where do we go from here? How can we move forward on these issues? What practical steps can we take? What is possible when we are dealing with such contorted and complex issues?

Clearly, improved communication between street children and adult supporters is central to this work. We must learn how to avoid paternalism, cultivate real dialogue, and listen to children with respect—all difficult processes, given the fact that most of us grew up with strongly hierarchical backgrounds. However, we also need to make sure that we do not make the fundamental paternalistic error of thinking that the task at hand involves learning useful communication skills and increasing staff sensitivity. Although these are important, the stakes are much higher.

Much, we suspect, hinges on our capacity to positively reorient the inevitable adult ambivalence toward children's sexuality. Preventing children's engagement in abusive sexual practices is extremely important. But children and adolescents are also sexual beings, with feelings of desire and connection, curiosity and lust. Sexuality and the license to deal with sexual feeling are rights and responsibilities for children as much as for anyone else. In denying this, adult-run NGOs may be doing the greatest disservice to the children and young people they aim to serve.

All too often, adults attempt to regulate children's sexual expression through fear and shame. But stigmatizing children's sexual expression does enormous harm. Can we free ourselves from such deeply held adult attitudes toward children's sexual practices? At *kuleana,* this is a constant battle (and sometimes a source of tension among staff): how easily we all slip into familiar patterns of adult-child power dynamics, how easily our imagination fails to come up with healthy alternatives to adult-child relationships that stigmatize children's sexuality.

And yet a positively recast framework for responding to children's sexuality is more likely to lead to effective HIV and STI prevention responses among children. Careful and exhaustive reviews of school AIDS programs, for example, have shown that open sex education generally leads to more responsible and safer attitudes toward sex and sexual relationships (Fine 1988; WHO 1992). Our own experience with the street children of Mwanza shows that recognizing street children's sexual desires as normal and healthy is an essential starting point for effective HIV and STI prevention. By making the discourse on sex open, honest, direct, and attractive, we may be able to encourage children's safe, healthy, and enjoyable sexual expression.

This means a critical shift in our language and emphasis. Can we at *kuleana* do it? Do we have the courage to talk with children, for example, about sexual desire being wonderful rather than sinful; about pleasuring safely rather than avoiding risk; about celebrating responsibly rather than preventing death? Do we have a powerful conceptual vocabulary to talk about what it takes to be a man (not aggression and machismo) and what it takes to be a woman (not docility and sexual satisfaction of men)?

In the end, our success at *kuleana* might hinge on our ability to be with children in a different way. Respecting children involves according them the right to participate in making decisions that affect their lives and the lives of their communities, including the right to share in the process of making decisions about their sexual well-being. Although it would be naive to think that children making their own decisions will solve everything, it is important to include their meaningful participation in constructing a healthy culture of their own sexual relationships. Possibly only through the institution of more democratic forms of children's participation will they be able to enter into a real partnership with adults and ultimately be in a position to safeguard their health and make responsible decisions in their own interests.

The balance between the terrifying work of rethinking our response to children's sexual expressions, the larger work of facilitating children's meaningful participation, and getting practical, important, day-to-day things done efficiently is extremely difficult. Perhaps these divisions are artificial, and there are useful ways of integrating them all. Regardless, however, the work of dealing with street children's sexual practices cannot be limited to a small subset of activities. The task is huge, and it demands enormous energy, imagination, and commitment. At *kuleana* and elsewhere, where many of us are overwhelmed with the nitty-gritty of daily responsibilities, whether we have the resources to do the job in more than a haphazard fashion remains a question.

The scenarios discussed above present particular challenges for HIV and STI prevention work with street children. We need to understand the types of sexual activity, the complexity of relational power dynamics, and the often mixed motivations of sexual engagements among street children. Entangled in the unhealthy web of relational dynamics described above, street girls' and boys' sexual experiences can entail extremely difficult negotiations with harmful consequences. But it would be a mistake to think of children's sexual experiences only in terms of danger or to characterize their sexual engagement as only risky, misguided, or requiring control. Street children's decisions to have sex in varying circumstances are probably based on potentially healthy impulses—for friendship and connection, for curiosity and desire, for practical gain. The real challenge is working with street children to turn these impulses into safe, healthy, responsible, and enjoyable choices that affirm their dignity.

Findings to Keep in Mind When Developing Sex Education Programs for Street Children

Editor' Note: Based on their years of experience at *kuleana*, Rakesh Rajani and Mustafa Kudrati offer the following thoughts on the possibility of HIV and STI prevention among street children.

1. Street children in Mwanza (and we suspect elsewhere as well), engage in higher levels of sexual activity among themselves, including homosexual activity, than stereotypical exploitation and prostitution. Although the "per act" risks from engaging in stereotypical prostitution and rape are higher, street children are at higher risk from sexual activity among themselves because this behavior is far more prevalent and because they typically do not classify this as sexual activity. An overemphasis on the dangers of sex with exploitative adults or prostitutes can be harmful if it inadvertently creates a false sense of security about sexual activities between children.

2. What adults call sex may not be "sex" for street children. As discussed above, street boys in Mwanza categorize what adults call sexual activi-

ties in three separate clusters, only one of which—vaginal sex—is classified as a "sexual" activity. In contrast, some of the *kunyenga* activities were seen as being part of the "violence" continuum ("Cool it, give him the money or he'll beat the hell out of you, or he'll fuck you if he is really angry"). Other activities, such as comfort sex, rubbing, and fondling, were perceived as being part of the "play" continuum ("That? . . . We were first playing cards and then playing hide and seek with our hands"). In other words, most "sexual" practices are not categorized as sex by these children! To refer only to "sex" in HIV and STI prevention interventions may therefore fail to address activities categorized by children as "violence" or "play."

3. The varieties and contexts of street children's sexual practices are deeply embedded in complex power and friendship dynamics. For boys, *kunyenga* represents a range of activities that are partly intimidating and violent and partly desired for offering affection and belonging. After the age of fourteen to fifteen, boys confirm their manhood through vaginal sex with women and girls who are on the margins of society. In their sexual relationships with men, street girls are often caught between seeking comfort, protection, connection, and practical gain and avoiding pain and domination. In seeking fulfillment within patriarchal norms, girls enter into nonmutual relationships in which they have little room to maneuver safer and healthier sexual lifestyles. Therefore, simply telling children to stop having sex or offering alternatives to money earned through sex is unlikely to work. Furthermore, HIV and STI prevention programs for young people often assume a desire on the part of sexual partners to strengthen their (monogamous) relationship. But this is not the case for both female and male street children, for whom sexual liaisons vary greatly. In this context, the notion of building mutuality—through learning to listen to each other, making joint decisions—may be wildly unrealistic.

4. HIV and STI prevention is simply not a priority or a major concern for most street children. Sex is not perceived as a major health issue or a source of risk. Virtually all the children in our study were aware of the fatal consequences of acquiring HIV, but this had little impact on changing behavior. In some of our education sessions, we learned that the children were much more interested in "virility" than "safer sex.". Teaching a boy how to refuse the invitation to serial rape on the rocks will not be enough if he sees this initiation as necessary for acceptance within the group. Avoiding a person with a history of violence may not be a priority if he has the clout to bail his favorite street children out of jail. In all these cases, sexual relations meet some of the street children's most critical needs.

5. The immediate is what matters, because that is where street children have to survive. Because one's life depends on a series of immediate daily negotiations, street children cannot afford to look toward the future. To children faced with harsh realities, AIDS and STIs are minor, peripheral issues. Concretely, this means placing immediate gains over long-term health consequences. When asked to consider the potentially harmful and painful effects of acquiring STIs, one girl typically responded, "Yes, but I have to make sure I have some money for food and movies, and also I have to pay Asha back her loan." One of our colleagues said it succinctly: "Consequences beyond twelve hours are out of range."

6. Children who have experienced violence often sense that they are unable to control their own lives or determine their futures. Violence pervades the lives of street children. As reported earlier, 89 percent of these children cited violence as one of their reasons for leaving home, and virtually all respondents said that they had experienced police brutality at least once on the streets (Rajani and Kudrati 1993). When children are violated, they get the message that they are bad and worthless. Without self-esteem, young people feel unable to make a difference in their lives and unmotivated to act to protect themselves. In this environment, there is little incentive for children to invest in their future or to practice safe sexual behavior. One child in Mwanza put it bluntly, "Who cares if I get AIDS . . . I'm gonna die when I'm gonna die."

How to Do HIV and STI Education with Street Children

1. Develop a relationship with street children. Sexual behavior is a personal and complex issue; dealing with it requires relationships of mutual trust. There are no shortcuts. Create a climate of open communication and confidence. Don't dominate or preach. Avoid patronizing. Don't pity. Learn to respect children and have them respect you. Listen. Learn to speak street language. Be patient. Be truthful. Take time and energy. Try to see the world from the children's point of view. Let them know that you care.

2. Begin with the children's priorities and give them your support. You have your agenda, and street children have theirs, and usually risky sexual behavior isn't high on their list. Deal first with issues that are important to the children because (a) they often know what matters

more, (b) these issues may affect sexual behavior, and (c) otherwise they won't pay much attention to you. Be open to working with other priorities before HIV and STIs. A range of support services, including health care, legal advocacy, income-earning opportunities, counseling, and safe refuge, may be needed. Find out what matters to children—what they really care about, what they worry about, what gives them their kicks. Get excited with them. Get involved in their projects. Support them in pursuing their dreams.

3. Encourage peer-based learning and action. Most street children spend considerable time with other street children. They feel more connection with and learn tremendously from one another. Use child-to-child approaches. Provide ongoing support, but do not dominate. Help them build up structures and habits of supporting one another—each member will be stronger in this way. When children participate, you receive input from the experts. Identify their strengths and innovations, especially among those who are resilient and make responsible choices about sex. Build on their experiences and help them teach one another. They will feel ownership and learn practical skills. It will give them a sense of belonging and excitement and perhaps restore a sense of having control over their lives.

4. Deal with power relationships. Sexual negotiations are all about power—power to have it your way, to have your views matter, to know what is happening, to articulate your situation, to determine your own self-image, to refuse. In our adult-dominated world, children need the power to be heard and share in decision making, especially when they come from violent households. In our male-dominated world, girls need the power to take care of themselves and shape their world. Talk about fairness and justice. Challenge unfair authority. Question stereotypical roles and images. Challenge machismo. Use the language of rights. Do exercises (such as role reversals) to help children understand what it feels like not to have power and what they can do about it. Talk about abuse, make it clear that it is unacceptable, and discuss how to avoid it. Teach conflict resolution. Make it cool to share power.

5. Focus on developing life skills. Providing information is useful, but information alone is not enough. (What good is it to know how to use a condom if your partner will beat you up at its mere suggestion?) Preventing HIV and STIs requires life skills—the power to turn information into reality. This means learning to make decisions, take responsibility, take care of yourself, understand how your body works, handle difficult situations, deal with peer pressure, be confident, be assertive, and find out new information. It means analyzing a situa-

tion, organizing, and finding strategies to change the circumstances that put you down and strengthen the relationships that lift you up. Skills are not acquired nor behavior changed overnight—it takes time, so support that process. Share experiences. Talk about relationships. Use role playing, picture codes, puppets, theater, forum theater, music, and individual and group discussion.

6. Keep up the motivation; make it fun. Promoting healthy sexual practices is long and hard work, and it won't last if children are not continually renewed, if they do not find pleasure in the process. Make children (and staff) feel special, feel that they are making a difference. Give plenty of encouragement. Acknowledge positive and healthy practices in a concrete way—give certificates, badges, T-shirts; organize special recognition ceremonies. Nobody endures boredom, no matter how serious the matter. Organize your activities in a way that lets children enjoy themselves. Make your work activity-based, move about, draw, sing, act, go on field trips, play games, be silly. Make it thrilling to be involved in HIV and STI prevention.

7. Organize ongoing staff training and reflection. Most of us (staff) grew up with little support to deal with sexuality. Damaging hierarchical relations, condescension, moralizing, and shame pervade adult discourse on sexuality. We need to learn how to talk about sex with children in a healthy and constructive way. Examine your feelings and deal with your own sexual hang-ups and gender stereotypes. Reflect on and evaluate your approach and your strategies. What works? What needs to be strengthened? Identify the skills you need. Learn to be creative and bold. Learn from others. Think of how you can keep learning. Build a support network for one another.

Notes

We would like to thank the many *kuleana* staff and volunteers who participated in this project for their relationship with the children, for their fierce commitment, for their thoughtful comments, and for consistently helping us keep our bearings. Special thanks go to Concilia John, Butolwa Justine, Pelagia Lugeleka, David Masele, Lemmy Medard, Theo Mshabaha, Dipak Naker, and Mary Plummer.

1. By stereotypical prostitution, we mean the selling of sexual favors to external clients (that is, persons with whom the children have no prior relationship and no present relationship other than a sexual one).

2. Incidents of rape have recently been significantly reduced after two interventions by *kuleana:* the provision of a temporary night shelter and legal follow-up, leading to the arrest of two young men involved in raping children.

3. However, the rate of STIs among older male youth aged seventeen to twenty-five who sleep on the street, with whom *kuleana* also works but who were not part of this study, is comparably very high. In a December 1994 survey, nineteen out of twenty-nine (65.5 percent) self-reported having symptoms of STIs.

4. It is easy to see how this is especially true for girls who have been sexually abused by their parents or respected members of the family. In this context, providing alternatives to sex in the form of educational opportunities, business support, or increased physical protection may not necessarily work, though there have been positive indications from some project experiences (see, for example, Vasconcelos 1992).

References

Aggleton, P., H. Homans, and I. Warwick. 1988. Young people, sexuality education, and AIDS. *Youth and Policy* 23.

Bond L., R. Mazin, and M. Jiminez. 1992. Street youth and AIDS. *AIDS Education and Prevention Supplement* 4:14–23.

Boyden, J., and P. Holden. 1991. *Children of the cities.* London: Zed Books.

Demographic and Health Surveys. 1986–89. Columbia, Md.: Institute for Resource Development.

Dixon-Mueller, R. 1993. The sexuality connection in reproductive health. *Studies in Family Planning* 24(5):263–82.

Fee, N., and M. Youssef. 1993. *Young people, AIDS and STD prevention: Experiences of peer approaches in developing countries.* Geneva: WHO/ Global Programme on AIDS.

Fine, M. 1988. Sexuality, schooling, and adolescent females: The missing discourse of desire. *Harvard Education Review* 58(1):29–53.

Luna, C., and M. J. Rotheram-Borus. 1992. Street youth and the AIDS pandemic. *AIDS Education and Prevention Supplement* 4:1–13.

Mbunda, W. 1988. *Adolescent fertility in Tanzania: Knowledge, perceptions and practices. Survey Report 2.* Chama Cha Uzazi na Malezi Bora Tanzania. Dar es Salaam: UMATI.

Rajani, R., and M. Kudrati. 1993. *Street children of Mwanza: A situation analysis.* Mwanza: kuleana/UNICEF.

Tanzania Media Women's Association (TAMWA). 1993. *Teenage reproductive health—the need for strategies: Action in Tanzania.* Dar es Salaam: TAMWA.

UNICEF. 1990. *Children and AIDS: An impending calamity.* New York: UNICEF.

Vasconcelos, A. 1992. Street girls in Recife. Presentation at a meeting of the Ashoka Foundation Fellows, Cambridge, Mass.

World Health Organization. 1992. *School health education to prevent AIDS and sexually transmitted diseases.* Geneva: WHO.

Listening to Boys

A Talk with ECOS Staff

Cecilia Simonetti, Vera Simonetti, and Silvani Arruda, with Debbie Rogow

E COS (Studies and Communication on Human Sexuality and Reproduction) is a nonprofit organization founded in 1989 and based in São Paulo, Brazil. Our mission is to help promote and transform values and behavior related to sexuality, health, and reproductive rights, and to do so in ways that help overcome discrimination based on gender, age, class, and race. We fulfill our mission through producing print and video materials; conducting research, seminars, and training workshops; and providing technical assistance.

In the past several decades, a range of educational programs has been developed to address the issues of teenage pregnancy and sexually transmitted diseases (STDs). Many of these programs have focused on girls. Some have tried to teach girls to say no to unwanted sex, some have tried to teach girls to say no to all sex, and some have tried to educate girls to use contraception. All these programs banked on girls' greater incentive to absorb and act on information, since they face disproportionate consequences from unwanted outcomes.

Other programs have aimed their efforts at "couples," perhaps optimistically hoping that by treating the adolescent couple as a functioning, communicating unit, it might become one. Unfortunately, that notion seems idealistic in light of the fact that girls often have very little say in whether or not and in what circumstances they become vulnerable to unwanted pregnancy; many girls have sex that they do not want and do not enjoy.

Almost no sexuality education programs have focused on boys—boys who often exert the primary influence over whether sexual activity occurs; boys who know little about bodies and sexuality but are desperately afraid to ask; boys who are facing confusing messages about what kind of males they should be in the modern world.

Our organization, ECOS, wanted to know: What are boys in Brazil thinking and feeling about the pressure to have sex? How can we help them sort out their conflicting feelings and values and prepare them for satisfying and respectful sexual lives? We were convinced that working with girls and mixed groups was not an adequate way to learn about boys' needs and not an adequate way to meet those needs.

So we set out to listen to boys and to record some of their reflections on a videotape. Over the course of several months, we met four times each with two different groups of fourteen- to eighteen-year-old boys. During these eight sessions, we listened to boys talk about how they make their way through the "thicket" of adolescence. We also produced a videotape based on the last sessions with both groups, focusing on their reflections about their entry into sexual activity.

Although these eight sessions and the videotape were really only a beginning for our work with boys, we think that they generated useful lessons to help in understanding adolescent masculinity. This chapter describes our initial experience, some of what we learned, and where we see ourselves going in the future.

Making a Video on Adolescent Male Sexuality

The idea of working with boys actually came out of our work with girls. We had been doing an occasional question-and-answer column in a popular girls' magazine called *Caricia*. From the questions girls wrote in to the magazine about sexuality, relationships, and reproduction, we learned that girls were not the "subjects" of their own sexual experiences. Girls were convinced that boys had all the answers and knowledge, and they depended on boys to tell them their own experiences. For example, one girl wrote that a boy told her he could tell that she wasn't a virgin. Despite her knowledge of her own sexual inexperience, she wanted to know how she could have lost her virginity! Another girl wrote that her boyfriend would tell her whether he had put his penis in just a little or all the way.

It was from this process that we began to think that we should know more about these boyfriends. Most of what we knew about them we had learned primarily through girls. However, when we decided to deepen our understanding about boys' worlds and boys' consciousness, there was virtually no material to guide us. So we organized two sexuality workshops with fourteen- to eighteen-year-old boys. We told the boys that we wanted to produce a video showing what they thought and felt about relationships, girls, sexuality, and being boys. They agreed to participate. In a series of four sessions with each group, we discussed a variety of issues.

In the first session, our purpose was to have the participants introduce themselves and learn the characteristics of the group. Everyone, including us, sat in a circle. One of the staff members wrote on the blackboard words such as "love," "wish," and "hatred" and asked each person to say his name, age, something he liked, something he hated, and a wish he would like to have fulfilled.

After this warm-up, we used a group dynamic technique to explore the group's interest in sexuality. The participants were asked to split into groups of five or six and to list the issues they would like to discuss with us. When the small group discussions were over, the groups wrote their issues in big letters on sheets of paper. One person from each group taped the sheets with the chosen issues on the board; if there were any repeat issues, the sheets of paper were taped over each other.

To establish priorities for discussion, participants were asked to vote by placing little colored adhesive balls on the sheet with their favorite issue. The three most popular subjects were relationships between boys and girls, virginity/the first time, and homosexuality. Since virginity/the first time was the one that stirred the most interest, we planned to videotape the discussion of that issue during the next session.

For that session, we prepared a list of questions about the first sexual experience: What were their expectations? How did these differ between boys and girls? and so forth. Questions about personal experience were avoided so as not to expose the participants to ridicule by others. We wrote these questions on slips of paper, placed them in a box, and asked each participant to draw one question from the box and respond. These responses were videotaped and gave us enough material for two videos: "Boys: The First Time" and "Virginity." The final tape includes cuts from both groups.

We had done occasional rap groups with boys before, and we had met with many boys in coed sex education classes, so we had a sense of how to make these groups work. For example, we knew how deeply boys' self-esteem is wrapped up in sexuality issues and how great peer pressure can be. Our first rule was to give them plenty of time to open up. We didn't ask them to talk about themselves in the beginning. We didn't want to put them in the position of behaving "perfectly" but dishonestly and then not being able to take back what they had said an hour earlier. And we didn't want them to feel defensive. During an earlier experience, we had asked boys too directly and too soon about the questions they had. They had been uncomfortable with the public admission of having any questions at all, of not knowing everything, and had responded with obviously hostile questions, such as What should we do when we get sick of our wives? So this time, when we wanted to get them to talk about themselves, we began with safer group dynamic techniques, such as anonymous questions written on paper.

Along with the information and support the process provided, the boys had an extra incentive: they knew that they were going to learn about video technology. It's hard to overestimate what a great tool video is. We work with videos in two ways: First, we use an independent production company with a highly qualified team to prepare excellent quality videos around a carefully defined audience and message. Second, with simple equipment, we utilize video as a learning process for both building production skills and deepening participants' awareness of thematic content. In this case, what really matters to us is the discussions during the course of the work rather than the final product.

Making videos can have a tremendous impact on adolescents. They look at the video immediately after taping; they often want to observe it several times, and they experience themselves intensely. They also learn along the way about creativity, technical production, and so on. They are surprised to find that a video can be edited, that we can record scenes that will be assembled not necessarily in chronological order but in a logical sequence that is connected by ideas. Also, the sequence does not have to be recorded through one lens. For example, imagine that we are recording a sequence with a boy and girl playing the parts of father and daughter, in which the father is forbidding his daughter to go out wearing a miniskirt. Various shots from different angles can help create the dramatic effect of the dialogue. Their experience in production helps them understand that much of what takes place on television programs has been edited or assembled to achieve a certain feeling or reaction.

Through process video, kids see the possibility of doing something creative, which can be critical to self-esteem. This is especially true for girls, who generally don't have other opportunities to experience power, but it is also true for boys. And we've seen some of the boys who participated in the workshops change. One boy, Roberto, was a very sensitive and vulnerable kid, and the other guys sometimes said that he was gay (which he wasn't). After the filming, Roberto came to talk to us. He said that he felt more respected and less isolated during the group discussions. Another boy, Gilberto, had difficulty expressing himself due to his extreme shyness. The workshop created a safe space for him, one in which he became motivated to work out his shyness. People noticed the change in Gilberto. Some of the boys said that they wanted the groups to continue, but we weren't able to do this because of our previous time commitments and funding limitations. Other boys came silently and left silently, so we don't know what the experience meant for them.

In addition to listening to boys, we tried to familiarize ourselves with the world these boys inhabited. As much as we could, we immersed ourselves in popular teen culture, including boy culture. Yes, we watched all their favorite TV shows and movies, read their magazines, listened to their music, everything! For a while, our office walls were covered with posters of our own favorite—and least favorite—stars.

What We Learned

Brazil is a country where machismo runs very deep. But in many ways, our culture is also very modern. And let's face it, men's and women's roles are changing rapidly. So adolescent boys are exploring their identity in a changing world, and their conflicts and confusion about what is appropriate for malehood are very close to the surface. But this conflict is positive—change grows out of the need to resolve conflict. All of us in the sexuality education field are hoping to see change.

One of the biggest conflicts boys feel is between the desire to be themselves and the desire to perform in the male world. They worry that girls want enchanted princes, and they don't feel like enchanted princes. They are conflicted about how "macho" to behave. For example, once when the boys were talking about relationships in the abstract, they spoke about their girlfriends' needs. They criticized machismo and wanted to seem enlightened. But then we showed them a video of girls talking about boys' machismo, in which the girls ask for equal gender treatment, that the boys be less jealous and stop picking on them because of short, tight, or low-necked clothes, and that they demonstrate their affection more openly. The boys changed before our eyes. Their body language became defensive. When the video was over, they told us, "We hated that film!" We asked them what they wanted to tell these girls. They answered, "Go learn to cook! Go home and wash dishes." And "These girls confuse machismo with superiority." Another said, "Hoje orgullo, amanha bagulha," which means "Today's pride is tomorrow's old hag."

They tell us that they are worried about penis size, being homosexual, and getting and keeping erections. We think that much of the unspoken reluctance about condoms—among men as well as boys—is not really about "loss of sensitivity" so much as about fear of losing their erections when they stop to put the condoms on. This fear reinforces their general attitude that contraception is an exclusively female responsibility. They complained that "the girls weren't buying their pills, then they get pregnant and make you get married." They told us that their first response when a girlfriend tells them she is pregnant is, "I want you to get a paternity test." One boy who had married his pregnant girlfriend was furious at her for not having taken the pill. Few of them even know what a condom costs. Yet despite their fears, attitudes, and ignorance, some have used condoms, and many have used withdrawal. So some of them do acknowledge some responsibility for contraception.

Moreover, they are caught between wanting information about sexuality and being afraid to bring up a question or a doubt in front of their friends. As a result, these boys don't have the slightest idea about menstruation or when women ovulate. Many don't know about a girl's clitoris. And they are afraid to admit that they are virgins.

Many of these conflicts stem from peer pressure or the pressure to meet a girl's expectations. But we have been most struck by how much pressure boys feel to meet the expectations of their fathers. They feel that their dads are anxious for them to become sexually active. Some of them think that this resolves fathers' fears about their sons being homosexual. In any case, "laying a girl" becomes a badge of success in the male world.

Along with feeling that they are getting pressure from their dads, the boys also have a lot of feelings about what they're not getting from them. Unlike girls, who complain about too much parental control—about skirt length, makeup, and behavior—the boys complain about the absence of their fathers. Some say that they have tried to talk to their fathers. They bring up AIDS, but the fathers tell them, "This is a gay thing." Or they might be worried about a cousin who is using drugs and they don't know what to do. They try to talk to their dads, but they find that their dads don't know what to say. Their words are so clear about how difficult it is to cry, to express their emotions, even to hug each other.

What's Next

We tried to learn as much as we could about the sources of "macho" feelings and how these feelings affect sexual behavior. It's a lot to figure out, but fathers and fathering are a big piece.

By now, we're very attracted to the idea of working with families. We've made a video about AIDS that is for fathers and sons called

"Um Abraco" (An Embrace). It was recently awarded first prize in a Brazilian national health videos contest. The video is also used in a training program for mostly male municipal health workers. We are told that it provokes a very emotional response. So far, we've sold about three hundred copies.

We've begun to give talks about AIDS and drugs to moms and dads who come to pick up their kids at a local child-care center. These parents are very interested.

And we're currently doing a five-day gender training course for public school teachers, half of whom are men. We go through a series of steps with them. We ask what kinds of girls or boys they appreciate as students—in terms of their behavior, their appearance, and so forth. We show them illustrations of everyday situations involving males and females and ask them to interpret what they see. We analyze case studies of family responsibilities by asking who carries out what tasks. We examine adjectives used for males as compared with those used to describe females.

These teachers come to see that they have far more internalized gender stereotypes than they had realized, that they are reproducing inequality in their day-to-day lives. For example, when they looked at a picture of a man caring for a child, they assumed that he was widowed. They learn to apply a critical lens to everyday life. The experience has been the most meaningful for the male teachers. Their evaluations are very emotional.

We'd like to start with preschool, to work with four- to six-year-old kids and their parents in child-care centers, but we don't have the funds yet. Actually, we want to start even younger: if we had financial support, we would work with expectant fathers.

The more attention we pay to the issue of masculine identity, the more we realize how much changing societies demand of young men. They must be strong, brave, and in control. Yet at the same time, we ask them to be sensitive and not to become violent or unemotional. It is not surprising that they feel confused and conflicted about their proper role.

Much more needs to be learned about how young men form their gender identity in contemporary societies, how they weigh their conflicts and alternatives related to masculinity, what rewards and costs go along with changing their sexual behavior and attitudes, and what kind of fathers and husbands they want to become.

We have so much to learn about male sexual identity—for example, how male socialization influences male contraceptive use, STD and HIV risk, notions about "love," and parenting practices.

Finally, we hope that more men begin working with boys. Men can provide important alternative models of "performance" in the male world. We need their help, and not just in Brazil.

When Sex Is a Job

An Interview with Chantawipa Apisuk of Empower

Ara Wilson

*F*ew places in the world are as well known for prostitution as Thailand. Indeed, even though it is illegal, the sex industry is so great in this Southeast Asian kingdom that, as Chantawipa Apisuk succinctly put it, "There are more brothels than schools."[1] With all the attention given to prostitution in Thailand, what remains rare is a real concern for the perspectives of the women in the trade. As founder and head of Empower, a grassroots advocacy organization for sex workers in Thailand, Chantawipa Apisuk has focused on these women's concerns. I talked with Chantawipa at Empower's headquarters in Nonthaburi about prostitution in Thailand, her own development as an activist on this issue, and the strategies and approaches that best address the needs and rights of the hardworking women in the sex trade.

The Birth of an Activist

From 1973 to 1983, Chantawipa was in the United States, furthering her studies. It was during this period that her interest in political

Empower

Empower's approach is conveyed in its name: Education Means Protection of Women Engaged in Recreation. Empower has three "drop-in" centers, two in Bangkok and one in the northern city of Chiang Mai. Its headquarters, which is located in Nonthaburi, about an hour north of Bangkok's sex industry areas, also functions as home to a sister organization that gives support to people living with AIDS. A woman coming to an Empower center can find classes in English and the requisite courses to obtain equivalency primary or secondary school diplomas from the government. Other instruction includes creative expression, such as batik and drama; health issues; and, when there is demand, skills such as sewing and typing. The organization also produces and distributes a free Thai-language newspaper that addresses the experiences and concerns of women in the trade. Empower includes projects to enforce workers' rights laws, which apply to bar workers. In addition, the friendly, nonjudgmental atmosphere of the centers offer a place for women to gather and develop a sense of community so that they can change their situation in the huge sex industry as people who are, traditionally, seen but never heard from. In all these efforts, Empower brings a sense of play and creativity. In 1994, the organization became an official foundation, which allows for easier fund-raising and smoother relations with the government, particularly in Empower's ability to offer its non-formal education program for equivalency certificates. In 1995, Empower celebrated its first decade.

involvement emerged. In solidarity with other anti-imperialist and human rights workers, Chantawipa worked for the release of political prisoners in Southeast Asian countries. "There were different nationalities, men and women working together on issues equally, not divided," she recalls, and this experience provided her with a model for working collaboratively and building coalitions. Chantawipa also kept an eye on dramatic new developments within Thailand and observed that although "there were outspoken women leaders in the political conflict, they didn't specifically address women's issues." Her interest in women's issues, specifically prostitution, emerged later. "In the United States, I came into contact with women activists working against the Vietnam War and in the late 1970s against the 'dumping' of U.S. products into other countries, like Nestle's baby formula [which can be dangerous for women who cannot read the instructions for use or do not have access to running or hot water] or Depo-Provera [which had not yet been approved for use in the United States by the Food and Drug Administration]." These international campaigns against practices that directly harmed women and children were a first step. "They made me involved, a little bit, in women's issues."

Perhaps most significant in raising her awareness about women's issues, however, was her travel experience as a Thai woman. "In the 1970s, when people saw a Thai woman abroad, the assumption was that she was educated and rich. In 1983, I noticed a difference, even in the response of people in Bangkok. Now they asked why I was leaving the country alone. Why was I leaving my husband? Outside of Thailand, because of my Thai passport, people assumed I was a drug trafficker or a prostitute. I saw other Thai women being asked the same questions or singled out for difficult treatment from consular or immigration officials." These experiences ignited her activist sensibility. She saw that this was a stereotype that applied to her as a Thai woman. She understood that "this problem was *my* problem as well." As a result, unlike many other Thai women, she does not stigmatize sex workers.

When Chantawipa returned to Thailand in 1983, Bangkok was transformed. Among the changes was a visible sex industry.[2] The most famous red-light area in Thailand consists of the few lanes that make up Patpong, an area smack in the middle of the downtown financial district, which caters almost exclusively to Western men (with the exception of one lane, Thaniya, which is devoted almost exclusively to Japanese clientele). "Before I left Thailand, Patpong was just a small drinking place filled with U.S. servicemen and foreigners, not well known to Thais." Now this neon-lit area is filled with dozens of go-go bars, some stacked on top of each other, interspersed with fast-food and foreign restaurants that cater mainly to Western tourists. Despite the change, Chantawipa says that she was not shocked by Patpong. As she points out, "Other cities have this. I thought it was like Times Square in New York."

Based on her international political experience, Chantawipa first understood the sex trade predominantly in terms of imperialism and exploitation of the third world; she saw the issue as "workers controlled by foreigners." "In the beginning, we thought that tourism was the problem, not prostitution. A lot of tours came. In Thaniya, we saw Japanese tour guides leading busloads with a flag. I can still see it in my memory." However, she also came to emphasize that women in the sex industry face a number of difficulties because of the stigmatization of their work and, consequently, of themselves. She describes their position with an analogy to her earlier political work: "I saw them like political prisoners in the sense that they are considered 'criminals' when in fact they have not done anything truly wrong but offend the status quo."

Stigmatization of Sex Workers

As in other countries, in Thailand, the attitudes toward prostitution are complex and often contradictory. For example, prostitution is accepted in part because "Thai society believes that men need sex more than women; therefore, men must have sexual outlets. It is also held that the sex business is needed because it prevents the problem of a husband taking minor wives."[3] And yet, despite the prevalence of prostitution and the comforting belief held by many foreign customers that sex work is an acceptable or integrated part of Thai culture, the women in the industry are stigmatized. Like elsewhere in the world, blame, criticism, and legal action are directed almost exclusively at the women workers rather than at the customers or the business owners. Chantawipa asserts that "mostly high-status and rich men" go to sex workers. "They feel, 'I've been working all day long, I have to relax and go to the massage parlor.'" These are powerful people, so "society won't say anything to them." The more powerful agents escape attention and repercussions. "Besides, a lot of people involved make a profit. They have to be doing this with 'protection' because the industry is illegal." The men who buy sexual services are elusive. "If you see a man walking into a brothel and ask 'Are you buying a woman to sleep with?' no one will say he is a customer. It's easy for men to pay money and not be responsible."

The women are another story; women working in the trade are more visible, therefore easier to name and target. In general, it is the women who are "scorned and treated like they are dirty, stupid, lazy, and promiscuous—like troublemakers. It is the women who are viewed by doctors as disease spreaders, and when men have STDs [sexually transmitted diseases] they call it 'women's disease.' As a result, when women ask for treatment for an STD or a gynecological exam, they are poorly treated by clinic staff. Social workers also see these women as poor, stupid, and silly; they are from the countryside and so are backward and ignorant. For development workers and NGOs [nongovernmental organizations], they are a 'target group,' the result of social failure of the national development plan. So they must be 'helped' or 'protected.' And researchers see them as being so different from themselves. They want to see where they eat, how they live; they think it's exciting."

Many people both within and outside of Thailand have called for government intervention to "solve" the problem of the sex industry. However, to date, the Thai government's approach to the industry protects business owners and clients. In "cracking down" on the industry, government has targeted the women. Indeed, "police see women as criminals to be punished, and they use loopholes in the law to take advantage of the women and get money from them. Once in a while, they raid the brothels to get a promotion. When this happens, the women and girls working in brothels and other establishments are put in 'rehabilitation' or homes for socially handicapped women, as they are called." In these homes, girls and women are confined to a kind of reform school, where they receive training in skills that ostensibly provide economic alternatives: skills such as hair cutting, mat weaving, and doll making. However, as Chantawipa points out, the potential income from these activities is not a viable economic alternative. Even if it were, there is a numerical limit: "about 800 to 1,000 women a year" are placed in these homes, "so hundreds of thousands" remain employed as sex workers

But the real problem with this kind of programmatic response, she argues, is that "rehabilitation doesn't help" because the Social Welfare Department "limits or controls the women. It treats them as unequal. It makes them feel guilty. The underlying message is, 'you are dirty, now we wash you so you become clean again.'" This judgmental attitude and regulation of behavior do nothing to help the women gain control of their own lives. Therefore, there is no long-term or even realistic solution to the problems sex workers face.

Chantawipa's Vision: Empower

Chantawipa takes the pain of the stigmatized "bad women" to heart and tries to foster a view of these women as complex and whole people, not solely in terms of their profession. Thai sex workers are usually providing for their children, their younger siblings, or their whole families. "At home, most of these women cook, wash, care for family members. Many times, they have to return home to take care of a sick family member. They are responsible leaders of the family." To her mind, most women do not "choose" to do sex work, rather, "some push-or-pull factor drives them to work in the industry. Indirectly, all the women were forced to become sex workers because of low education, life conditions, and low self-confidence."

She acknowledges that women's involvement in sex work, usually from their teenage years, is physically and emotionally difficult. "Teenagers and young people have sexual feelings and want to be near someone—but someone they choose, not everybody, not just anyone." But these women have to have sex with and spend time with men not of their choosing, and all the while "they have to do what the customer wants to do. They have to act happy, otherwise they're not providing good service. As a profession it's difficult; to have sex with someone we don't know is painful."

Though realistic about the nature of the job, to Chantawipa, the constant focus on sex is a mistake and reflects a limited analysis of sex workers' situations and needs. "I think we should ignore the word 'prostitution' and promote anything that helps women be accepted in society to make them equal to other women. Sex workers must be considered as workers." Concentrating on sex reinforces the stigma of prostitutes and ignores other problems that are more pressing to the women themselves. As Chantawipa points out, "there are other problems—between women and owners, between women and society"—that are more central to helping women tackle the challenges in their lives. "We have to ask, what is the highest level of exploitation these women face? Is it economic exploitation, social exploitation, or sexual exploitation?" She finds the size and organization of the industry compelling evidence that the economic dimension should be seen as dominant: "It's a business on every corner. People make money from selling women." She puts the sex industry in a broader perspective of tourist marketing and consumption: "Sex selling is a promotion to have more people come to Thailand; the government promotes tourism to earn foreign currency. It's like shopping, like trying this group's music or food."

The goal of Empower is to protect women throughout the entertainment industry from the dangers of their jobs. These include the physical dangers of being beaten by their bosses or customers; health dangers, including STDs, poor nutrition, lack of sleep, and poor living quarters; economic exploitation, such as the practice of fining women for not being made up on time or not going out with men the required number of times or, if bar owners can get away with it, keeping the women at work beyond 2 A.M., when bars officially close; and societal attitudes. It is perhaps the latter that is the most debilitating.

Empower's approach to working with these women is pragmatic. Its response is based on an understanding of women's day-to-day problems and needs as workers in a large, even international, industry that exploits them. "The women who come to our centers have limited education, don't read newspapers, and are isolated from society. It's sad. They are nineteen, twenty years old and they don't know Bangkok except for the bars. They don't even know how to get around Bangkok. They want to put money in the bank and their children in school, have letters translated, read the daily paper. They need education to be able to sign their names in the bank." Chantawipa notes, however, that these are not problems limited to prostitutes; rather, they are citizens' rights.

Perhaps the major obstacle to women's organizing and self-help is society's condemnation of them; the stigma against sex work sometimes reduces the women's capacity for self-protection or assertion. Chantawipa believes that "sex workers have a sense of guilt for being in the profession," and because of that, "they feel

they have to do whatever their clients ask for. Society offers no protection to the women." Judgmental or even hostile treatment of
these women by society, business owners, clients, and even those
who are supposedly in a position to help them can deepen the
women's isolation, compounding the serious risks of working in
the sex industry. For example, Chantawipa interprets the common
practice of self-medicating as a consequence of the prejudice these
women encounter in clinics. For example, one of Empower's
clients went to the leading university hospital and was treated
badly. She complained, but the nurse said something like, "You'd
think you'd be used to pain like that by now. Don't complain."

One of the ways Empower challenges this stigma is by accepting
sex work as the women's current reality; Empower does not try to
get the women to leave sex work. "We try to enable the women to
take control of their lives and of their work conditions, and repair
their pride," Chantawipa states. Learning English is a key part of
the empowerment process. This has a practical goal of helping
women negotiate with clients and employers. There is also a more
ambitious, and perhaps political, goal: "We teach English to
women to help them express their wants and their rights. We try to
raise women's confidence and consciousness about themselves."
Many in Empower's circle view the organization more in terms of a
process than in terms of measurable ends, and Chantawipa tells
how one student described Empower as a train: "You can get on
and ride for one stop, or for the whole way." Although Empower
does not suggest to the women that they leave the industry, it
understands that women's time in this job is limited because of
health risks and customer demand for younger women. So
Empower tries to help women plan for the future.

Empower's Reception

One characteristic that sets Empower apart from other projects is
its nonjudgmental approach. The model for relationships in
Empower is not a professional one of social service provider and
client, or rescuer and victim, but rather one of friends, often
expressed in sibling terms, which are used freely in Thailand.
"Empower tries to understand people no matter who they are,"

Chantawipa explains. "We don't say the profession is bad or a sin. We say you are doing what is good for you." As Chantawipa explains, "These women send money home. We try to say, 'You're a leader in your family,' and strengthen their pride. We don't say bad things about the work; this discourages their ability to enter society."

This nonjudgmental approach disturbs some people who are concerned about prostitution, and Empower has been criticized for it. The focus on women as workers does not completely mesh with the common critical view of the industry, which typically passes judgment—explicitly or implicitly—on the women and their work. And in the early years, many were not clear about Empower's aims. Chantawipa recalls, "People criticized me as promoting prostitution by educating prostitutes to be 'clever' sex workers, to bargain for more money."

Other NGOs do not necessarily understand sex work or the work of Empower. "Empower is seen as 'great' for bringing 'witness' to international conferences." But Chantawipa and other representatives are aware of the unspoken questions: "People wonder, 'how do these women do what they do?'" Chantawipa observes that although NGO representatives who come to visit sometimes "exhibit routine thinking, we try to use these exchanges as an opportunity for education. For example, when they ask about a prostitute's salary, we raise issues of salary cutoffs" (when a woman has her salary docked or is fined for not fulfilling certain requirements, such as not taking on enough clients or not being on time). In working with NGOs and health care providers, Chantawipa tries to spread her humanistic understanding of these women as multidimensional people like ourselves: "NGOs need to recognize that yes, these women are sex workers, but they are also mothers, daughters, family members."

Chantawipa has seen a change in her position as the organization has continued to grow. "In the beginning, I was more like a friend or a relative, but now I'm seen as a leader." She suggests that she has been entrusted with representing the women's concerns to a larger public. It is in this arena of public advocacy that Empower has carved out a new role for itself and has introduced the viewpoints of sex workers into the manifold discussions of prostitution. In its ten-year existence, Empower has been actively involved with other NGOs and networks in Thailand, and its representatives have attended many international conferences. "The network is important. This issue is global, not just Thai. But we have to improve local conditions, protect Thai women, and also expose the issues to the world. Our local experiences can affect international attitudes, and international pressures can affect local conditions."

Notes

1. Guesstimates of the numbers of women in the sex trade vary from 75,376 to 2 million. The estimates are so divergent because of the difficulties of measuring an illegal business and differences in both the interests and the methods of different counters. A 1991 middle-range count of 150,000 to 200,000 commercial sex workers, including children under eighteen, is widely accepted.

2. There are many different forms of the sex industry in Thailand, ranging from escort services to sex shows to businesses thinly masked as massage parlors, tea shops, coffee shops, and even barber shops to outright brothels. "Locked brothels" effectively enslave the workers, who do not have the freedom to come and go, to choose customers, or to insist on condom use. Usually the arrangement is that these women, who are often procured from minority groups or neighboring countries, work until they have paid back a "debt"—often "loans" to the girls' parents. In Bangkok, Empower concentrates on the go-go bars, pubs, and services catering to foreigners, where the women have a greater ability to negotiate with customers than do women in brothels or massage parlors.

3. Having more than one wife is technically illegal, but the law is not enforced, and the practice remains fairly common. Because of the drain on family resources presented by a man maintaining additional households for mistresses or minor wives, it is said that wives prefer that their husbands go to prostitutes.

Changing Attitudes toward Violence against Women

The Musasa Project

Sheelagh Stewart

Rape is nothing more or less than a conscious process of intimidation by which all men keep all women in a state of fear.
—Susan Brownmiller[1]

Chibaro *is being forced to do something that you really don't want to do by someone who is stronger than you.*
—Policeman at Zimbabwe Republic police training course, 1989

The Musasa Project is a nongovernmental organization that was established to tackle the problems of rape and domestic violence in Zimbabwe. Its approach has been one of fostering change from within various institutions in Zimbabwean society. In particular, the founders of the Musasa Project worked closely with various branches of the Zimbabwe Republic Police (ZRP) to help institutionalize an effective response to violence against women.

Beginnings

The idea for the Musasa Project began in early 1988 when I and another Zimbabwean woman, Jill Taylor, a psychologist, started to discuss possible ways to address violence against women as it was

343

manifested in Zimbabwean society. Our immediate goal was to work within the legal and law-enforcement systems to alleviate the problem. Our undertaking began in earnest when we received funding in May 1988 to conduct a nine-month pilot project to establish an appropriate model for a follow-up project that would actively attempt to change commonplace attitudes—among Zimbabweans in general and the ZRP in particular—about violence toward women in Zimbabwe.

Initially, Jill Taylor was employed part-time as the coordinator of the Counseling and Research Project on Violence against Women, as Musasa was then called, and I worked as a volunteer. We trained twenty-two women in counseling and training techniques; they became the initial core members of the project. In 1989, we decided to call the project Musasa, meaning "a favorite resting place for tired and weary travellers . . . a temporary shelter put up by a family while they build a permanent home" (MATCH 1993, 2). The Musasa Project has two main activities: (1) public education and outreach, which includes one-on-one talks with women who have been raped, training courses for Musasa counselors, and workshops for the ZRP and representatives of other agencies who deal with rape and violence; and (2) counseling (including legal advice) for survivors of rape, domestic violence, and incest.

As of this writing, the Musasa Project has 600 members, decentralized regional committees all over the country (Musasa 1994), and a full-time paid staff of seven, including a consultant-director, public educator, counselor, legal practitioner, administrator-accountant, and support staff. In 1993 alone, 699 clients were counseled.

The Pilot Project

Musasa's pilot project was an internal process that attempted to establish whether there was a problem with violence against women in Zimbabwe, and if so, how best to approach it. Our approach was to interview more than seventy Zimbabweans who were interested in and concerned about rape and domestic violence and appropriate ways of dealing with these problems. Interviewees included officials of the Ministry of Women's Affairs, doctors, lawyers, government officials, health professionals, academicians, and members of the ZRP.

The pilot project also included training sessions that utilized participatory research in the form of workshops and "training exchanges" for Musasa counselors and future trainers. (A workshop uses participatory training methods—that is, it invites the trainees' active involvement through, for example, role playing—but it involves less individual interchange and has a more clearly defined agenda than a training exchange.)[2] The input from the participants in the training exchanges was crucial in determining the ultimate nature of the project and our subsequent work with the ZRP.[3] All the interviewees were prepared to discuss domestic violence, but no one really wanted to talk about rape. At the end of the nine-month pilot period, we still had not ascertained whether there was a word in Chishona for rape. Then, in the last training discussion group, the word *chibaro* cropped up.

Chibaro, apparently, is the word used for "rape" in Chishona. It is also the word used to describe the labor that the colonialists imposed on the local populace in lieu of a tax, when the populace could not pay in cash. Such a definition presented us with a perfect way to introduce the issues of rape and domestic violence in subsequent training sessions, because of its emphasis on power and the abuse of power. That is, central to any attempt to change ideas and attitudes about rape and violence against women is the understanding that such behavior involves the abuse of power. *Chibaro* also implies a powerful commonality between men and women, providing a bridge to greater understanding and ultimate change: men who rape women are no different from the colonialist government that "raped"—exploited the labor of—black Zimbabweans. Practically everyone with whom we worked was able to relate to such an analogy, and it became the jumping-off point for all the subsequent work we did around the issue of rape.

Rape Culture

In order to tackle the problem of violence against women, the members of the Musasa Project team set out to examine and understand "rape culture" as it exists both universally and in Zimbabwe.

An interesting example of this convergence between universal and local rape culture occurred when I showed *The Accused* (an American movie in which a woman is raped by several men while other men look on and cheer) at the beginning of a five-day workshop on rape and domestic violence. In Zimbabwe, it is not uncommon to watch movies interactively: everyone participates, shouting warnings and the like during the film. During the gang-rape scene, the audience identified with the rapists by clapping and cheering. This incident seemed to me to illustrate a deep-seated and perhaps even universal identification with ideas about who gets raped and whose fault it is. The end of this story is somewhat more encouraging. By the end of the film, the trainees were deeply embarrassed by their "participation," and the workshop turned into an excellent exchange of views that, in many ways, became the cornerstone of Musasa's future work—creating a space that allows people to speak freely and challenge their own assumptions from within.

At Musasa, we define rape culture as an environment in which traditional assumptions and attitudes about men and women quietly nurture behavior that leads to or supports rape and domestic violence. These assumptions remain unchallenged in a rape culture, and they penetrate into every corner of society, even its medical, judicial, and legal systems. Such attitudes are so deeply ingrained and so insidious that most people are unaware of the ways in which they permit—sometimes even encourage—violence against women to thrive. The result is that women are left feeling vulnerable and frightened of men, but either they don't know why or they are not always aware of those feelings, and they blame themselves when they are abused. Moreover, their attackers as well as those who are supposed to be "protecting" them (that is, the judicial and legal systems) also tend to blame them for their victimization.

Most elements of rape culture throughout the world fall into recognizable patterns—for example, blaming the victim for "bad" behavior, invoking male needs when abuse occurs, or claiming that the victim consented to sexual activity or other abuse. Most legal systems collude with the prevailing rape culture by having in place various impediments to the successful prosecution of rape—for example, the admissibility of the victim's previous sexual history.[4]

Rape Culture in Zimbabwe

Rape culture in general swings on the twin pivots of male sexual needs and blaming the victim, but the particular expression of these pivots in Zimbabwe is molded by Zimbabwean culture and history. One of the important facets of this particularity is the role played by colonialist authorities in the subjugation of women who were outside the cash economy and were therefore potential revolutionaries. In essence, I would argue that the British South African Police (BSAP) allowed the black male community to "police" black women by imposing on them the fear of rape as a way of controlling their mobility and autonomy. Thus, the attitudes and behavior that were encouraged during colonialist rule helped foster the rape culture that exists in Zimbabwe today.

Blaming the Victim

A common belief is that women get raped because they "ask for it," as evidenced by the following comment:

> *"I can understand that birds who go to nightclubs alone and wearing miniskirts get raped, but I was out with my boyfriend."*
> *—Zimbabwean rape survivor counseled by Musasa*

As evidenced by this statement, it is frightening for a woman to make the link between one mentally deranged man in a dark alley or one "badly behaved" miniskirted woman who "asked for it" and the idea of rape as an institutionalized form of control over women. It is common for rape survivors to look for evidence that they themselves have contributed to the assault—partly because this is such a widespread belief, and partly because the implications of a generalized rape culture are so frightening.

At various workshops that we conducted, the following reasons emerged for why women in Zimbabwe are raped:

- They smoke cigarettes.
- They have "permed" hair.
- They walk alone at night (and this in a country where the transportation infrastructure is poor and it is not culturally acceptable for women to ride bicycles).
- They live alone (a euphemism for being a prostitute).
- They wear miniskirts.
- They wear trousers. (Trousers were worn by many of the female "comrades" during the struggle for Zimbabwean liberation, and

this attitude about women who wear trousers is part of a wide-spread devaluation of their contribution from that of fighters to that of camp followers and prostitutes.)

Prostitution

A more general reason advanced for raping a woman in Zimbabwe is that she is a "prostitute." In Zimbabwe, as in many other cultures, the use of the word "prostitute" says more about the rapist than it does about the woman he attacks. The types of women who are *not* considered prostitutes are much fewer than those who *are* considered prostitutes. In essence, only women who are unmarried and living with their parents, or women who are married and living with their husbands, are *not* prostitutes—although they, too, may earn this label. It is also generally believed that a woman who wants to have sex is a prostitute, whereas a woman who does not want to have sex is respectable. (See "She Consented," below.)

In Zimbabwean society, to be a "prostitute" is to be utterly marginalized and cut off from all sources of support, both social and material. Thus, regardless of the fact that prostitution should never be a justification for rape, the label is a potent weapon in the armory of rape culture. Social ostracization is particularly crippling in a family-, clan-, and community-oriented culture such as the one in Zimbabwe.[5]

Male Entitlement, Male Need, and the Abuse of Power

In Zimbabwe, as in other parts of the world, rape has a two-part justification, which runs: (1) "She was smoking [wearing a miniskirt, etc.], and I am not responsible for my actions"; (2) "I was overcome and I had to have sex with her."

> *"Men need sex; they get sick if they don't have sex, so if I see a woman, I can't help myself, I have to have sex." —trainee in a ZRP workshop*

In Zimbabwe, there is an additional twist that complicates the story, as suggested earlier: a history of the exploitation of black labor by white colonialists.

> *"He would send my husband away to work. Then he came that night and told me that my night work was with him. He came every day till my husband came back."* —*Zimbabwean rape survivor and seasonal harvest worker, raped by employer and then fired*

Black women have traditionally been both the most vulnerable and the most threatening in the colonialist scheme of things—most vulnerable because they faced the double oppression of race and sex, but most threatening to the colonialist order because they historically operated outside the cash economy and were therefore beyond direct colonialist control. This situation had two results: the frequent rape of black women by white men, supported by the belief that black women existed to service white male needs; and the refusal by the BSAP to take black women's complaints of rape— whether by black or white men—seriously, and the BSAP's laissez-faire attitude of letting the community manage its own problems.[6]

The Power of Virgins

Myths about the power of virgins appear in numerous cultures.[7] There are two Zimbabwean manifestations of this idea. One is the young virgin as healer of sickness in general and of sexually transmitted diseases in particular. (This myth has had dreadful consequences in light of current HIV infection rates.) In the recent past, men who were ill and visited a *nyanga* (witch doctor) were advised to sleep with a virgin as a cure. Similarly, men who experienced bad rainfall or a bad crop, or—in the urban context—who had bad luck in business were advised to sleep with a virgin to improve their luck.[8]

Second, the Apostolies—a Christian religious sect in Zimbabwe—advise their followers that sleeping with virgins draws them closer to God and that sleeping with their daughters has a biblical precedent.

> *"When he had finished he told me that God only made Adam and Eve and that we had come from Adam sleeping with his daughters and that was why he slept with me."* —*Zimbabwean incest victim*

She Consented

"Women say 'no' when they mean 'yes.'" This is the father of all old chestnuts. This belief is particularly problematic when the lines between yes and no are blurred—that is, in situations where there *is* consent on the woman's part. In Zimbabwe, this blurring of yes and no is extreme and women sometimes say no when they mean yes, because they are afraid of seeming "loose."[9] The all-encompassing definition of a "prostitute" in Zimbabwe has already been considered, and most—possibly all—Zimbabwean women fear the label. The effect of this fear on women's behavior is that, even in a relationship of mutual respect, when both parties wish to have sex, a woman generally says no several times (in a ritualized fashion) before intercourse takes place. Saying no indicates respectability and is an essential part of the exchange, as is the use of (ritualized) force or at least coercion, which is taken as proof of masculinity.[10]

The Colonialist Legacy: A Dual System of Justice

A further legal-political issue that has contributed to the confusion over "consent" is the legacy of a dual legal system in which the colonialist, white-run jurisdiction dealt with criminal offenses and a traditional jurisdiction, operated by village chiefs, dealt with civil offenses. Criminal offenses, such as theft and murder, are generally more serious than civil offenses, such as defamation of character. Whereas criminal offenses may carry a prison sentence or a fine paid to the state, civil offenses are most often rectified through payment of damages to the individual who has sustained the harm. Sex offenses can be either criminal, as in the case of rape, or civil, as in the case of "seduction" (see Armstrong and Ncube 1987). Seduction, during the time of colonialist rule, involved a situation in which a young man who could not afford to pay the *lobola* (bride wealth) would "seduce" a young woman, often with her consent, pay nominal damages to her father, and then pay the *lobola* over a period of time. Although more expensive in the long run, such an approach to marriage relieved the prospective groom of the need to pay the *rusambo* (down payment) normally required before the marriage commenced, therefore bringing marriage within the reach of younger and less well-off men.

A resulting problem was that many "rapes" (sexual relations without the woman's consent) were called "seductions," for two reasons. First, the people wanted to administer their own legal system as much as possible, as part of a general system of resistance against the colonialist power (with unfortunate results for women).[11] Second, damages were paid to the woman's father in the case of seduction, presenting obvious temptations and also appearing to satisfy the requirements of local justice. Again, the consequences for the woman were severe, in that she could well end up married to a man who had raped her. In cases of rape, which were handled by the colonialist criminal jurisdiction, the perpetrator would go to prison, which was generally perceived as not doing anyone any good.

Although the state now handles all offenses, whether criminal or civil, Zimbabwe's recent history of mislabeling rape as the more innocuous seduction has exacerbated the confusion and helped further blur the distinction between yes and no. Rape is viewed as an act of violence without consent, whereas seduction—which is, in fact, often the same as rape—is considered an offense in which the father's financial interest in his daughter is damaged and to which the woman has given her consent.[12]

Strategizing around Rape in Zimbabwe: Musasa and the Zimbabwe Republic Police

Musasa's initial strategy for breaking down Zimbabwe's rape culture was to attempt to institutionalize an effective response to rape and domestic violence in the police force and various arms of the legal system. The project's early objective in this process was to change the way in which the police behaved in a professional context. Although it was obvious that the police were part of the problem of violence against women, in that they dealt badly with victims of rape and domestic violence, they were also enthusiastic about addressing their problems with and improving their treatment of these cases. During the pilot project, we established an excellent rapport with the ZRP's community relations liaison officers (CRLOs), which we believe made them more responsive to us as the project progressed than they might otherwise have been.

Once the Musasa Project itself was under way, the ZRP continued to express an interest in learning how to handle rape and domestic violence cases.

Historical Context for the ZRP Training Sessions

In order to understand Musasa's work with the ZRP, an understanding of the context in which it developed is necessary. Zimbabwe became independent in 1980 and, consequently, the ZRP has been metamorphosing from a much feared and hated state tool under the Smith regime to a force that has sought closer links with the people it serves. The CRLOs were given the specific task of changing this image. In general, then, the Musasa Project was working in an environment where everyone welcomed change away from the previous regime. More specifically, this desire for change meant that the parallel between the Rhodesian regime's oppression and control of men and men's oppression and control of women was easier to invoke, as evidenced by the two meanings of the word *chibaro*. It is probably true to say that an opening existed in Zimbabwe that enabled us to address the basic power issues that underlie acts of rape—an opportunity that might not exist anywhere else.

Our strategy involved a process of analyzing the legal system, choosing levels through which that system could be accessed, and then working from one level within the system to the next. As described above, the first step was a series of workshops, or training sessions, held with the CRLOs of the ZRP. From this group we ascertained that it would be important to train the specific department in the ZRP dealing with criminal offenses. Our strategy was to get the CRLOs to invite officers from the criminal section to the next workshop. It soon became clear, however, that training the ZRP without also focusing on parts of the judicial system was ineffective. The ZRP officers themselves took responsibility for inviting some of the prosecutors from the Harare Magistrates Court to the next training session. A direct spin-off from this was a workshop mainly for senior prosecutors, facilitated by top-ranking members of the ZRP.

The ZRP training sessions always began with a discussion of the problems that the police faced in dealing with rape as an organized institution. These discussions were often accompanied by the use of visual tools of analysis: organizational "maps" were used to initiate discussions about places in the system where the police experienced difficulty when dealing with rape cases. Such discussions almost always indicated common problem areas that became the basis for more in-depth discussion and, ultimately, action.

A training session typically ran for five days and included two days on rape, two days on domestic violence, and one day of liaison with other useful community organizations. Five days is a long time for a workshop, so it was crucial to keep the sessions lively, interactive, and fun for everyone. Controversial comments such as "there is no such thing as rape within marriage" were always opened up for general discussion, and with encouragement and support, other attitudes and alternative opinions emerged. Other controversial topics included the characteristics that do and do not define a "prostitute" and men's responses to women whom they say "lead men on."

Of particular interest in this context was the role played by the female members of the police. During the early training sessions, they seldom expressed opinions and, if they did, they were usually extremely conservative and unsympathetic to the position of other women in Zimbabwe. As the training sessions progressed, this began to change, and two years into the process a gender distinction in opinions began to emerge. On an issue such as "women like to be beaten; otherwise, they feel unloved"—a common topic for debate—all the women and some of the men believed that women did *not* consider beating to be a sign of love. This subject often led to interesting discussions at teatime, with some of those who believed that women enjoy beatings making comments such as, "So you really don't like being beaten?"

Discussions at tea breaks and in small groups often became journeys of self-discovery—a key objective of the Musasa Project, because they represented the potential for changing behavior and attitudes from the inside. They were indicative of an environment in which the trainees felt free to challenge long-held assumptions and traditions associated with rape culture. Because the participants were encouraged to engage in *self*-examination and *self*-criticism, as opposed to enduring criticism from outsiders, they were less likely to become defensive and more open to new ideas—with the result that their behavior and attitudes were more likely to change.

Our Results

Musasa's work with the police began to make a difference in the way the ZRP treated rape victims in the police stations and in the prosecution of rape cases. A typical problem, for example, was that complainants in rape cases often withdrew their charges, which meant that the clear-up rate for rape was low. Consequently, police officers felt that it was easier to ignore the woman when she first came in than to open a docket that was almost definitely going to impose a drag on their clear-up rates. The identification of this problem immediately opened possibilities for discussion about why women withdraw their cases. As a result, almost all rape survivors now give their statements in a separate office, which provides some privacy, and the police treat them with much more sympathy than they did before the project started (Meursing 1993, 30).

Musasa's approach—which fostered a relationship of mutual respect and cooperation with the police force—was also instrumental in speeding up the complaints procedure normally used by the police in cases of rape. When we were helping a rape victim, we would phone the police from Harare and ask that the case be handled quickly. The police response to our requests was excellent.

As the police training sessions progressed, our networking improved, and individual police officers who did not follow the new procedures—that is, attending to rape cases quickly, providing privacy for the complainants, and treating rape victims with greater sensitivity—began to feel the effects of complaints against them. Eventually, this more sensitive procedure for handling rape cases was applied throughout Zimbabwe. At first, the improved response to rape cases helped only those women who were represented by Musasa, but one of the goals of the project has been to broaden this sensitivity to the position of women in general.

There are, of course, more intransigent problems that have proved to be difficult to change, such as the overall legal definition of rape in Zimbabwe (that is, sexual intercourse by a man with a woman without her consent) and the continued existence of the double-jeopardy rule in our law (the rule that permits judges and magistrates to treat with caution the evidence of certain categories of individuals—accomplices to a crime, children,

Training Sessions

Generally the training sessions were great fun, and everyone thoroughly enjoyed them. The exchange that follows illustrates both the tone and the issues in Musasa's interchanges with the police:

Trainee: Excuse me, but do you know what happens if you have two bulls in one *kraal*? [A *kraal* is an enclosure for cattle made out of thorns, to keep cattle in and intruders (such as lions) out.]

Trainer: No, what?

Trainee: They fight—you can't have two bulls in one *kraal*, so if your wife is trying to be a bull, you must beat her.

Trainer: Do we have two bulls in the Zimbabwean *kraal*?

Trainee: No, only one—the president.

Trainer: And does anyone challenge this bull?

Trainee: No.

Trainer: And does he beat the vice-president?

Trainee: No! [Much hilarity, but an acceptance of the idea that real men with real authority don't need to beat.]

and female complainants in cases of a sexual nature). However, in instances in which the police feel at a loss and in the grip of a system that they cannot change, they have formed working groups with prosecutors to tackle these more intransigent issues. This type of dialogue between law-enforcement officials and lawyers is significant, and it is hoped that legal reform will follow.

One unanticipated effect of this work was that the police themselves began to feel empowered to better deal with cases of rape and domestic violence. Eighteen months into the process, during a discussion of legal issues in one of the training sessions, which was being conducted by a state prosecutor, a number of police officers argued vociferously for a change in the legal definition of rape, to include an element of power abuse.[13] This new confidence in their position and role seemed to be significant in ensuring better treatment of rape victims. Their new attitude was strengthened with the publication of a manual, distributed by the ZRP, that clearly specified the legal position on rape and the best procedures for handling it.

Musasa's Changing Strategy

As described earlier, we began by trying to change the police officers' professional behavior only. In the early stages of the project, overall behavioral change seemed too daunting an objective to take on. For one thing, it would have meant challenging basic precepts about the position of men and women in Zimbabwean society, and this was perceived as being too risky—perhaps even radical. At that time, issues were cautiously framed and cautiously acted upon, and there was a general reluctance to challenge the patriarchal power structure that underpins violence against women. Recently, however, the Musasa strategy has become far more radical, directly challenging the traditional patriarchal system. The Musasa Project now addresses gender issues directly through a series of gender workshops with health, legal, and education professionals and other interested parties that aims to make all elements of Zimbabwean society aware of "how patriarchy works within all structures of our society" (Musasa 1994, 12).

The project is also taking on broader issues concerning the traditional position of women in society, such as the right to own land and the payment of the bride wealth. Although not, on the face of things, directly related to domestic violence, a woman's right to own land may have an impact on battering, because her dependence on a man increases her vulnerability and makes it difficult or impossible for her to leave him if he is abusing her. Likewise, the practice of paying *lobola*, discussed above, "has become instrumental in controlling and battering women," since women "become devalued when *lobola* is paid for them because they are reduced to the equivalent of a commodity" (Binks 1994, 3). Once a man pays for a woman, he believes that beating her is within his rights, since he "owns" her.

Lessons Learned

The success of the Musasa Project in improving the ZRP's handling of rape cases is a function of the successful institutionalizing of concerns about and problems with rape in the police force and various arms of the legal system. In the final part of this chapter, I examine the strategy employed by Musasa overall, considering which elements have been successful and which have been problematic, and extract general principles that may be of use to other activists.

It is important to begin with a disclaimer. The much-vaunted concept of replicability—the idea that if an approach is sound it will work in other parts of the world—is problematic in the context of rape and domestic violence. Although it is clear that the Musasa approach has made a difference in the way the ZRP deals with rape and violence against women, it is equally clear that the success depended on a specific confluence of values and history, both in the country at large and within institutions, such as the police force, with which we worked. That having been said, some useful principles and ideas have emerged from the work that was done.

1. *It is crucial to know and understand the workings of the system with which one is engaging.* Two examples make this clear. First, our initial sense of success with the CRLOs was misplaced, as they lacked the power to make actual changes in the procedures employed for approaching crime within the ZRP. They did, however, provide the link to the Criminal Branch, which does have the power to make these changes. Second, with a system such as the ZRP, which has a clear division between the upper and lower ranks, it is important to work with all levels—both the top-ranking officers and the police in the stations who actually deal with rape survivors.

2. *It is easier to foster change from within the system than from outside it.* The Musasa Project worked with one part of the system—the ZRP—to get it to acknowledge the need for change, and then to call on other parts of the system (prosecutors within the legal system) to start working on similar changes. This approach leads to wide-ranging change that a small agency such as the Musasa Project could never achieve from outside the system.

3. *The specifics of each approach must be planned carefully.* Training legal professionals is very different from training police officers. Lawyers have a tendency to listen only to other legal professionals, and credibility—in terms of knowledge of the law—has to be established from the outset. Someone with a good working knowledge of the law may be able to suggest innovative legal solutions. In addition, he or she may be able to counter standard legal mythology—for example, the notion that if caution were not exercised in rape cases, thousands of innocent men would now be languishing behind bars, or the belief that women who bring charges of rape are likely to be lying.[14]

4. *There are always gaps in the system, and seeking and plugging such gaps is an important part of any strategy to change the system.* Women in Zimbabwe often fall through vast "cracks" between doctors who do not know the legal definition of rape and lawyers who have to prove in court that a rape took place.

5. *These same gaps can be used to promote improved practice throughout all parts of the system.* Doctors can be invited to workshops by prosecutors, for example. Once a project is "inside" one part of a system, the possibilities are endless.

6. *There are limits to this type of change, and these limits need to be acknowledged.* The sort of progress made by the Musasa Project may depend on a belief among the police and other participants that the project does not pose any threat to the status quo. When the political nature of antirape activism becomes obvious, this type of internal change may become impossible. In addition, there is always the danger of being co-opted into a "cozy" relationship in which superficial changes are made but the fundamental changes required to free women from the threat and fear of rape do not materialize. There are clear differences, for example, between strategies that aim to protect women from the all-pervasive threat of sexual assault and strategies that seek to remove the threat. Strategies falling into the second camp require radical change and are unlikely to succeed within existing systems.

7. *This is hard work.* In 1992, I wrote that this type of work "requires endless patience in dealing with tenaciously held negative attitudes about women and endless repetition of offensive and obnoxious jokes condoning violence" (Stewart 1992, 170). This remains true.

In conclusion, the Musasa Project strategy has been effective in changing the way the police deal with rape cases and in raising awareness about power issues and their relation to violence against women. However, the extent to which there has been an actual change in the "rape culture" remains to be seen. What continues to be demonstrated by Musasa's experience is that it is possible, under certain circumstances, to work effectively through the existing system to bring about change. One observer familiar with the project summed it up well when she said, "At best, the system will change itself from the inside; at worst, there is a breathing space within which women can be empowered to take the issue further."

Notes

1. Brownmiller's well-known text on rape refers to the generalized existence of what I have called "rape culture." Recent writers in the United States have debated the "*all* men" (emphasis added) component of this definition; nevertheless, there is no doubt that all women fear rape (with reason), and that legal and social changes that would ease these fears have not been implemented to any great degree, let alone to a degree where the fear is unnecessary. I would, therefore, argue for the continuing validity of Brownmiller's statement.

2. The idea of the training exchanges was both to teach the trainees how to better deal with rape and domestic violence and to provide a forum in the classroom where the trainees could contribute their own ideas and knowledge—among themselves and for the benefit of the trainers—about these issues in the Zimbabwean context. In order to allow for the exchange of knowledge and experiences among trainers and trainees, the structure of the training exchanges involves longer tea breaks, more extensive group discussions, and plenty of time for and facilitation of sharing appropriate personal experiences.

3. See Stewart (1992) for an in-depth description of when and how the ZRP became involved with Musasa and the details of Musasa's police training.

4. These impediments vary, from the double-jeopardy rule to the prohibition against charges of rape within marriage, and have been discussed at length elsewhere (see Commonwealth Secretariat 1987).

5. This is such a depressing picture of catch 22–type social control (only prostitutes get raped; therefore, if you were raped, you must be a prostitute; therefore, you consented; and therefore, it isn't rape) that it is worth citing an example of one of the most advanced case laws on

this issue in Zimbabwe. In an appeals court case, *The State v. Adam Bwanasi* (HC-B-48-87), the judge ruled that a woman's presence alone in a bar late at night is no indication that she is a prostitute; that even if she is a prostitute, that fact is irrelevant; and that a "prostitute in circumstances of this nature should be treated like any other complainant."

6. In general, complaints by white women were also not taken particularly seriously unless the accused was a black man. Such a phenomenon is described, albeit in the form of fiction, in Harper Lee's *To Kill a Mockingbird*, in which a married white woman accuses an innocent black man of rape. In fact, it was the accuser who tried unsuccessfully to seduce the black man, and her father beat her for it (see also Vogelman 1990).

7. The Jungian myth of capturing the unicorn relies on both the unicorn as a symbol of purity and virginity and the use of a virgin as the "bait" that attracts the unicorn, who submits and lays his head (and horn) in her lap. This myth is about rites of passage and acquiring strength, and whichever way you turn it, the message is clear: the (young) virgin-woman is the door, the route, and the way. She is nothing in herself except transitorily beautiful, and the rite of passage for the man involves loss for her.

8. The Zimbabwe Traditional Healers Association (ZINATHA) has denied that its members recommend such a practice and claims that unregistered healers are responsible. Whoever is the culprit, the practice persists (Taylor and Stewart 1991; Stewart 1992; Meursing et al. 1993).

9. Although this is something that happens in other parts of the world, campaigns on the issue of "no means no"—although understandable—do not leave room for the complexity of cultural norms that surround sexual exchanges. I am not for a moment suggesting that such complexities or cultural norms excuse rape—rather, that if women working against rape do not open the discussion to consider the complexity of responses to a request (or demand) for sex, particularly culture-specific responses, rape survivors may again be in the position of blaming themselves for not giving clear enough messages.

10. The fear of being perceived as a prostitute is further evidenced by women's use of herbs that dry out the vagina; a wet vagina is indicative of wanting sex and implies prostitution (Runganga 1990; Meursing et al. 1993).

11. Rwezaura (1985) has noted a similar phenomenon in Tanzania and observes: "The development and transformation of customary law during the colonial period was underlined by a process in which custom and tradition became a means by which the local rulers and fam-

ily heads bargained with the colonial state for retaining a part of their political power in their communities" (4).

12. However, it is important to note in the context of this discussion that the notion of "consent" under African customary law is extremely problematic, because, as noted by Armstrong and Ncube (1987), "customary law marriages are frequently group or family marriages. . . . As such, the notion of free individual consent is often subsumed by the larger interests of the family alliance." That is, the degree of a woman's actual "consent" regarding matters sexual and otherwise is questionable in a society that does not permit women to have the final say over their own destinies.

13. Conversely, the issue of rape within marriage, though taken up by Musasa and hotly debated within the workshops, was never really accepted as a valid issue by the police officers.

14. The response to the latter myth is that false reporting is highest in cases of theft because of the insurance implications, and there is no evidence that false reporting of rape is any higher than in any other class of crime.

References

Armstrong, A., and W. Ncube. 1987. *Women and Law in Southern Africa.* Harare: Zimbabwe Publishing House.

Binks, M. 1994. Violence against women. *Taurai, Speak Out, Khulumani, 3.*

Brownmiller, Susan. 1993. *Against our will: men, women and rape.* New York: Fawcett.

Butegwa, F. 1993. Limitations of the human rights framework. In *Claiming our place: Working the human rights system to women's advantage,* edited by M. Schuler. Washington, D.C.: Institute for Women, Law and Development.

Chirume, L. 1989. A study of the phenomenon of wife beating: Zimbabwe as a case study. Bachelor of laws diss., University of Zimbabwe.

Commonwealth Secretariat. 1987. *Resource manual on violence against women.* London: Commonwealth Secretariat.

Cotton, A. 1993. Proposal for funding the Cambridge Female Education Trust—educating girls to secondary school level in Zimbabwe. Unpublished manuscript.

MATCH International. 1993. *End to violence against women: African women's initiatives.* Harare: Zimbabwe Electricity Supply Authority Training Centre, Musasa Project.

Meursing, C., et al. 1993. *Child sexual abuse in Matabeleland*. Bulawayo, Zimbabwe: Matabeleland AIDS Council.

Musasa. 1994. *The Musasa Project, sixth annual report, 1993–94*. Harare: Musasa Project.

Njovana, E. 1993–94. Gender-based violence and sexual assault. *African Women* 8:17.

Runganga, A. 1990. The use of herbal and non-herbal agents in sexual intercourse by a sample of Zimbabwean women. Ph.D. diss., University of Zimbabwe.

Rwezaura, B. 1985. *Traditional family law and change in Tanzania: A study of the Kuria social system*. Baden-Baden: Nomos Verlagsgesellschaft.

Schuler, M., ed. 1992. *Freedom from violence: Women's strategies from around the world*. New York: UNIFEM.

————. 1993. *Claiming our place: Working the human rights system to women's advantage*. Washington, D.C.: Institute for Women, Law and Development.

Stewart, Sheelagh. 1992. Working the system: Sensitizing the police to the plight of women in Zimbabwe. In *Freedom from violence, women's strategies from around the world*. Edited by M. Schuler. New York: UNIFEM.

Taylor, J., and S. Stewart. 1989. *Musasa: A project for Zimbabwe*. Ottawa: MATCH International.

————. 1991. *Sexual and domestic violence: Help, recovery and action in Zimbabwe*. Harare: A. von Glehn and J. Taylor, in collaboration with Women in Law in Southern Africa.

Vogelman, L. 1990. *The sexual face of violence*. Johannesburg: Raven Press.

Sexual Reality

The Gap between Family Planning Services and Clients' Needs

Gill Gordon

Much discussion of the future of family planning programs, at both policy and practical levels, has involved the extent to which family planning services and AIDS prevention services can and should be integrated. Many, if not most, service providers continue to view family planning services and AIDS prevention services as separate issues. Overcoming that perception will no doubt go a long way toward overcoming the barriers to promoting safer sex. However, without a realistic assessment of the safer-sex options currently on the table and of providers' attitudes about, willingness to address, and skill in discussing these options with their clients, efforts to train family planning staff to provide counseling and education in HIV prevention will not have a significant impact on changing people's actual behavior.

In 1987, on the mandate of its member family planning associations (FPAs), International Planned Parenthood Federation (IPPF) established an AIDS Prevention Unit (APU) to assist program planners and policymakers in exploring how HIV prevention services might be incorporated into each component of their programs. In 1988, APU staff began conducting HIV prevention workshops with FPA staff. The experience of the APU has revealed a gap that often exists between social norms and providers' values in relation to sexual behavior on the one hand and clients' needs on the other. Often providers do not sufficiently understand or communicate the precise ways in which HIV infection can be transmitted and the safer sexual behavior options that are available to clients, with the result that the services and education provided are irrelevant. Based on information that was gained from training workshops for key staff in three West African FPAs and a 1992 needs assessment among selected FPAs in each of the regions,[1] this chapter describes the nature of this gap. It also offers some insights into how to bridge the differences between providers' attitudes and clients' needs regarding sexual behavior.

Sexual Options and HIV Prevention: Provider Perceptions versus Client Reality

The primary options for HIV prevention promoted within IPPF and its FPAs are condom use, abstinence, fidelity within marriage, and nonpenetrative sex. This section looks at how these options match the realities of the attitudes and sexual lives of various groups of clients; how effective they are likely to be in preventing HIV infection; to what extent providers are helping clients determine the best HIV prevention strategy for themselves; and whether providers are helping clients overcome the gender inequalities that put them at risk of HIV infection or simply reinforcing gender stereotypes. The experiences described in this chapter and the quotations from individuals and groups are taken from the HIV and sexuality needs assessment and review visits, unless otherwise stated.

Condom Use

FPAs promote condom use mainly through community-based distribution (CBD) programs, male involvement projects, social marketing, and specialized projects for young people. Condom application is demonstrated on bottles, fingers, wooden penis models, and, in one case, a man. Some staff show pictures while describing how to apply a condom. In most programs, condoms are promoted as having the dual benefit of pregnancy and disease prevention. However, many family planning workers are not enthusiastic about condoms because they have to be used at the time that sex takes place, and their use-effectiveness rate is lower than for other provider-dependent methods.

Also, condoms are not popular with clients for a number of reasons. Many people with whom APU staff spoke described the experience of condoms breaking and their resulting lack of credibility. Breakage may be due to badly stored or expired condoms (they can be seen on display in the sun), incorrect application (they may be pulled on like socks or torn by rough nails), excess friction caused by dryness in the vagina, vigorous or prolonged activity, or use of petroleum jelly as a lubricant. For some people, condoms are too costly to be used every time one has sex. Although one condom may cost a small amount, a person who has sexual intercourse four times a night needs four condoms.

Condoms can also directly affect sexual practices. If the woman is not aroused or is dry, the condom can cause pain and discomfort. The delay in ejaculation may be welcomed, or it may cause dismay in situations in which one or both partners want to complete the sexual act as quickly as possible. This might be the case if sex is being carried out in a hurry without privacy, if the woman is not enjoying it, or if the sex is a purely commercial transaction. Some men are unable to maintain an erection while wearing a condom (in which case the FPA staff advise the woman to stimulate the penis). Both men and women can feel that "sex is quite tasteless and soundless using a condom."[2]

Another problem with condom use is that it is often seen as appropriate for casual sex or having sex with girlfriends, but not with wives: "With us the man expects to have natural sex, the full flesh to flesh," said one wife. For this reason, the introduction of condoms in a relationship is seen as a sign of infidelity or a lack of commitment. Indeed, FPAs provide condoms to young men or older men "mainly for extramarital sex." Some married men said that although they would not mind their wives suggesting condoms if they were being used for birth spacing, they would throw their wives out if they suggested using condoms as a way to prevent AIDS.

For women, condom use raises slightly different issues. Most importantly, the women themselves say that they have no control over their husbands. Indeed, many women who have been counseled about the benefits of condom use for disease prevention still prefer a form of contraception, usually Depo-Provera, that can be used surreptitiously. For women who feel that there is no point in having sex if there is no chance of conception, the fact that condoms also prevent pregnancy increases the impression of a lack of commitment.

For both men and women, condoms may signify profanity in a sacred place (the vagina), lack of trust (that is, implied promiscuity), prostitution, or denial of nourishment that comes from the semen. Another negative aspect is that men and women may have anxieties about ill health associated with the use of condoms. For example, some fear that the condom might slip off and migrate inside the woman, its removal requiring an operation, or that the condoms have been contaminated with HIV by the Americans to reduce African populations.

Although there are a number of difficulties with condom use—both practical and sexual—at a field level, there is some indication of condom acceptability. For some people, condoms may have positive sexual meanings; they might indicate a relationship that is caring, comfortable, safe, or protected, and some users described them in these terms. One man "really loved condoms now [that he] had got used to them." CBD agents promote condoms as a way to delay ejaculation, thereby pleasing women. Condoms can also be erotic for some people, and some staff in clinics suggest making them a part of love play.

FPA staff need to be aware of men's and women's fears regarding condom use so that they can respond to them effectively. They also need to talk with men, educate them about and convince them of the dangers of HIV, and provide them with condoms. Finally, FPA staff need to be aware that if condoms are used correctly every time, their failure rate as a contraceptive is comparable to that of other methods.

Abstinence

In the FPAs, abstinence is vigorously promoted for all unmarried young people, especially young women, and sometimes for married women whose husbands are away. However, abstinence is an effective option in preventing HIV infection only if both partners come together as uninfected virgins. This presents a problem in cultures in which girls and young women marry men who are sometimes ten years their senior and who almost always have prior sexual experience. Moreover, with the growing fear of HIV infection, older men are seeking younger and younger girls in the belief that they will be uninfected.

Furthermore, with puberty occurring earlier and marriage later, abstinence would be necessary over a period of perhaps ten years, at a time of maximum sexual energy and maturation into adulthood. Many—if not most—people view sexual activity as positive and essential for both physical and mental health after a person has matured, at around the age of sixteen. Thus, abstinence might not be viewed as a sexually healthy option.

Advising women to abstain from sex is not always realistic, because women often do not have control over when they have sex, with whom they have it, and the type of sex they have. Many young women and some boys have their first sexual experience against their will; they may be raped or coerced into sex by an older relative or neighbor. A married woman who refuses sex may be beaten, even if the man has an infection (although, in some cultures, a husband's infection would be a legitimate reason for a woman to refuse sex). Finally, for both girls and women, money to pay school fees, to learn a trade, even to eat and dress can come from sexual relationships. In poor families, in particular, difficult economic circumstances may push girls into early sexual activity.

Finally, some FPA staff equate sexual activity in young people with delinquency. For example, an FPA staff member claimed that prostitutes had visited the clinic. When asked how he knew that they were prostitutes, he replied that they admitted to being unmarried. In this culture, women are considered to be prostitutes for any number of reasons; certainly any unmarried woman who is sexually active would be considered a prostitute. (See Stewart's chapter in this volume for further discussion of this issue.) In another clinic, sexually active young women were told that, as "spoiled goods," they would not be respected in marriage even if they were fortunate enough to get husbands. Passages from the Bible were quoted, and the nurse on duty proudly announced to visitors that the majority of unmarried clients left without contraceptives.

This emphasis by FPA staff on abstinence for women means that young women's contraceptive and sexual health needs are often not met. For example, one young woman of eighteen who was doing petty trading had a lover who helped her pay her apprentice fees. She came to the clinic for contraception because she did not want to get pregnant while still at vocational school. Instead of receiving contraceptive services, she received a lecture on "the dignity of adolescent chastity" and was asked if she could not pay her apprentice fees through her petty trading. When she insisted that she needed contraceptives, she was asked to return with her partner for a discussion. She never came back. Not only did this resourceful and responsible young woman encounter barriers to contraception when she went to the clinic for help, but she was not given any safer-sex options other than abstinence.

Nonetheless, several workers said that they would give contraceptives to a single woman if she had a "proper" reason for wanting them—for example, if she was engaged and wanted to finish school before she conceived. However, if they found that the woman wanted contraceptives just so that "she could be promiscuous," they would lecture her on the right road to take and would withhold the contraceptives unless she absolutely insisted.

FPA staff also tell their clients to reduce their number of partners in order to avoid HIV. Most clients interpret that message to mean that they should have only one sexual partner *at a time*. For example, a leaflet aimed at truck drivers showed a man with three "wayward" girls under his arm while another stood with one more sober-looking girl. The man with three partners died of AIDS, whereas the man with one partner remained strong and healthy. In populations with a high prevalence of HIV, unprotected sex with one partner, particularly when serial monogamy (that is, having one partner at a time, but not necessarily the same partner forever) is practiced, still puts people at risk of HIV infection.

Sexual Fidelity within Marriage

For the most part, during the workshops and in the needs assessment, neither the FPA staff nor the community members perceived married women as a group at risk of HIV; they were more likely to mention truck drivers, young people, and street hawkers as being at risk. Discussions with community members revealed that a number of people thought that condoms would protect a man from sexually transmitted diseases (STDs) and HIV and that staying with one partner would protect a woman. During a session in which market women were being trained as health promoters, the participants composed a song about STDs that mentioned wives' fidelity as their only protection.

Not surprisingly, "stay faithful to your spouse" is the safer-sex option that the majority of FPA staff most vigorously promote to married women. This may not be realistic in a setting in which married women are the fastest growing group with HIV infection. Is this, in fact, a realistic strategy for prevention when FPA staff give these admonishments to women but not to men?

The FPA staff say nothing about the importance of the husband's fidelity in preventing HIV infection because they believe that he is entitled to have more than one woman or because this advice might make him angry. As a result, it is usually the condom, not fidelity, that is promoted in male involvement programs, and in one program it was promoted as a means of protecting only the man—not his wife—from infection.

At the same time, married women are often held responsible for their husbands' fidelity. "Keeping your husband from straying" has been flagged as an additional benefit of using a modern contraceptive, because it allows a woman to be sexually available at all times, even during traditional abstention periods. FPA staff have been known to advise female clients who complain of unhappy sexual relationships to dress in sexy nightwear, cook a nice meal, send the children next door, and seduce their husbands. "After all, if you don't make the effort to do this, you have only yourself to blame if he goes to other women," one FPA staffer told a client. In group discussions, women point out that although they are faithful, their husbands are not. "No matter how loving the wife, the man will have other women. There is nothing we can do," said one participant. In this case, FPA staff simply affirm the behavior of women who put condoms in their husbands' bags if they travel, "like a caring wife so that at least he won't bring disease home to the family."

Divorce and separation have the same effect as extramarital sex in terms of multiple partners and HIV prevention. This is also true for polygynous cultures. Divorce and separation rates are high in many West African countries. In a rural Muslim area of Gambia, over one-fifth of the women had been married more than once, and just over half had been co-wives. Polygynous marriages themselves are inherently unstable because the often older man, who might be impotent, is married to several younger wives, who are likely to look for lovers outside the marriage in order to meet their own sexual needs. Likewise, it is unusual for a woman or man to remain unmarried after widowhood.

The fairly common occurrence of extramarital sex—whether it is done willingly or involuntarily—is a reality that flies in the face of FPA providers' advice to practice fidelity within marriage. Over a lifetime, a woman may have a series of sexual relationships that play a major role in her economic strategy for survival and progress. Evidence in Nigeria and Ghana shows that women have extramarital liaisons to meet economic needs that their husbands are unable to satisfy. Even couples in stable married relationships may be obliged to live apart if one is transferred to another area, which leaves both partners vulnerable to extramarital sexual relations. Finally, another reality of life that runs counter to fidelity in marriage is that some ethnic groups have annual festivals in which migrants return to their hometowns and it is permissible to drink and have sex with anyone one fancies.

The reality of multiple sexual partners (at one time or over a period of time, directly or indirectly) also has significant implications for contraceptive choices—implications that providers do not seem equipped to help their clients address. For example, in one FPA, women fitted with IUDs are advised not to have affairs because doing so can result in serious infections. Although this advice makes the husbands happy—because it reassures them that using this contraceptive will not make their wives promiscuous—it does nothing to address the equally harmful consequences of the husbands' potential infidelity.

Providers also have to acknowledge that married clients who engage in extramarital sex wish to practice contraception privately, regardless of the risk of HIV infection. For example, in one rural outreach clinic, where a group of six women had a discussion about AIDS, three of them were vulnerable to HIV infection: a widow involved in a new relationship; a trader traveling to the north to buy her produce, who sleeps wherever she can, usually with a man; and the wife of a traveling businessman who does not send money home, who obtains her needs from other lovers. The nurse was aware of their dilemma and suggested condoms in a perfunctory way, without much conviction. She did not discuss how they might persuade their men to use condoms or the possibility of using them in extramarital relationships. As a result, only one woman accepted the condoms, and all three chose Depo-Provera as a family planning method because their men need not know about it.

Nonpenetrative Sex

Nonpenetrative safer-sex practices include any activity that does not involve penetration of the vagina, rectum, or mouth and in which semen or vaginal fluids do not make contact with the mucous membranes—for example, masturbation, massage, kissing, simulated sex in the armpit or between the thighs, or erotic dancing. Although many providers are reluctant, even embarrassed, to discuss nonpenetrative sex options with their clients— often asserting that these are examples of "perverted Western practice"—participants in workshops and small-group discussions generated long lists of inventive activities that do not involve penetration. These activities were discussed with no evident embarrassment as viable options for safer sex. In fact, in some ethnic groups, young people used to be socialized to have nonpenetrative sex before marriage in order to avoid pregnancy.[3]

At a meeting with FPA staff and two young people, the problem of young girls presenting with vaginal infections—allegedly from the use of bananas as sex toys—came up for discussion. The seventeen-year-old girl present displayed no embarrassment whatsoever, informing the group of giggling adults that she and her friends used bananas, that of course they did not share them, and that "if one wished to do it ten times, one would of course buy ten bananas." This incident seemed to highlight an acceptance of such behavior in this culture, despite FPA providers' discomfort with it.

This is also true in the case of masturbation. Most FPA staff agree that masturbation is natural, that people do it—particularly sexually active young people who are in school—but that they would not feel right about promoting it as a safer-sex option or even acknowledging that it is a good thing. "It is a natural thing—even small children do it—but it is addictive and can lead to homosexuality and [in men] the inability to have intercourse with a woman; therefore, it is best avoided." Some workshop participants expressed a fear that if one child reported to his or her parents that masturbation was being taught in school, the school would be closed down.

Although nonpenetrative sex is an option for safer sex, there are limitations that need to be frankly acknowledged. For example, one nurse explained that when she talked about such acts with a group, it proved to be too much for her clients; she said that they got excited and "in the mood" very easily, so she stopped at telling them about condoms.[4] Furthermore, some people have risky encounters in a hurry. "They are stealing each other, so they have to be quick so that no one catches them." Such encounters are not good situations for nonpenetrative sexual experimentation. Others thought that a man would not have the self-control to stop before penetration. Indeed, some mothers advise girls not to allow boys to touch them because the boys will become too excited to stop, and the girls will get pregnant. Finally, hygiene might be a problem if the man has dirty hands.

Another commonly held belief is that people engage in nonpenetrative sex as "romance" or foreplay leading to intercourse but that it does not constitute "real sex." One participant commented, "Of course people do rub themselves against each other until they come. But sex has meaning beyond relieving yourself, and most men and women would feel cheated, as if they hadn't done anything." Other men thought that nonpenetrative sex simply takes too long; in one discussion, for example, a man said that he would prefer to use jelly as a lubricant rather than "waste time" arousing the woman. The response of some young men to the suggestion of nonpenetrative sex was, "It's not real sex, but go ahead and tell us about it anyway." In another discussion, an FPA volunteer was initially adamant that men and women would not be satisfied with nonpenetrative sex, that it was not a viable option in Ghanaian culture. However, on reflection, he recalled that he and his girlfriend used exactly that practice to get through university without pregnancy. He also remembered that girls in boarding schools would have sexual relationships—the "Dear-Dear thing" (lesbianism)—and in those days there were no problems with pregnancy and STDs.

Nevertheless, some FPA staff have been including nonpenetrative sex as an option for safer sex, especially in talking to young people; they believe that clients are grateful for a new alternative and that more educated people might try it. One FPA service provider promoted sexual activities other than intercourse as being beneficial to sexual pleasure, particularly for women. She presented people with a vision of how sexual relationships might be creative, caring, and loving. In a men's group discussion, one participant said that if he shared these ideas with his friends, he "might get a slap and a kick, but others would like it."

Strategies for Change

Several significant obstacles that emerged through the work of the APU need to be acknowledged and overcome. First, service providers bring their own long-standing attitudes, biases, and perceptions to the clinic, which affect their interaction with clients and the advice they give on how to practice safer sex. The messages that the FPA staff give to their clients often do not match the reality of either the HIV epidemic or people's sexual lives.

Second, the APU and FPAs address counseling and education as if their clients and groups have a free choice in deciding what to do about sex. The "informed choice" concept that is promoted within IPPF implies providing people with information on options so that they can make the most suitable choice for themselves. However, FPA staff are offering safer-sex options without taking into account the context in which clients make these choices. Does the client have even the fundamental choice about whether to have sex and with whom, much less whether to use condoms or avoid penetration? If a woman has no choice herself, how can she expect to influence her partner's behavior? Does sex take place in a private place with time to try out new ways of pleasing each other? Are condoms available? Can a girl or young woman afford to say no to sex in the short or long term?

Third, during the HIV prevention training, it became apparent that many FPA staff are concerned not only with physical aspects of sexual health but also with social and moral well-being. One or two participants even complained that there was a lack of moral teaching and that the sessions were, at times, profane. Before colonialism, sexual cultures varied among ethnic groups, with some having severe sanctions against sex outside of marriage and others being more permissive. Religion still plays a central role in the daily lives of the majority of Africans, with traditional sexual values overlaid with Christian or Muslim values. In fact, FPAs have attracted employees who have a religious motivation to "develop" society. In one FPA, for example, counseling training was provided by the Christian Council. Some staff have Bibles on their consulting tables.

The Christian or Muslim outlook is often greatest in the most highly educated individuals, who are also highest in the FPA hierarchy. Senior staff and managers believe that they have the right not only to impart scientific knowledge to community workers and groups but also to "correct" values. For example, whereas community workers may believe that premarital sex is a good and essential behavior for sexual and general health and well-being, senior staff and trainers believe that it is right to wait until marriage before engaging in sex, even if that does not occur until one's mid-twenties.

Finally, service providers may experience a conflict between the contraceptive targets they are asked to meet and the mandate to provide clients with the information they need to make informed choices about reproductive and sexual health. Many FPA staff perceive their role as that of providing information, advice, and technology to people who are less informed than themselves and who need to be told what is best for them. They do not appreciate the expertise and experience that their clients bring to a counseling or education session. Indeed, until recently, this perception was created by IPPF and donors who were concerned about population growth. FPA staff were told to increase the numbers of people using modern contraceptives by explaining the benefits and minimizing potential costs. If people had concerns about the use of contraceptives, they were politely informed that these were "misconceptions."

IPPF's strategic plan, Vision 2000, approved in 1992, embraces a radically different ideology. Women's empowerment, information and services for youth, responding to unmet needs, and sexual and reproductive health are major pillars of the strategy, and the plan aims to "advance the basic human right of all women, men and youth to make free and informed choices regarding their own sexual and reproductive health and advocate for the means to exercise this right."

Lessons Learned

The workshops organized by APU were designed to allow FPA staff to explore some of these issues. The goal was to train FPA workers to help clients explore their own situations in relation to HIV, to look at their options for risk reduction, and to act on their own *informed* decisions. A key message of the workshops was that HIV and AIDS cannot be isolated from sexual practices and behavior. The training acknowledged that few of us feel entirely comfortable talking about sexuality and used a variety of activities to help participants explore their feelings, share difficulties, and practice service provision skills. (The objectives and activities of the workshop are summarized in on the next two pages; all are based on experiential methodologies.)

The workshops emphasized that information plays a small, albeit vital, part in the process of behavior change and that the information must be relevant to the person's life. Attitudes, skills, and social and economic factors are equally—if not more—important in determining behavior, sexual or otherwise. The value of respect and equality between family planning worker and client, whatever the difference in education and wealth, was also stressed. Clients should be acknowledged as experts on their own situations and sexual lives, with the service provider acting as a facilitator in problem solving and providing information and new perspectives only as they become relevant and helpful in the discussion.

The HIV prevention workshops enabled FPA staff to internalize the problem of HIV, to talk more comfortably about sexuality, to facilitate group discussion on safer sex, and to become more aware of their own attitudes. However, three five- to ten-day workshops held over a period of four years and isolated from ongoing program development cannot be expected to make a major impact on staff practices. Concomitant changes are needed in general work practice, management, and supervision to support the use of the knowledge and attitudes gained in the workshops. Staff need to be supported and rewarded for using participatory approaches, addressing the underlying causes of sexual ill health in the community, and taking the difficult step of providing contraception to unmarried youth. They need structures to regularly

Workshop Training Objectives and Activities

Objective	Activity
To increase knowledge of HIV and AIDS	Methods demonstrated the importance of building on and clarifying the current knowledge and opinions of participants and exploring the relationship between facts and feelings
To explore one's own attitudes and values about sexuality	We used values clarification activities and provided opportunities for participants to look at their own sexuality history
To separate fact from opinion in relation to sexuality and avoid imposing one's own values on the client	We used an activity called "think, feel, do," in which participants were presented with a difficult situation in relation to sexuality (For example, you go into your thirteen-year-old son's bedroom and find a packet of condoms, with one missing, by the bedside. At that moment your son comes into the room. What do you think? What do you feel? What do you do?)
To understand the risk of acquiring HIV through different sexual practices	Small groups brainstormed and listed all the sexual practices they could think of, and these were classified as no risk, low risk, and high risk in relation to HIV infection
To understand a range of different options for reducing the risk of HIV	In small groups, people generated a list of options; these included abstinence, reducing numbers of partners, mono-gamy or polygyny, nonpenetrative sex, and use of condoms
To develop skills in counseling individuals and groups on options for safer sex	Participants practiced counseling skills in integrating HIV and STD concerns with contraceptive counseling

Workshop Training Objectives and Activities (cont.)

Objective	Activity
To develop skills in holding small-group discussions in the community to explore the problem of HIV and options for prevention	Participants practiced the skills of listening, asking questions, using pictures and stories to stimulate discussion, group dynamics, focusing, reflecting back, challenging, and summarizing in the classroom; they then held small-group discussions with different groups living in the locality—for example, truck drivers, schoolchildren, hairdressers—on the topic of safer sex
To develop skills in promoting condom use and demonstrating how to use them	Participants worked in pairs with a model penis and condoms to practice counseling each other on condom use, particularly focusing on the impact of condoms on sexual relationships; they addressed feelings about pleasure, meanings, and level of commitment in a relationship
To understand the determinants of sexual behavior and the barriers to practicing safer-sex options	We asked people to brainstorm and list all the reasons they could think of that people might find it difficult to use a condom or to stay with one partner; they then classified the reasons into knowledge, feelings, skills, social and cultural, economic, and physical (This activity graphically demonstrated the small part that knowledge plays in determining behavior); participants then suggested ways that the FPA might address the different types of barriers to change
To develop audio-visual materials for the promotion of safer sex	We encouraged staff to develop audiovisual materials with the active participation of community groups, and to use drama, storytelling, and pictures in an interactive way rather than to disseminate print materials to audiences with mostly low levels of literacy

discuss progress and problems, since this way of working is emotionally and physically more demanding and risky.

In order to change behavior, an FPA needs to work with the community to find practical ways of addressing sexual health problems as well as acknowledging the limited power of many clients to act on information. This implies changing from information dissemination and service delivery programs to a participatory community development approach, which requires the development of a new set of skills and attitudes among service providers.[5] The following steps can be taken to address the problems identified in this chapter, and to try to modify the behavior of both FPA staff and clients and thus bridge the gap between their goals and perceptions:

1. Include structured sessions on gender issues in FPA staff training and actively challenge gender discrimination and attitudes that result in sexual ill health. Seek ways of addressing gender issues and train staff in the necessary skills—for example, conflict resolution.

2. Include structured activities on religion, the traditional sexual culture, and sexual health in FPA staff training. This could lead to policy formation and a group agreement or contract that says that clients' needs should be met even if their lifestyles are not consonant with the values of the service provider.

3. Initiate pilot projects that test the feasibility of FPAs using a participatory community development approach in the broader area of sexual health. Move from the clinics into the community. Analyze the costs and effectiveness of different approaches. Hold dialogues with a range of groups in the community—not only women—and encourage different groups to talk to one another and resolve conflicts. IPPF is currently carrying out this step through the Sexual Health Project in six FPAs over three years. As Vision 2000 becomes internalized and operationalized within the IPPF system, it should become easier for FPAs to adapt their programs to include many aspects of sexual health.

4. Network with groups and organizations, such as women's groups, credit agencies, agricultural departments, and vocational training schools, that have the resources to address some of the underlying determinants of sexual health.

Despite the IPPF's training efforts and the establishment of the AIDS Prevention Unit, it seems clear that a gap remains between FPA services and clients' needs. This gap reflects a larger one between the attitudes of FPA staff and the reality of their clients' sexual lives. As IPPF steps up its efforts to integrate AIDS prevention and sexual health services with family planning services, it is hoped that the gap explored in these pages will eventually be bridged.

Notes

1. The workshops were conducted by the APU of IPPF and were part of a larger strategy to improve the provision of services in FPAs in Africa and Latin America. In 1992, staff from the APU and region carried out a needs assessment in relation to HIV and sexuality in selected FPAs. The methodologies used were individual interviews and small-group discussions with staff, volunteers, and community groups and observations. Program officers from the APU and regions also visited FPAs to review their needs and progress.s
2. This quote comes from focus-group discussions held in rural Zimbabwe prior to the production of a mini feature film on AIDS by Development for Self-Reliance.
3. It should be noted that this teaching was heavily based on the fear of death or banishment from the community for those who practiced premarital sex and could be crippling to later sexual enjoyment.
4. This is not an insubstantial concern. Female CBD workers in particular can experience harassment and unwanted proposals from men who interpret talk about sexuality as implying free sexual behavior in women.
5. APU developed a manual entitled *Preventing a Crisis* that focuses on participatory approaches to health promotion and training. The manual is premised on the understanding that behavior is not determined by knowledge alone but by attitudes, values, skills, social support, and environmental factors related to power and wealth. *Talking AIDS,* a simple guide for community workers, has also been developed to promote discussion on options for protection against HIV.

Appendix 1
Relevant and Related Readings

We asked the contributors to this volume to recommend reading and materials related to their work. This list does not claim to be representative of the topic of sexuality and gender. Rather, it is an attempt to put people in touch with materials that they may not otherwise know about.

Gender and Sexuality Theory

Abu-lughod, Lila. 1986. *Veiled sentiments: honor and poetry in Bedouin society.* Berkeley: University of California Press.

Butler, Judith. 1990. *Gender trouble: Feminism and the subversion of identity.* New York: Routledge.

Clatterbaugh, Kenneth. 1990. *Contemporary perspectives on masculinity: Men, women, and politics in modern society.* San Francisco: Westview Press.

Cornwall, Andrea, and Nancy Lindisfarlane. 1993. *Dislocating masculinity: Comparative ethnographies.* New York: Routledge.

D'Emilio, John, and Estele B. Freedman. 1988. *Intimate matters: A history of sexuality in America.* New York: Harper.

Early, Evelyn. 1993. *Baladi women in Cairo: Playing with an egg and a stone.* Boulder, Colo.: Lynne Reinner.

Hutchins, Loraine, and Lani Kaahumanu. 1991. *Bi any other name: Bisexual people speak out.* Boston: Alyson Publications.

Jejeebhoy, Shireen J., and Sumati Kulkarni. 1989. Reproductive motivation: A comparison of wives and husbands in Maharashtra, India. *Studies in Family Planning* 20(5):264–72.

Moore, Kirsten, and Debbie Rogow, eds. 1994. *Family planning and reproductive health: Briefing sheets for a gender analysis.* New York: Population Council.

Rotundo, J. Anthony. 1993. *American manhood: Transformations in masculinity from the revolution to the modern era.* New York: Basic Books–Harper.

Rugh, A. 1984. *Family in contemporary Egypt.* Syracuse, N.Y.: Syracuse University Press.

Segal, Lynne. 1990. *Slow motion: Changing masculinities, changing men.* New Brunswick, N.J.: Rutgers University Press.

Wallace, Michele. 1979. *Black macho and the myth of Superwoman.* London: John Calder.

Weeks, Jeffrey. 1985. *Sexuality and its discontents: Meanings, myths and modern sexualities.* London: Routledge.

The Biological Basis of Sexuality

Bleier, Ruth. 1984. *Science and gender: A critique of biology and its theories on women.* New York: Pergamon Press.

Fausto-Sterling, Anne. 1993. The five sexes: Why male and female are not enough. *The Sciences* 33(2):20–25.

Harlow, Sioban. 1995. *What we do and do not know about the menstrual cycle; or questions scientists could be asking.* New York: Population Council.

Horgan, John. 1993. Trends in behavioral genetics: Eugenics revisited. *Scientific American* 268:123–31.

LeVay, Simon. 1993. *The sexual brain.* Cambridge, Mass.: MIT Press.

Methodological Issues in Sexuality Research

Bozon, Michel, and Henri Leridon. 1994. Sexuality and the social sciences: What can be learned from a survey. A presentation. *Population: An English Selection* 6:195–202.

di Mauro, Diane. 1995. *Sexuality research in the United States.* New York: Social Science Research Council.

Elias, Christopher J., and Ruth Simmons. 1993. *The study of client–provider interactions: A review of methodological issues.* Population Council Programs Division Working Paper no. 7. New York: Population Council.

Hemmings-Gapihan, G., and C. I. Niang. 1983. *Dimension sociologique des opérations de recherches sur les soins de santé primaires* (Project 83-AID-319). Washington, D.C.: United States Agency for International Development.

Leslie, Joanne. 1992. *Women's lives and women's health: Using social science research to promote better health for women.* New York: Population Council; Washington, D.C.: International Center for Research on Women.

Parker, Richard G., and John H. Gagnon. 1995. *Conceiving sexuality: Approaches to sex research in a postmodern world.* New York: Routledge.

Ramos-Jimenez, Pilar, and Patricia Monina P. Yadao, eds. 1993. *Gender, sexuality and reproductive health in the Philippines: Participatory research in sexuality and reproductive health.* Manila: De La Salle University.

World Health Organization. 1992. *A study of the sexual experience of young people in eleven African countries: The narrative research method.* Geneva: World Health Organization, Adolescent Health Programme, Division of Family Health.

Aspects of Reproductive and Sexual Health

Baker, Jean, and Shanyisa Khasiani. 1991. *Induced abortions in Kenya.* Population Council East and Southern Africa Regional Office Working Paper, Research Program on Abortion, Series no. 1. Nairobi: Population Council.

Bruce, Judith. 1992. Women's interests: How can family planning managers respond? In *Managing quality of care in population programs,* edited by Anrudh Jain. West Hartford, Conn.: Kumarian Press.

Coeytaux, Francine, Ann Leonard, and Erica Royston. 1989. *Methodological issues in abortion research: Proceedings of Population Council seminar, December 12-13, 1989.* New York: Population Council.

Elias, Christopher J., and Lori Heise. 1993. *The development of microbicides: A new method of HIV prevention for women.* Population Council Program Division Working Paper no. 6. New York: Population Council.

George, Annie, Shikha Mallik, and Usha Sethuraman, comps. 1993. *Women's reproductive health and sexuality: An annotated bibliography.* Bombay: Tata Institute of Social Sciences (unpublished).

Gittelsohn, Joel, Margaret E. Bentley, Pertti J. Pelto, Moni Nag, Saroj Pachauri, Abigail D. Harrison, and Laura T. Landman, eds. 1994. *Listening to women talk about their health: Issues and evidence from India.* Delhi, India: Har-Anand Publications.

Gupta, Geeta Rao, and Ellen Weiss. 1993. *Women and AIDS: Developing a new health strategy.* Washington, D.C.: International Center for Research on Women. (Additionally, this organization produced reports on fifteen projects as part of its Women and AIDS Research Program. Featured countries include Brazil, Guatemala, India, Jamaica, Malawi, Mauritius, New Guinea, Nigeria, Senegal, South Africa, Thailand, and Zimbabwe. For more information on the Women and AIDS Research Program, contact Dr. Geeta Rao Gupta and Ms. Ellen Weiss, ICRW, 1717 Massachusetts Avenue, Suite 302, Washington, DC 20036 USA. Telephone: 202-797-0007. Cable: INTERCENT. Fax: 202-797-0020.)

Indian Journal of Social Work. 1994. Special issue: *Sexual Behaviour and AIDS in India* 55(4).

International Women's Health Coalition (IWHC). The IWHC publishes the following materials; contact the coalition for availability: IWHC, 24 East 21st Street, New York, NY 10010 USA. Telephone: 212-979-8500. Fax: 212-979-9009. Email/Internet: IWHC@igc.apc.org.

☐ Germain, Adrienne, and Rachel Kyte. 1994. *The Cairo consensus: The right agenda for the right time.* New York: IWHC.

☐ Sen, Gita, Adrienne Germain, and Lincoln Chen. 1994. *Population policies reconsidered: Health, empowerment, and rights.* Boston: Harvard University Press. (A limited supply of these books is available for free to colleagues in Asia, Africa, and Latin America from IWHC. Others may purchase the book from Harvard University Press, 79 Garden Street, Cambridge, MA 02138. Fax: 1-800-962-4983 (USA); 617-495-8924 (international).)

☐ Germain, Adrienne, King K. Holmes, Peter Piot, and Judith N. Wasserheit. 1992. *Reproductive tract infections: Global impact and priorities for women's reproductive health.* New York: Plenum Press. (A limited supply of these books is available for free to colleagues in Asia, Africa and Latin America from IWHC. Others may purchase the book from Plenum Press, Attn: Pat Vann, 233 Spring Street, New York, NY 10013, USA.)

☐ Dixon-Mueller, Ruth, and Judith N. Wasserheit. 1991. *The culture of silence: Reproductive tract infections among women in the Third World.* New York: IWHC. (Available in Spanish and Portuguese.)

☐ Germain, Adrienne, and Jane Cottingham, eds. 1991. *Creating common ground: Report of meeting between women's health advocates and scientists on women's perspectives on the introduction of fertility regulation technologies.* Geneva: World Health Organization.

☐ ———. 1994. *Reproductive health and justice: International women's health conference for Cairo '94.* New York: IWHC and Cidadania, Estudos, Pesquisa, Informaçáo, Açăo (CEPIA). Available from IWHC in English. Available in Portuguese and Spanish from CEPIA, Rua do Russel, 694-2 andar, Gloria CEP 22210-010, Rio de Janiero, RJ, Brazil. Telefax: 55 21 225 6115.

□ ———. 1994. *Challenging the culture of silence: Building alliances to end reproductive tract infections.* New York: IWHC.

Khattab, Hind. 1992. *The silent endurance: Social conditions of women's reproductive health in rural Egypt.* Amman: UNICEF; Cairo: Population Council.

Laumann, Edward O., John H. Gagnon, Robert T. Michael, and Stuart Michaels. 1994. *The social organization of sexuality: Sexual practices in the United States.* Chicago: University of Chicago Press.

Olowo-Freers, Bernadette P. A., and Thomas G. Barton. 1992. *In pursuit of fulfillment: Studies of cultural diversity and sexual behaviour in Uganda: An overview essay and annotated bibliography.* Kisubi: Marianum Press.

Population Council, comp. 1994a. *Reproductive health approach to family planning: Presentations from a panel on professional development day at the USAID cooperating agencies meeting.* New York: Population Council.

Population Council. 1994b. *Policy Series in Reproductive Health* (available in English and Arabic):

□ Zurayk, Huda, Nabil Younis, and Hind Khattab. 1994. *Rethinking family planning policy in light of reproductive health research.* Cairo: Population Council.

□ Younis, Nabil, Karima Khalil, Huda Zurayk, and Hind Khattab. 1994. *Learning about the gynecological health of women.* Cairo: Population Council.

□ Khattab, Hind, Huda Zurayk, and Nabil Younis. 1994. *Field methodology for entry into the community.* Cairo: Population Council.

Rogow, Debbie, and Sonya Horowitz. 1995. Withdrawal: A review of the literature and an agenda for research. *Studies in Family Planning* 26(3):140–53.

Winikoff, Beverly, Christopher J. Elias, and Karen Beattie. 1992. *Special issues of IUD use in resource-poor settings.* New York: Population Council.

Winikoff, Beverly, and Barbara Mensch. 1991. Rethinking postpartum family planning. *Studies in Family Planning* 22(5): 294–307.

World Health Organization. 1993. *Sexually transmitted diseases amongst adolescents in the developing world: A review of published data.* Geneva: World Health Organization, Adolescent Health Programme, Division of Family Health.

Zeidenstein, L. 1990. Gynecological and childbearing needs of lesbians. *Journal of Nurse-Midwifery* 35(1):10–18. To get a copy, please write to Laura Zeidenstein at 16 Fuller Place, Brooklyn, NY 11215 USA.

Sexual Abuse and Coercion

Boyer, Debra, and David Fine. 1992. Sexual abuse as a factor in adolescent pregnancy and child maltreatment. *Family Planning Perspectives* 24(1):4–10.

Heise, Lori L., with Jacqueline Pitanguy and Adrienne Germain. 1994. *Violence against women: The hidden health burden.* Washington, D.C.: World Bank.

Heise, Lori, Kirsten Moore, and Nahid Toubia. 1995. *Sexual coercion and women's reproductive health: A focus on research.* New York: Population Council.

Matabeleland AIDS Council. 1993. Child sexual abuse in Matabeleland.

Purewal, Jasjit, and Naina Kapur. n.d. Sexual abuse, female sexuality and the language of violence against women. Unpublished.

Taylor, Jill, and Sheelagh Stewart. 1991. *Sexual and domestic violence: Help, recovery and action in Zimbabwe.* Harare, Zimbabwe: A. von Glehn and J. Taylor.

Training and Program Information

Armstrong, Ewan McKay, and Peter Gordon. 1992. *Sexualities: An advanced training manual.* London: Family Planning Association.

AVSC International. 1992. *Family planning counseling: The international experience meeting report, Istanbul, Turkey, April 20–24, 1992.* New York: AVSC International.

Centre for Health Education, Training and Nutrition and Awareness (CHETNA) and Rajasthan Voluntary Health Association (RVHA). 1994. *Training on health and development of adolescents.*

Dixon, Hilary, and Peter Gordon. 1990. *Working with uncertainty: A handbook for those involved in training on HIV and AIDS, second edition.* London: Family Planning Association.

ECOS videotape series. For more information, contact Cecilia Simonetti, ECOS, Rua dos Tupinahambas, 239 São Paulo, SP CEP-04104, Brazil. Fax (55) (11) 573-8340.

☐ *Boys: The first time.* Focuses on the sexuality issue from the point of view of values and attitudes of male teenagers, bringing in as a counterpoint the opinions of female teenagers.

☐ *Virgin age.* Aimed at adolescents and/or professionals in the areas of education, health, and communication. Focuses on the values and attitudes of youngsters in relation to virginity.

☐ *Camera in hand I—message to parents* (videotape and brochure kit).

☐ *Camera in hand II—message to boys* (videotape and brochure kit).

☐ *Great sex* (videotape and brochure kit).

☐ *A hug* (videotape and brochure kit). Emphasizes the relationship between parents and children in the time of AIDS.

☐ *Is it or isn't it?* (videotape and manual). On adolescence and psychotropic drugs and AIDS; made to promote reflection among teenagers, parents, and educators.

☐ *Família dá Samba*. Deals with the diversity of family arrangements.

☐ *Legal abortion*. Registers the experience of the Hospital Jabaquara in establishing legal abortion services.

International Planned Parenthood Federation (IPPF). IPPF publishes a magazine called *Challenges: Issue on Sexual and Reproductive Health* and the following videos. Both are available from IPPF, Distribution Unit, Regent's College, PO Box 759, Inner Circle, Regent's Park, London NW1 4LQ.

☐ *Preventing a crisis* ($8.00, in English, French, Spanish, Arabic, Portuguese).

☐ *Talking AIDS* ($4.00, in English, Spanish, Portuguese).

☐ *Counselling and sexuality*. A video-based training resource. A set of four videos and a manual for use by trainers of counseling skills in the field of sexual health. (Cost: $35 each or $100 for the set for developing countries; $55 each or $200 for the set for others. Available in English, Arabic, and French.)

☐ *Unmasking AIDS*. A video and two guides intended as a training resource for people involved in sex education and STD and HIV prevention. (Available in English and French.)

Jiménez, Elisa. 1984. *Reflexiones en torno a la sexualidad y a la educación*. Caracas: AVESA.

———. 1986. *Salud sexual y socialización*. Ponencia presentada in the Third Latinamerican Congress of Sex and Sexual Education and the Second Venezuelan Congress on Sexuality. Caracas: AVESA.

———. 1988. La educación sexual frente a los roles y estereotipos sexualex. In *Manual de Formación de Multiplicadores del Proyecto de Educación Sexual y Planificación Familiar del Ministerio de la Familia*. Caracas: AVESA.

———. 1991. Consideraciones en torno a la salud sexual y reproductiva. Presented at the Second Venezuelan Congress of Women. Caracas: AVESA.

Leonard, Ann, ed. 1994. *Community-based AIDS prevention and care in Africa: Building on local initiatives.* New York: Population Council.

PROFAMILIA. To obtain these booklets, contact PROFAMILIA, Calle 34 No. 14-52, Bogotá, Colombia. Fax (571) 338-3159.

☐ *Cartilla adolescentes preguntas y respuestas sobre sexualidad.* 1991.

☐ *El lenguaje de la sexualidad en tu adolescencia,* by Elizabeth Garcia-Restrepo and Margarita Maria Cardona Jimenez. 1994.

Quality/Calidad/Qualité booklet series on quality of care. To receive back issues or to be added to the mailing list, write to Ann Leonard, Population Council, One Dag Hammarskjold Plaza, New York, NY 10017 USA.

☐ *Celebrating mother and child on the fortieth day: The Sfax Tunisia postpartum program,* by Francine Coeytaux. Introduction and afterword by Beverly Winikoff, M.D. 1989. (Available in English; text in Spanish and French available in typewritten format.)

☐ *Man/hombre/homme: Meeting male reproductive health care needs in Latin America,* by Debbie Rogow. Introduction and afterword by Judith Bruce and Ann Leonard. 1990. (Available in English and Spanish.)

☐ *The Bangladesh women's health coalition,* by Bonnie J. Kay, Adrienne Germain, and Maggie Bangser. 1991. (Available in English.)

☐ *By and for women: Involving women in the development of reproductive health care materials.* Case studies by Barbara Ibrahim and Nadia Farah (Egypt), Blanca Figueroa (Peru), Margaret Winn (South Pacific). Introduction and afterword by Valerie Hull, 1992. (Available in English.)

☐ *Gente joven/young people: A dialogue on sexuality with adolescents in Mexico,* by Magaly Marques. Introduction by John M. Paxman and afterword by Judith Bruce. 1993. (Available in English.)

☐ *The Coletivo: A feminist sexuality and health collective in Brazil,* by Margarita Diaz and Debbie Rogow. Introduction by José Barzelatto. 1995. (Available in English and Portuguese.)

☐ *Doing more with less: The Marie Stopes Clinics in Sierra Leone,* by Nahid Toubia. Introduction by Grace Eban Delano. 1995. (Available in English.)

World Health Organization. 1993. *Natural family planning: What health workers need to know.* Geneva: World Health Organization, Family Planning and Population Division of Family Health.

Appendix 2

A Guide for Screening and Counseling Women Who Are Abused

Domestic abuse is most commonly the abuse of a woman by a man. Therefore this guide refers to the perpetrator as a male and the victim-survivor as a female. However, one should never rule out abuse simply on the basis of gender—women can hurt women (for example, mothers abusing daughters) and, more rarely, women can hurt men.

Screening for Abuse

All patients should be screened for abuse, especially if:

- The woman presents with chronic, vague complaints that have no obvious physical cause (more sexually and physically abused women seek care because of persistent headaches, chronic pain, sleep disturbance and other vague symptoms than because of injury).
- She is pregnant.
- She has had a miscarriage or an abortion.

Reprinted with permission of Lori Heise. This guide appeared as Appendix II in *Sexual Coercion and Reproductive Health: A Focus on Research,* by Lori Heise, Kirsten Moore, and Nahid Toubia (New York: Population Council, 1995). It was adapted with permission from Marian Sassetti, Domestic violence, *Primary Care: Clinics in Office Practice* 20(2)(1993):289–305.

- Her injuries don't match her explanation of how she sustained them.
- Her husband is overly solicitous or controlling.
- She is suicidal, or has a history of attempted suicide.

Because abusers often accompany women to the doctor in order to keep them from disclosing, always separate a woman from her husband or kin before probing for abuse. Generally, this can be done by asking others to leave "until the patient is examined." If your facility cannot accommodate private interviews or examinations, do not put a woman in greater danger by refusing to believe her story, no matter how implausible. If her abuser is with her, her life may depend, quite literally, on you accepting her explanation of her injuries.

Conducting the Interview

Follow these guidelines:

1. *Don't be afraid to ask.* Contrary to popular belief, most women are willing to disclose abuse when asked in a direct and nonjudgmental way—indeed, many are secretly praying for someone to ask. You can gently state: "Being in relationships is often very difficult and can cause us lots of pain and suffering. Many women who feel the way you do are suffering from violence in their homes. Could this be happening to you?" or "Can you tell me if anyone is hurting you or making you feel bad about yourself?"

2. *Create a supportive environment.* Let her tell her story. State very clearly that she is not crazy and that no one deserves to be beaten or raped no matter what the circumstances. This reassurance is crucial and cannot be overstated, as simplistic as it may sound. Acknowledge her feelings and let her know that she is not alone. Commend her for taking the first step toward improving her life and her children's lives. Affirm that she did the right thing by telling someone about the crime that is occurring in her life.

3. *Remain nonjudgmental and relaxed.* Most battered women are exceedingly good at picking up nonverbal cues as to how people are reacting to them. (Indeed, many women try to escape episodes of battering by learning to "read" the mood of their partners.) Remember, the most important step to ending the violence is achieved the moment you allow the woman to tell her story.

4. *Explain that she has medical and legal rights.* The penal codes of almost all countries criminalize rape and physical assault, even if there are

no specific laws against domestic violence. Try to find out what legal protections exist in your country or state for victims of abuse and where women and children can turn for help in enforcing their rights. Most legal systems have some type of restraining order or peace bond that can be used to order a man to stop abusing his partner. In a growing number of jurisdictions, special legislation has been passed that permits judges to order a wider range of remedies, including barring the man from the conjugal home, mandating that he pay maintenance and child support, and mandating that he seek treatment. Be especially sensitive to a woman's fear of "losing" her children should she leave her partner. Investigate local child custody laws so that you can allay these fears, if the law is on her side.

5. *If pressed for time, establish an alliance and schedule a return visit in the very near future.* Tell the woman that you are glad that she has told you about the problem and that you want to spend more time with her addressing this very serious issue. Find out whether she is in immediate danger and needs urgent intervention. If there is no emergency, tell her that you are concerned about her health and well-being and that you want a follow-up visit with her to fully discuss and address the issue. Make sure that she leaves with, at the very least, the number of a local crisis center she can call.

Ask the following questions:

1. *Is she in immediate danger?* Ask if she is afraid to go home. If so, help her plan for her safety. Is there a friend or relative she can call? Offer to contact the local women's shelter or crisis center.

2. *Are there children involved in the abuse?* If there are, make sure that you evaluate them now or in the immediate future. If abuse has occurred, you may be mandated to report it (depending on the laws in your state or country), but you must provide for the safety of the woman, because reporting child abuse may exacerbate the battering situation.

3. *Does her partner use drugs or alcohol?* Drugs and alcohol do not *cause* violence, but some women are more at risk of attack when their partners are under the influence. Ask her whether she associates her partner's violence with his drinking or drugging. If so, her partner's condition can provide an important cue for her to take protective measures, such as spending the night with friends or family. Generally, it is unwise to try to discuss any issue of import when a man is drunk or high; encourage her to wait until he is sober to bring up issues, especially concerns regarding his drinking or drug use.

4. *Does she use drugs or alcohol to help her cope?* These drugs can blunt women's ability to make rational decisions and can lead to addiction. The drugs can also be used for suicide.

5. *Has she ever attempted or thought of suicide?* Make sure to ask if she has a plan if she says that she has thought of suicide. The situation becomes urgent once an individual has formulated a plan for suicide, because he or she typically acts on it in the near future.

6. *Does her partner have or use a weapon? Has he threatened to kill her?* These are *not* idle threats. The woman must understand that threats of harm or death are good predictors of future behavior.

Providing Acute and Long-Term Care of Battered Women

1. *Avoid the pitfall of "rescuing."* You cannot direct a woman's life or tell her what to do. Remember, she is the expert on her own particular situation. What you *can* do is help her see that she *does* have choices and options and offer to support her in whatever course of action she chooses to take, *including the decision to return to the batterer.* Let her know that she is always welcome to come back to you, and avoid judging the choices that she makes.

2. *Beware of prescribing psychotropic drugs.* Even women who appear to be depressed or otherwise psychologically compromised are often reacting sanely to the insane circumstances of their lives. If you prescribe medication that limits a woman's capacity to react with clarity, you may actually increase the danger that she is in. Most often, battered women are not mentally ill and should not be treated as if they were.

3. *Provide her with literature and information about community resources.* Contact your local women's crisis center or shelter and familiarize yourself with services available locally for victims of physical or sexual abuse. Always provide the name and number of a local resource group to any woman who discloses abuse, even if she does not express the need for immediate assistance. Consider writing the referral on a business card or prescription pad so as not to attract attention. Inform her that she may encounter prejudices and difficulties when she attempts to access the resources to which she is entitled, but encourage her to persevere. Without forewarning, she is likely to retreat into hopelessness and inaction if she encounters victim-blaming attitudes on the part of social service workers, the police, and others.

4. *Clearly document the woman's history and physical findings.* Record as many details of the woman's history and physical condition as possible; these facts may prove crucial later if she decides to prosecute. Record, for example, "Patient states that she was hit in the face with her partner's fist, punched in the stomach two times, and hit with a screwdriver" or "Patient states that her husband said three times that he was going to kill her." Upon examination, you would record "a 3-cm swollen ecchymotic area on the left shoulder, consistent with a wound from a punch; three linear ecchymotic areas on each side of the neck, consistent with strangulation marks." Laboratory examinations should be recorded in the same way, even if they yield negative results. Illustrate the location of the injuries on a body map and photograph the injuries whenever possible.

5. *Encourage her to join a support group.* Participation in support groups has been shown to have a positive impact on the health and psychological well-being of victims of abuse. Consider making space available in your facility where victims of abuse can meet.

Taking Care of Yourself

1. *Beware of feelings of failure.* The goal of the office or clinic visit is not to get the woman to leave her abuser. The goal is to identify women who are living in abusive situations and to help them connect with available services and support.

2. *Recognize the good that you have done.* You have made an important contribution simply by breaking the silence around abuse. You may well be the first person in this woman's life who has been concerned enough to ask about her well-being.

About the Authors

Sondra Zeidenstein is coauthor with Tahrunnessa Abdullah of *Village Women of Bangladesh: Prospects for Change* and editor of *Learning about Rural Women*. She has done research and evaluation of women-focused projects in Thailand, the English-speaking Caribbean, and Bangladesh.

Kirsten Moore is program manager at the Population Council. She recently edited a series called "Briefing Sheets for a Gender Analysis of Family Planning/Reproductive Health" with Debbie Rogow and is coauthor of *Sexual Coercion and Reproductive Health: A Focus on Research* with Lori Heise and Nahid Toubia.

Kamran Asdar Ali is a medical doctor by training and a Ph.D. candidate in the Anthropology Department of Johns Hopkins University. He has done anthropological fieldwork in Mexico and Egypt and received a Population Council fellowship to conduct doctoral research on local attitudes about the family planning program in Egypt.

Ana Amuchástegui is professor of psychology at the Universidad Autónoma Metroplitana-Xochimilco in Mexico City. She has done research on the social construction of sexuality and gender with the Population Council since 1992. Along with Marta Rivas, she has published works on sexuality that focus on young people and AIDS prevention, first sexual experiences, and abortion. Her latest work, *Culturas híbridas: El significado de la virginidad y de la iniciación sexual,* will be published as a chapter in *Sexualidad: Vivencias Mexicanas.*

Murray Anderson-Hunt is a psychiatry registrar and Ph.D. candidate at the University of Melbourne, Australia. His research interests include the experience and psychobiology of women during reproductive, maternal, attachment, and sexual behavior throughout the life cycle. He also has a particular interest in the psychoneuroendocrinology of oxytocin.

393

Silvani Arruda of Brazil coordinates the training department at ECOS. She also edits the monthly bulletin, *Transa Legal,* for teenagers and educators and is coauthor of the series of videos produced by ECOS.

Adriana Baban is a senior lecturer in health psychology. She has done research on stress and coping, sexuality and reproductive behavior, and cross-cultural psychology and has published more than twenty-five papers. She is coauthor with Henry P. David of *Voices of Romanian Women: Perception of Sexuality, Reproductive Behavior and Partner Relations during the Ceaușescu Era* and *Stress in Health and Illness* (Dacia, 1992).

Rani Bang and Abhay Bang are wife and husband who hold master's of public health degrees and have completed medical studies in obstetrics-gynecology and internal medicine, respectively. They have founded a volunteer organization, SEARCH, that provides rural health care and conducts research in Gadchiroli, a remote district in India. They spearheaded a mass movement on a variety of health issues, including alcohol abuse, sexually transmitted diseases, child mortality, and primary health care.

Henry P. David is director of the Transnational Family Research Institute, Bethesda, Maryland. His more than three hundred publications include *Reproductive Behavior: Central and Eastern European Experience* with R. J. McIntyre (Springer, 1981) and *Born Unwanted: Developmental Effects of Denied Abortion,* edited with Prague colleagues (Springer, 1989). He is presently preparing a volume *From Abortion to Contraception, 1920–1995: Changing Currents in Women's Rights, Health, and Reproductive Behavior in Central and Eastern Europe.*

Lorraine Dennerstein is director of the Key Centre for Women's Health at the University of Melbourne, Australia. She is the author or editor of twenty books and the author of two hundred papers or chapters in books. She was awarded the Order of Australia for her contributions to the teaching of women's health.

Margarita Diaz is the head of the Training, Education and Communication Unit of CEMICAMP. She has worked intensively in research and training in family planning and sexual education during the last ten years and has developed information, education, and communication materials and training curricula in both areas. She is coauthor of *Ensinando a Ensinar* (Teaching to Teach), a book that is being used as a training manual in sexual education in the schools of Brazil.

Ruth Dixon-Mueller, former professor of sociology at the University of California at Davis, has served as a consultant for several United Nations agencies and for the International Women's Health Coalition. She is the author of *Population Policy and Women's Rights, Rural Women at Work: Strategies for Development in South Asia,* and *Women's Work in Third World Agriculture.* She now lives and works in Costa Rica.

Julia A. Ericksen is a member of the sociology faculty at Temple University in Philadelphia. Her research interests are in the area of sexuality and gender. She is coauthor, with Sally Steffen, of a forthcoming book on sexual behavior surveys, *Kiss and Tell: The Revelations of Sexual Behavior Surveys*, to be published by Harvard University Press.

Gill Gordon was information, education, communication program officer in the AIDS Prevention Unit at International Planned Parenthood Federation and is now a consultant in sexual health and a tutor in education for primary health care and development at the Institute of Education, London University. She has carried out training and needs assessment in AIDS education and sexual health mainly in West Africa and India. She has coauthored a number of articles on gender and sexual health and produced a video-based training manual on counseling and sexuality with Peter Gordon.

Napaporn Havanon received her Ph.D. in sociology from Brown University. She is deputy dean of the Graduate School at Srinakharinwirot University, Thailand, and is also a consulting associate at the Population Council's Bangkok office. She has conducted research on women's decisions to terminate unwanted pregnancies; appraisal of quality of care; adherence to reproductive rights in family planning programs in Thailand; and production, reproduction, and family well-being in Vietnamese households.

Warren Hedges recently taught as a Visiting English Professor at Duke University. He has written about gender and fiction in journals that include *masculinities* and *Texas Studies in Literature and Language,* and about "White Men in the United States" for a forthcoming *Men's Studies Encyclopedia.* He is currently at work on a book manuscript titled *Death and Breeding: Reproduction and Gender in American Fiction.*

Elisa Jiménez Armas was one of the founding coordinators of AVESA and was an important figure in the Venezuelan women's movement. She was also a leader of the Latin American feminist health movement. Elisa died in March 1994.

Olfia Kamal is the senior research assistant for Social Research Delta Consultants and was the field operations manager for the Giza morbidity study. She is coauthor of a policy paper entitled "Field Methodology for Entry into the Community." She is also coauthor of "Comparing Women's Reports with Medical Diagnoses of Reproductive Morbidity Conditions in Rural Egypt."

Hind Khattab is an anthropologist with extensive experience in field research on women, particularly issues related to health. She is the director of Social Research Delta Consultants, a consultant to the World Health Organization in countries of the eastern Mediterranean region, most recently with a focus on reproductive morbidity and AIDS. She is also the author of a book on the Giza reproductive morbidity case studies, *The Silent Endurance: Social Conditions of Women's Reproductive Health in Rural Egypt,* and coauthor of "Field Methodology for Entry into the Community."

Mustafa Kudrati is director of the *kuleana* center for children's rights in Mwanza, Tanzania. He is coauthor of *Life First! A Practical Guide for People with*

HIV/AIDS and Their Families, published in English, Swahili, and Kinyarwanda. At *kuleana,* he is involved in promoting street children's rights through the provision of essential services, health care, nonformal education, and legal advocacy; he is also in the process of developing a new initiative on marginalized girls. He is the team leader of a World Health Organization–sponsored study on street children and substance abuse in Mwanza.

Cheik Ibrahima Niang is professor of environmental anthropology at the University Cheikh Anta Diop in Dakar, Senegal. He has worked with the Global AIDS Programme at the World Health Organization, the Women and AIDS Project at the International Center for Research on Women, and the International Development Research Centre and is conducting research on sexual behavior, AIDS and other sexually transmitted diseases, and AIDS prevention strategies.

María Isabel Plata is an attorney and executive director of PROFAMILIA, the family planning association of Colombia, and a member of the Women's Advisory Panel of International Planned Parenthood Federation.

Rakesh Rajani is coordinator of the *kuleana* center for sexual health in Mwanza, Tanzania, where he is involved in youth advocacy. He is coauthor of *Life First! A Practical Guide for People with HIV/AIDS and Their Families* and several briefing papers on children's rights. He is also the team leader of a social science study on sexually transmitted infections and health-seeking behavior, with a special emphasis on gender analysis.

Ann Robbins is a staff scientist at the Center for Biomedical Research of the Population Council. She conducts research on the development of female and male contraceptives as well as basic research on the effects of hormones on the brain and on the sexual behavior of rodents.

Debbie Rogow is a senior consultant to international reproductive health organizations. She recently authored "Women's Health Policy: Where Lie the Interests of Physicians?" and "Withdrawal is a Choice: A Review of the Literature and an Agenda for Research." She is currently teaching a fertility awareness class to staff of the Population Council.

Jason Schultz has spent the last five years founding and leading profeminist men's groups on college campuses across the United States, including Men Acting for Change at Duke University. He specializes in discussions of male diversity, sexual assault prevention, sexuality, and rethinking masculinity. He now works for Stir-Fry Productions, a California company that specializes in diversity training and resolving racial conflict within organizations, campuses, and communities.

Cecilia Simonetti has been working with adolescents in Brazil since 1978. She edited a series of educational materials (pamphlets and videos) on adolescent sexuality. For the last five years, she has also done gender training and project evaluation.

Vera Simonetti has taught photojournalism at the Pontificia Universidade Católica de São Paulo in Brazil since 1980. She coordinates the communication department at ECOS and has been producing videos and audiovisual material for the last ten years.

Sally A. Steffen is coauthor with Julia Ericksen of *Kiss and Tell: The Revelations of Sexual Behavior Surveys,* forthcoming from Harvard University Press. She has done research on the congressional response to teenage pregnancy and on sex education and the law. She is currently a law clerk for Federal District Court Judge Raymond J. Broderick.

Sheelagh Stewart, a Zimbabwean lawyer, was director of the Musasa Project, an NGO set up to target the problems of rape and domestic violence in Zimbabwe. She is now a research officer at the Institute of Development Studies in Brighton, U.K.

Ninuk Widyantoro is a consulting psychologist with a major interest in women's reproductive health issues. She is founder and consulting psychologist of FENOMENA, a psychological consulting bureau. She has been working for many years in clinics and villages, in both urban and rural settings, and has written articles on abortion, contraceptive choice, and women's reproductive rights.

Ara Wilson volunteered her services at Empower from 1993 through 1994. She is a Ph.D. candidate at City University of New York and is writing a dissertation about how Bangkok's commercial development is affecting Thai women.

Dooley Worth initiated the first AIDS risk-reduction program for women in New York in 1986, in cooperation with the New York City Department of Health. She has conducted extensive research on the links between women's drug use, their childhood experiences, and their HIV status. She directed the ethnographic research component of the National Institute on Drug Abuse's five-site Sexual Partner's AIDS Prevention Project (WHEEL) and has evaluated AIDS services for both the Health Resources Services Administration (HRSA) and the U.S. Conference of Mayors (Centers for Disease Control prevention programs). Currently, Dr. Worth works with the Henry Street Settlement Mental Health Program, which has developed a three-generational approach to working with families with AIDS.

Nabil Younis is professor and chairman of the Department of Obstetrics and Gynaecology at Al-Azhar University. He is the author of "A Community Study of Gynecological and Related Morbidities in Rural Egypt" and a policy paper entitled "Learning about the Gynecological Health of Women," which deals with the subject from both a medical and a social perspective.

Huda Zurayk is senior associate with the Population Council's Cairo office. She coordinates a regional research group on reproductive health and has been involved in the multidisciplinary research on reproductive morbidity in the Giza villages in Egypt. She is also a visiting professor at the American University of Beirut.

Index

Emotional abuse, 9, 125, 304
Empower (organization), 13, 333–34, 338–42
Empowerment, 4; of women, 174, 200, 209, 261, 334, 338–42, 376
Endocrine, 254–55
English language lessons, 334, 340
Erection, penile, 59, 281–82, 291–92, 294–95 n.4, 329, 365
Ericksen, Julia A., 8, 73–85
Eros, 270–76. *See also* Sexuality
Erotica, 164, 211–12, 215–16, 255, 294 n.1
Estrogens, 256, 257, 273, 280
Ethiopia, 141
Ethos, 270–71, 273–74. *See also* Culture; Social institutions
Exchange: protocol of, 214–15; sexual, 212–13, 216–18, 314, 350, 361 n.9
Exploitation, 263, 270–71, 274–75, 339
Extramarital sex, 144–45, 365, 369–72; in Senegal, 218, 220; in Thailand, 112, 116

False reporting, rape survivors suspected of, 359, 362 n.14
Families, 5, 76–77, 80, 131, 170 n.3, 304; ECOS' work with, 330–31; life of women at high risk of HIV, 119, 121–25, 126–27; provided for by Thai sex workers, 338, 341; in Romania, 27, 28, 29
Family Planning Associations (FPA), IPPF, 363–80
Family planning services, 1–6, 87, 98, 148–51, 158, 223; attempts to impose values on community, 96, 227, 247, 364, 367–72, 374; bringing sexuality into, 9–11, 137–53, 158–70, 195–209; fertility awareness taught by, 180, 182–91; gap between programs and clients' needs, 14, 363–80; sexuality and gender in literature of, 138–39, 151 n.1, 152 n.2. *See also* Contraception
Femininity, 27, 143, 316. *See also* Gender; Identity, gender/sexual
Feminism, 80, 87, 261. *See also* Women's movement
Fertility, 181, 255; making decisions about, 5, 8–9, 98, 100, 101–6
Fertility awareness (FA), 10, 180–92; basal body temperature, 254–55
Folk body imagery, in Egypt, 104–5

Folklore, represented by *mythos,* 270–71
Follicle-stimulating hormone (FSH), 256, 285
Forced (Coerced) sex, 3, 143, 201, 350, 367. *See also* Rape; Sexual abuse
Ford Foundation, 172, 179, 226
Freedman, Ronald, 79–80

Gambia, 370
Gay culture. *See* Homosexuality
Gender, 83, 87, 137–38, 331, 364; discussed in fertility awareness training, 187–89; issues of recognized by PROFAMILIA, 172–77; place in sexual initiation, 87, 89–90; sexuality in framework of, 139–51; training on for family planning providers, 207, 379
Gender differences, 1–2, 8, 39, 75, 99, 293; in control over unwanted sexual acts, 137–38, 313, 367; in division of labor and activities in Senegal, 212; inequalities, 7–8, 20–24, 26–27, 34, 38–39, 364, 379; among members of Zimbabwe Republic Police, 354; in perceived responsibility for sexual problems, 201; in timing of sexual initiation, 89–90, 141
Gender identity. *See* Identity, gender/sexual
Gender roles, 1–6, 11, 33, 139, 158, 329; assumptions on in Mexican culture, 89–90; challenged by Musasa, 357; and dangers of ideal of romantic love, 128–29; Egyptian men's attitudes toward, 101–7, 108 n.7; well-defined for street boys and girls, 312, 313–15, 318, 321. *See also* Men; Women
Genitals, female. *See* Cervix; Clitoris; Vagina
Gestagens (Progestagens), 287–91, 294 n.2, *table* 286. *See also* Progestins
Ghana, 370, 373
Girls, 188, 304–8, 311–17. *See also* Children; Youth
Gonadotropin hormone-releasing hormone (GnRH; Luteinizing hormone-releasing hormone; LHRH), 285, 287, 291–92
Goodson, Patricia, 195
Gordon, Gill, 14, 363–80

Gynecological disease/morbidity, 11–12, 234–35, 237 n.2, 238–50, 249 n.1; studies in rural villages, 11–12, 223–24, 226–37, 238–50. *See also* Reproductive health
Gynecological (Pelvic) examinations, 7, 19, 237 n.2, 337; as part of rural studies, 11, 224, 231, 238–41, 243–46, 248–49

Hatton, Lyn, 264
Havanon, Napaporn, 9, 110–18
Healers, traditional Zimbabwean, 350, 361 n.8
Health, 65, 103–5, 107 n.4, 228, 267–68, 324; conditions of Thai sex workers, 337, 339–40. *See also* Reproductive health; Sexual health
Health (Medical) care, 130–31, 241, 306, 337, 340, 346; for diseases discovered during rural studies, 230–31, 239; screening women for abuse during, 388–89; services for rape victims in Zimbabwe, 359
Hedges, Warren, 8, 45–69
Heroin addiction, 120–21, 127, 132 n.1
Heterosexuality, 46, 48, 57, 90, 210
HIV, 46, 120
  ☐ infection with, 110–11, 118, 301–2, 350; studies of women at high risk of, 9, 119–32
  ☐ prevention, 363–80; as part of *kuleana*'s work, 303, 305, 316–17, 318–22; use of Laobe women in Senegal project, 11, 213–15, 219–21
  ☐ risk factors, 3, 9, 110, 119, 121, 162, 332; in Africa, 210, 211–12, 216–21, 307–15
  ☐ *See also* AIDS
Homophobia, 3, 46, 53, 56, 310
Homosexual encounters: between otherwise heterosexual individuals, 6, 115, 142–43, 373; of street boys as "play" not "sex," 310, 318
Homosexuality, 7, 46, 74, 81–82, 142–43, 254; adolescent boys' concern about, 326, 329, 330; Kinsey data on, 78; masturbation seen as leading to, 372; relationships in the Middle East, 99; risk of HIV infection, 110
Hormones, 63, 159–60; effect on male sexual behavior, 12,